iversity Committee Recommendation
Graduate School of Education
June 2013

Springer Series on Rehabilitation

Myron G. Eisenberg, PhD, Series Editor
Veterans Affairs Medical Center, Hampton, VA
Thomas E. Backer, PhD, Consulting Editor
Human Interaction Research Institute, Los Angeles, CA

Kristofer J. Hagglund, PhD, ABPP, is the Associate Dean of Health Policy and Academic Affairs and Professor of Health Psychology and of Public Affairs at the University of Missouri–Columbia. He is also the codirector of the Center for Health Policy, a nonpartisan research and policy analysis organization committed to improving health and health care. He was a 2000–2001 Robert Wood Johnson Health Policy Fellow in the Office of Senator Tom Harkin (D-IA), where he worked on legislation addressing mental health parity, the health care safety net, rural health care, and patients' rights. Dr. Hagglund was President of the Division of Rehabilitation Psychology of the American Psychological Association in 2003–2004 and was awarded the James Garrett Early Career Achievement Award by the Division in 1997. Dr. Hagglund has an active research program and has published more than 50 manuscripts in the areas of chronic illnesses and disability, health care delivery systems, and health policy. He is the co-principal investigator of the Missouri Model Spinal Cord Injury System and a co-principal investigator of the Missouri Arthritis Rehabilitation Research and Training Center, both funded by the National Institute on Disability and Rehabilitation Research. He is also the co-principal investigator of a project addressing racial and ethnic health disparities that is funded by the Missouri Foundation for Health. Dr. Hagglund obtained his doctoral degree in clinical (medical) psychology from the University of Alabama at Birmingham. He is a diplomate of the American Board of Professional Psychology and a Fellow of the American Psychological Association.

Allen W. Heinemann, PhD, ABPP, completed his doctoral degree in clinical psychology at the University of Kansas with a specialty focus in rehabilitation. He completed an internship at Baylor College of Medicine in Houston and was an assistant professor in the Department of Psychology at Illinois Institute of Technology. Since 1985, he has worked at the Rehabilitation Institute of Chicago where he directs the Center for Rehabilitation Outcomes Research, a rehabilitation-focused health services research unit. He is also associate director of research at RIC and professor in the Department of Physical Medicine and Rehabilitation at the Feinberg School of Medicine, Northwestern University. He serves on the Coordinating Committee for Northwestern University's Institute for Healthcare Studies. He is the author of more than 110 articles in peer-reviewed publications and is the editor of *Substance Abuse and Physical Disability*. He is the recipient of funding by the National Institute on Disability and Rehabilitation Research, the National Institute on Alcohol Abuse and Alcoholism, Centers for Disease Control, and the Social Security Administration. During 2004 and 2005, he served as president of the American Congress of Physical Medicine and Rehabilitation and the Rehabilitation Psychology division of the American Psychological Association. He is the recipient of the Division 22 (Rehabilitation Psychology–of the American Psychological Association) Roger Barker Distinguished Career Award.

Handbook of Applied Disability and Rehabilitation Research

Edited by

Kristofer J. Hagglund, PhD, ABPP and
Allen W. Heinemann, PhD, ABPP

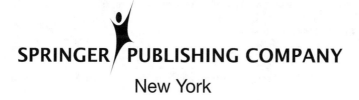

SPRINGER PUBLISHING COMPANY

New York

Springer Publishing Company, Inc.
11 West 42nd Street
New York, NY 10036

Acquisitions Editor: Sheri W. Sussman

Production Editor: Emily Johnston

Cover design: Joanne E. Honigman

Composition: Apex Publishing

06 07 08 09 10/ 5 4 3 2 1

Library of Congress Cataloging-in-Publication Data

Handbook of applied disability and rehabilitation research / edited by
    Kristofer J. Hagglund and Allen W. Heinemann.
        p. ; cm. — (Springer series on rehabilitation)
    Includes bibliographical references and index.
    ISBN 0-8261-3255-3
    1. People with disabilities Rehabilitation. 2. Rehabilitation—Research.
I. Hagglund, Kristofer J. II. Heinemann, Allen W. III. Series: Springer series on
rehabilitation (Unnumbered) [DNLM: 1. Disabled Persons—rehabilitation.
2. Health Services Research. 3. Rehabilitation—methods.
    WB 320 H2355   2006]
    RC451.4.H35H36 2006
    362.4—dc22   2006015370

Printed in the United States of America by Maple-Vail Book Manufacturing Group.

Contents

Contributors

Rosalie J. Ackerman, PhD
ABackans DCP, Inc.
Akron, OH

Amy J. Armstrong, PhD, CRC
Virginia Commonwealth University
Richmond, VA

Martha E. Banks, PhD
ABackans DCP, Inc.
Akron, OH

Allan I. Bergman
Brain Injury Association of America
Alexandria, VA

Kacie Blalock, PhD, CRC
North Carolina A & T State University
Greensboro, NC.

Margaret Brown, PhD
Mount Sinai School of Medicine
New York, NY

Susanne M. Bruyère, PhD
Employment and Disability Institute
Cornell University
School of Industrial and Labor
Relations–Extension Division
Ithaca, NY

Jane Burke, MS
University of Illinois
Chicago, IL

Rebecca P. Cameron, PhD
California State University
Sacramento, CA

Fong Chan, PhD
University of Wisconsin–Madison
Department of Rehabilitation
Psychology and Special Education
Madison, WI

Judith A. Cook, PhD
University of Illinois
Chicago, IL

Franklyn K. Coombs, MS, PE
Assistive Work Technology Services
Georgia Department of Labor
Rehabilitation Services
Atlanta, GA

Barbara Du Bois, PhD
Private Practice
Prescott, AZ

William A. Erickson, MS
Cornell University
Ithaca, NY

Laura Farah, PhD
Law, Health Policy & Disability Center
University of Iowa
College of Law
Iowa City, IA

Martin Forchheimer, MPP
University of Michigan
Department of Physical Medicine
and Rehabilitation
Ann Arbor, MI

Michael Frain, PhD, CRC
Florida State University
Boca Raton, FL

Robert T. Fraser, PhD, CRC
University of Washington
Seattle, WA

Amadee J. Fuentes, BS
California State University
Sacramento, CA

Wayne A. Gordon, PhD
Department of Rehabilitation Medicine
Mount Sinai School of Medicine
New York, NY

Elaina Sitaras Hirsch, BS
The Johns Hopkins School of Medicine
Baltimore, MD

Sharon R. Johnson, MS, CRC
Minnesota Division of Rehabilitation
Services

Joseph C. Kvedar, MD
Harvard Medical School
Boston, MA

Catherine A. Marshall, PhD, CRC
Department of Educational Psychology
Northern Arizona University
Flagstaff, AZ

Mary McAweeney, PhD
SARDI—Wright State University
School of Medicine
Kettering, OH

Charles T. Merbitz, PhD, BCBA, CRC
Chicago School of Professional
Psychology
Chicago, IL

Nancy Hansen Merbitz, PhD
Mental Health Resource Center
(MHRC), Inc.
Pontiac, IL

Susan M. Miller, PhD, CRC
Florida State University
Tallahassee, FL

Linda R. Mona, PhD
Veterans Affairs, Long Beach
Healthcare System
Behavioral Health
Long Beach, CA

Dennis Moore, EdO
Wright State University School of
Medicine
SARDI Program
Dayton, OH

Michael Morris, JD
University of Iowa
Iowa City, IA

Steven R. Pruett, PhD, CRC
University of Florida,
Gramsville, FL

Priscilla R. Sanderson, PhD, CRC
Research Department of Health
Sciences
College of Health Promotion
Native American Cancer Research
Partnership
Northern Arizona University
Flagstaff, AZ

Marcia J. Scherer, PhD, MPH
Institute for Matching Person &
Technology
Webster, NY

Tom Seekins, PhD
The Rural Institute
Department of Psychology
The University of Montana
Missoula, MT

Ralph William Shields
New York, NY

Denise Tate, PhD, ABBP
University of Michigan
Department of Physical Medicine
and Rehabilitation
Ann Arbor, MI

Dale F. Thomas, PhD, ABPP
University of Wisconsin–Stout
Menomonie, WI

David Vandergoot, PhD
Center for Essential Management
Services
Long Island, NY

Sara A. VanLooy, BA
Cornell University
Ithaca, NY

Christopher C. Wagner, PhD, CRC
Virginia Commonwealth University
Richmond, VA

Seth Warschausky, PhD
Department of Physical Medicine
and Rehabilitation
Ann Arbor, MI

Introduction: The Maturation of Psychology in Disability and Rehabilitation Research

Few research fields are as closely tied to promoting the well-being of their consumer stakeholders as rehabilitation psychology. The field grew out of clinicians' desire for information and evidence about how to best treat clients or patients in a variety of rehabilitation settings. Practitioners and scientists recognized that the unique circumstances of rehabilitation made the unquestioned application of standard diagnostic protocols and therapeutic techniques risky. For example, applying standard diagnostic criteria for affective disorders to individuals who had sustained trauma was recognized to contribute to over-diagnosis of depression. Over time, rehabilitation psychology has contributed to and captured the best of psychological theory and practice, and applied them to rehabilitation practice and policy. One need only consider the recent applications of social psychology, such as learning theory, life course development, or stress and adaptation, to appreciate the translational nature of rehabilitation psychology research. In fact, rehabilitation psychology emphasized research that was translational before the term *translational* came into vogue.

Rehabilitation psychology research continues to develop rapidly. More than ever, the field involves the individuals it is designed to help, including persons with disabilities and chronic illness, their families, and their loved ones. Research programs are focused on involving communities and society at large and interventions are designed to make fundamental changes in communities to promote full participation by persons regardless of sensory, physical, or cognitive capacity. In addition, rehabilitation psychology has begun to address central concerns in health care delivery and health policy. These developments provide cause for celebration. Nevertheless, many fundamental and applied questions remain unanswered. In this book the authors review varied aspects of rehabilitation psychology research and practice and offer insightful recommendations for future research programs, policy changes, and clinical interventions.

HISTORICAL PERSPECTIVE

The "Princeton Conference" of 1958 provided the "launching platform for a new field of psychological research and practice" in rehabilitation (Wright, 1959). Those meeting in Princeton sought to document the progress made since the Second World War, summarize the current state of knowledge, describe the problems encountered by clinicians in serving persons with disabilities, and provide a foundation on which future research and practice could be built. A second conference, held 13 years later in Monterey, California, served to coalesce the diverse elements of rehabilitation psychology. The conference was sponsored by the Board of Professional Affairs of the American Psychological Association and funded by the Rehabilitation Services Administration. Eleven major papers were commissioned in preparation for the meeting, and invited delegates discussed and revised the papers. The collected papers from the 1970 Monterey Conference reflect the proud traditions of the field of addressing individual, societal, and environmental factors in disability and rehabilitation (Neff, 1971). The invited contributions reflect the concerns of an emerging specialty: motor and cognitive aspects of impairment, disability, and personality, social psychological aspects of disability, behavioral interventions, employment and economic issues, racial and ethnic disparities, client relationships, research issues, roles and functions of psychologists, and manpower and training issues. For example, Franklin Shontz (1971) emphasized that "Research on the psychological aspects of disability must move to a higher level of scientific sophistication" (p. 62). Leonard Diller called for further work on evaluation of service recipients and treatment programs, as well as adequate indicators of treatment outcomes (1971). In the aggregate, the authors called for increased volume and quality of research in rehabilitation.

The 35 years since the Monterey conference provide evidence that the call for enhanced rehabilitation psychology research was taken seriously. The journal *Rehabilitation Psychology* recently marked its 50th volume and will complete a transition from a divisional journal to an official American Psychological Association journal in 2006. In an editorial acknowledging the end of his tenure as editor, Bruce Caplan noted that rehabilitation psychologists are integrally involved in, and are often directing, federally funded model systems in traumatic brain injury, spinal cord injury, and burn injury rehabilitation (Caplan, 2005). Rehabilitation psychologists are integrated in the enterprise of rehabilitation research within the National Institutes of Health, United States Department of Education, the Veterans Administration, the Centers for Disease Control and Prevention, the Social Security Administration, the Centers for

Medicare and Medicaid Services, and in universities, private foundations, and organizations that consult with federal and private entities.

This book continues the tradition of providing a periodic update of the field in critical aspects of rehabilitation research and practice. Whereas the 1971 collection of papers helped define the focus of a nascent field, the current works address a diverse set of problems and opportunities, including assistive technology, health policy, cultural diversity, employment, and the future of rehabilitation research. Of course, many other works critical to rehabilitation have been published since 1971 and one only need complete a simple literature search to find seminal work in research, clinical care, policy, and education in rehabilitation psychology. It is a testament to the growth and vibrancy of the field that so much is now being written in rehabilitation psychology. This is one of the few volumes that focuses solely on rehabilitation psychology research.

This book was originally conceived during the conference "Bridging Gaps: Refining the Disability Research Agenda for Rehabilitation and Social Sciences," held in Washington, DC, in May, 2002. The conference was cosponsored by the National Institute on Disability and Rehabilitation Research (NIDRR), the Division of Rehabilitation Psychology of the American Psychological Association (APA), and the Public Interest Directorate of the APA. The conference brought together a diverse group of stakeholders to discuss the future of rehabilitation research around the themes of NIDRR's core areas of research: Employment Outcomes, Health and Function, Technology for Access and Function, and Independent Living and Community Integration (Menz & Thomas, 2003). These domains have been maintained for this volume and for most of the authors presented at the "Bridging Gaps" conference. The chapters in this volume extend the dialogue from this conference and the previous conferences addressing the evolving field of rehabilitation psychology.

CONCLUSIONS

Collectively, the chapters demonstrate that the rehabilitation research paradigm is evolving to incorporate consumer participation in addressing problems relevant to consumers in an ecologically valid manner. The traditional approach of using nomothetically based studies to develop individually based interventions is complemented increasingly by other research methods. The authors demonstrate the ability of rehabilitation psychology and related disciplines to use community-based research to address environmental barriers. Collectively, the contributions of these authors demonstrate rehabilitation psychology's potential as an important contributor to the field of public health. As the number of people with disabilities and chronic illnesses grows, rehabilitation psychology researchers and practitioners will improve their population-based sophistication. But, the lessons of the past will have been learned: Population-based approaches will be used increasingly to address community problems, and consumers will be involved in, and increasingly lead, the development of interventions to change the mutable environment.

The next 35 years are likely to witness continued evolution of rehabilitation theory and research that informs practice and policy. While speculating about the specific contributions may be off-target, what is likely to characterize rehabilitation research is the importance of interdisciplinary collaboration. Tension among various perspectives and values exist and are likely to continue in rehabilitation research. Continued growth in health services research, and integration of rehabilitation psychology research focused on outcomes within this larger venue, are likely to continue. The application of rehabilitation psychology principles to policy discussions is apt to increase. The importance of including stakeholders from diverse perspectives is the bedrock of rehabilitation values. The emphasis on diverse values and perspectives and fully integrating consumers into research will afford rehabilitation psychologists the opportunity to contribute to the advancement in related fields. For example, rehabilitation psychologists will adeptly contribute to the growing research, education, and practice initiatives to reduce racial and ethnic health disparities. In addition, rehabilitation psychology will continue to participate in health services research and public health. By eschewing paternalistic practices of traditional health care and focusing on patient-centered care (Institute of Medicine, 2001), rehabilitation psychology will help individuals achieve increased participation in desired activities and improved quality of life. Also, by incorporating the concept of community into research and practice that has traditionally focused primarily on individuals, rehabilitation psychology will facilitate the removal of societal barriers to full participation among persons with disabilities and chronic illness.

REFERENCES

Caplan, B. (2005). "Golden" editorial. *Rehabilitation Psychology, 50*(1), 3–4.

Diller, L. (1971). Cognitive and motor aspects of handicapping conditions in the neurologically impaired. In W. S. Neff (Ed.), *Rehabilitation psychology* (pp. 1–32). Washington, DC: American Psychological Association.

Institute of Medicine. (2001). *Crossing the quality chasm: A new health system for the 21st century.* Washington, DC: National Academy Press.

Menz, F. E., & Thomas, D. F. (2003). *Bridging gaps: Refining the disability research agenda for rehabilitation and the social sciences*. Menomonie: University of Wisconsin–Stout.

Neff, W. S. (Ed.). (1971). *Rehabilitation psychology*. Washington, DC: American Psychological Association.

Shontz, F. C. (1971). Physical disability and personality. In W. S. Neff (Ed.), *Rehabilitation psychology* (pp. 33–73). Washington, DC: American Psychological Association.

Wright, B. A. (1959). *Psychology and rehabilitation*. Washington, DC: American Psychological Association.

Acknowledgments

The Editors would like to thank Drs. Dale Thomas, Fred Menz, and Connie Pledger for their consultation on this book and their leadership in the "Bridging Gaps" conference. We would also like to thank Ms. Nicole Whyte for her excellent assistance in preparing the book for publication. In addition, we sincerely appreciate the guidance and support of Ms. Sheri W. Sussman of Springer Publishing Company. The development of this book was supported, in part, by grant H133N000012 to the University of Missouri from the National Institute on Disability and Rehabilitation Research, United States Department of Education. The contents of this book do not necessarily represent the opinions of the U.S. Department of Education.

SECTION I

Community Integration

INTRODUCTION TO SECTION I: COMMUNITY INTEGRATION

Wayne Gordon and his colleagues make a compelling argument for new models of research into community integration for persons with disabilities. They build on the sage advice of Justin Dart, the renowned independent living movement leader, who tirelessly emphasized that rehabilitation research must focus on developing the full potential of each person. They describe an approach to rehabilitation research that resolves the dilemma posed by the methodological need for sample-based quantitative studies and the real-world need for studies that maximize the quality of life of unique individuals. Their work extends what has become known as "participatory action research" to involve the consumers of that research in all of its components.

Gordon and colleagues also describe a second element for successful rehabilitation research: better "case finding," that is, clearly identifying the characteristics of consumer participants needed to answer specific research questions, instead of relying on "convenience samples," which are typically drawn from researchers' clinical populations and rarely reflect the population on important characteristics. Relatedly, recognition of the substantial diversity within otherwise seemingly homogeneous samples of persons with disabilities is critical to producing research results that are meaningful to both populations and individuals. Finally, and perhaps most importantly, the authors call on researchers to establish research agendas that are important to people with disabilities. Rehabilitation psychologists have the luxury to work with a diverse population, but not the luxury to set research goals that are irrelevant to the needs and desires of this population.

Catherine Marshall and her coauthors emphasize the need for cross-cultural competency among rehabilitation psychology researchers and providers. They argue that class, as defined by education and income, is an essential component of our culture that must be considered if persons with disabilities are to have full access to rehabilitation services and achieve community integration. Furthermore, culture should be regarded as a positive force in rehabilitation research and service provision. Echoing the concerns of Edmund Gordon in his contribution to the Monterey conference (1971), the diverse and dynamic nature of rehabilitation service recipients' cultural context affords rehabilitation psychology the opportunity to advance the lives of persons with disabilities through research and intervention.

Martha Banks and Rosalie Ackerman address issues related to the inclusion of people who have been overlooked in the disability literature, including people of color, women, members of sexual minorities, and older adults with disabilities. They emphasize that research and policy should address the rates and types of disability across groups, multiple layers of disability, cultural differences in experiences of disability, cross-cultural concerns, access to employment-relevant quality education, financial resources, laws and policies, and sociocultural barriers to employment for people who are marginalized.

CHAPTER ONE

Community Integration Research: An Empowerment Paradigm

Wayne A. Gordon
Margaret Brown
Allan I. Bergman
Ralph William Shields

In the chapter on community integration (CI) within the Long-Range Plan of the National Institute on Disability and Rehabilitation Research (NIDRR, 1999a), the opening quotation from the late Justin Dart urges a shift in our values and in our thinking (as a society):

> Whether or not we have a disability, we will never fully achieve our goals until we establish a culture that focuses the full force of science and democracy on the systematic empowerment of every person to live to his or her full potential. (NIDRR, 1999a, p. 61)

How does Dart's charge to "establish a culture" in which people can achieve their "full potential" apply to the culture of CI research? For researchers in the field, achieving Dart's vision may require a paradigmatic shift in their conception of both research goals and methods. With respect to goals, "systematic empowerment" of people with disabilities in this new research culture becomes the bottom line in research activities and in developing a research agenda.

5

Two components suggest themselves as defining qualities of such an empowerment agenda. First, the voice of people with disabilities must not only be heard in defining the needs that are addressed through CI research but also be given primacy. And second, the output of research must provide the basis for taking action (aimed at the person and/or at the environment) to address the defined needs. Empowerment, in this view, flows both from hearing the voices of those who are the focus of research and from doing research designed explicitly to address their voiced needs.

Dart points to two sets of supports for creating a culture that nurtures the potential of individuals: the first is science. But what does it mean that the "full force of science" is used in the pursuit of empowering individuals? Clearly, science can only play a strong role if adequately funded. Also, science at "full force" requires that research activities meet the highest methodological standards. As will be discussed later in this chapter, these standards need to go beyond technical excellence, as it is usually evaluated, to also reflect research designs and models that avoid the simplistic and instead acknowledge the complexities of living life with a disability. The efficacy of scientific activity in expanding the power of people with disabilities in reaching their "full potential," as Dart terms it, also depends upon the processes used in planning and in choosing the priorities that better reflect what Seekins (2003) refers to as social validity. Finally, the "full force" of science requires not only our bringing to bear adequate financial resources and methodological acumen but also our working within a supportive paradigm in which the most highly valued outcome is providing the building blocks to improve lives of people with disabilities.

The second tool that Dart cites is democracy. In a democracy, we respect the individual's rights and voice, which are protected under the rule of law and become manifest through the power of democratic institutions, such as the right to vote and guarantees of freedom of speech. In shifting to an empowerment culture in research and in defining the values we incorporate into our work, researchers need to ask: Are we democratic, or autocratic, in our methods and goals? Does our research, in effect, support service and research models that are less than democratic, in the tradition of "one size fits all" or "we scientists know best"? Do we democratically respect the person who is the subject of research and is the focus of services, or do we autocratically rule over our research empire?

Interestingly, Dart's words explicitly reject the separation often insisted upon in thinking about people with and without disabilities. In his saying, in effect, that people are people, one implication is that although disablement is a necessary criterion in defining the focal population of our research, disablement is not necessarily the target of research.

Instead, in shaping a research agenda within a new paradigm, we need to focus with a lens that sees people with disabilities as people first, with disability as a (sometimes) distant second. Are we doing research that is narrowly focused on reduction of disablement, to the exclusion of defining our mission more broadly, in advancing our knowledge of how best to address the needs of people (who happen to have a disability)? If people are people, our role as scientists within an empowerment paradigm is to pinpoint personal and environmental barriers that prevent people from achieving their goals, as well as to add to the tool chest methods for eliminating such barriers.

In sum, Dart's words imply that doing science within this new paradigm means that its full force is focused on research that is action-oriented, person-centered, and aimed at helping each individual with a disability to reach his or her full potential within the community. The shift is away from nomothetic, disablement-focused research that may not be directly related to the needs of people with disabilities that are preventing them from achieving their potential.

Before proceeding further, two notes about language: First, NIDRR in the late 1990s advanced the New Paradigm, in which disablement was no longer conceptualized as residing within the person (the Old Paradigm), but instead as resulting from the interaction of the person and the environment (NIDRR, 1999a, 1999b). Although this way of thinking was historically a part of the education and training of many disability researchers, for example, rehabilitation psychologists (Brown &Heinemann, 1999), it *was* new for those researchers whose view of people with disabilities was based on their being trained within the medical model. The (lowercase) "new paradigm" being discussed in this chapter focuses not on issues of conceptualization of disablement (although it is compatible with the concepts of the New Paradigm), but instead on new ways of thinking about the methods and purpose of disability research: What are the roles of the researcher and of the person with a disability when working within democratic versus autocratic assumptions? What are the goals of our research? This focus and shift of values is embodied in what we refer to as the empowerment paradigm.

A second note about language: We use the term *insider* to refer to individuals with disabilities, in the sense that insiders are those who directly experience disablement from the inside. People who surround them—such as family members, clinicians, researchers, and policy makers—are *outsiders* to disability (this terminology was suggested more than 40 years ago by Tamara Dembo [1964]). The point is to emphasize a difference in perspective—outsiders versus insiders—which is not stressed when using terms such as *consumer* and *researcher*. The term *measured insiders* refers to insiders at the point of their participation in research-based or clinical assessments.

This chapter will address five areas relevant to advancement of the empowerment paradigm in the context of CI research: (a) definitions of CI, (b) empowerment of insiders within the research process, (c) empowerment of insiders specifically at the point of assessment/measurement, (d) optimizing research methods in an empowerment paradigm, and (e) sampling/inclusion issues. Because the authors have in-depth experience with research on CI of individuals with traumatic brain injuries (TBI), we trust that many, if not most, of the ideas and concerns we discuss in that context will be widely applicable to CI of other disability groups.

DEFINING COMMUNITY INTEGRATION

Community integration is a concept residing at the core of deinstitutionalization efforts within the worlds of developmental disabilities and mental health (Carling, 1990; Kruzich, 1985; Racino, 2002; Sullivan, 1992; Wherley & Bisgaard, 1987). The concept is also a focus in community-oriented research documenting the well-being of individuals with a variety of physical disabilities (Corrigan, Smith-Knapp, & Granger, 1998; Felmingham, Baguley, & Crooks, 2001; Fuhrer, Rintala, Hart, Clearman, & Young, 1992; Heinemann & Whiteneck, 1995; Millis, Rosenthal, & Lourie, 1994). The concept of CI has been defined primarily in terms of the measures used to gauge its success. For example, within the research literature focusing on CI of individuals leaving institutions, successful CI is often viewed in terms of an individual's being able to be maintained in a noninstitutional, community-based residence (e.g., Schalock, Harper, & Genung, 1981). Alternatively, successful CI has been assessed using indicators of frequency of engagement in activities in the community and in the household (e.g., Felce & Emerson, 2001; O'Neill, Brown, Gordon, O'Neill, Schonhorn, & Creer, 1981; O'Neill, Brown, Gordon, & Schonhorn, 1985; Salzberg & Langford, 1981;).

Within the world of TBI research, historically CI is often viewed loosely in terms of independence of functioning in community settings and expanded participation in expected community roles and activities (e.g., Gordon, Hibbard, Brown, Flanagan, & Campbell-Korves, 1999; Willer, Rosenthal, Kreutzer, Gordon, & Rempel, 1993;). In many community integration studies of TBI insiders, CI has come to be defined in operational terms reflecting participation in three areas (home, productive activity, and social engagement), as many researchers have adopted the Community Integration Questionnaire (CIQ) (Willer et al., 1993) to assess CI outcomes. The CIQ has the built-in assumption that more—income, participation, independence in functioning, and so forth—is better. When using the CIQ, a person's scoring below the normative mean is viewed as less successful CI than scoring above the norm.

However, within an empowerment paradigm, use of measures such as the CIQ to gauge success makes little sense, as the CIQ assumes that outsiders know best the variables that define success for people with TBI and that they can be normatively scaled. Measures such as the CIQ are not empowering, person-centered, nor, in Dart's words, "aimed at helping each individual with a disability to reach his or her full potential within the community." In fact, they disempower the voice of insiders with their nomothetic assumptions that substitute for the individual's own goals those valued by societal representatives.

Alternatives to normative definitions of CI are of more recent origin. The Community Integration Measure (CIM) comprises one example of a more empowering approach to assessing CI (McColl, Davies, Carlson, Johnston & Minnes, 2001), as its item content is based on suggestions made by TBI insiders within a focus group (McColl, Carlson, Johnston, Minnes, Shve, etal., 1998), and evaluative responses by measured insiders are sought. The CIM defines successful CI in terms of the insider's feeling positive about 10 areas of community living, for example, feeling "like I belong here." The developers of the CIM have shown that the CIM and CIQ are not significantly nor substantially correlated with each other, and that only the CIM is substantially correlated with a measure of subjective well-being (Minnes et al., 2003).

As a second example of defining CI nonnormatively, the Research and Training Center on Community Integration of Individuals with TBI (hereafter, RTC) at Mount Sinai School of Medicine, with which three of the authors are affiliated, has adopted a person-centered, subjective approach to measurement of CI (further discussed in the next section). In this measure, we adhere to the view that the CI concept covers a certain territory—being housed, occupied, and engaged in the community, and, within that territory, each insider needs to define what he or she values in these areas. This approach to defining CI has arisen from the model of participatory action research (PAR) (Krogh, 1998; White, 2002; Whyte, 1991) that the RTC adopted in 1993. As the RTC has practiced PAR, individuals with TBI participate with professionals in all aspects of planning, implementing, and disseminating the results of a broad range of research activities. In the RTC's evolution, empowered insiders, through their exercising their voices in the PAR context, demonstrated to the RTC's professionally trained researchers the disempowering assumptions built into measures such as the CIQ and the need for measures of CI that give greater voice to *measured* insiders, just as PAR amplifies the voices of *its* insider participants.

It is our view that PAR and nonnormative/subjective conceptualizations of CI and measures of CI are parts of the same paradigm. This connection has been discussed at length elsewhere (Brown & Gordon, 2004) and is summarized in the next section.

EMPOWERMENT OF INSIDERS WITHIN RESEARCH

Within all phases of the research process (i.e., planning, implementation, analysis, dissemination), power relationships between disability insiders and outsiders play out in two ways. First, power resides in *control,* which is held by those making decisions that give shape to the research in each of its phases. In terms of empowerment of insiders, an important consequence of having control (as in PAR) is in having the power to decide the degree to which the insider's or outsider's *perspective*—the second element of power within the research process—is incorporated into assessment.

The insider's perspective in research can be revealed in several ways. First, when it is PAR-based, the selection of a purpose to be addressed within a research activity at least in part reveals the insider's perspective on what is *important,* as does the selection of constructs and variables viewed as means for addressing the overall purpose. For example, in the RTC's early years, a group of women with TBI met regularly at Mount Sinai as a support group. In their monthly discussions, they recognized the theme emerging of their having numerous health problems in common, the advent of which they associated with brain injury. They suggested to RTC researchers that a study to document post-TBI health complaints was needed, and they provided numerous examples of areas to be explored (e.g., endocrine problems), based on their own "pilot data"—that is, their observations of their common health trends. Through PAR, they were empowered within the planning process; their involvement led to modification of the RTC's research, which in turn led to publications on post-TBI health issues (e.g., Hibbard, Uysal, Sliwinski, & Gordon, 1998a), which some of the PAR insiders coauthored.

The insider's perspective is also revealed in the degree to which the insider's *evaluations* are incorporated into measurement, in place of normative evaluations or evaluations by an outsider. Thus, measured insiders vary in the degree that a variable such as income is important to their lives and may also vary in the degree to which they endorse the normative assumption that more is better. In this example, an empowering question would focus on the insider's ratings both of importance of and satisfaction with income rather than (solely) on the level of his/her current income. Both subjective and objective data may be important to the outsider/researcher, but only subjective evaluations (e.g., of importance and satisfactoriness) tap unequivocally into the insider's perspective.

In sum, disempowerment in CI research occurs whenever the outsider's values and preferences are incorporated into a study, to the exclusion of mechanisms for tapping into those of the insider. This power imbalance is of concern because the insider's perspective can vary significantly from the outsider's. Thus, when measurement is fully controlled by outsiders who choose to measure solely within the perspective of outsiders, the needs and life situation of disability insiders may be misconstrued or otherwise misunderstood. On the other hand, when the story is told fully from the perspective of insiders, the purposes that outsiders bring into research may not be realized. A balance needs to be achieved between respecting the needs of outsiders to do measurement effectively and the needs of insiders to be heard. In this spirit, power can be shared by outsiders by opening decision-making processes to the insider's input.

Efforts to empower insiders have emerged (sporadically, over several decades) within *clinical* rehabilitation contexts. This is evident in the implementation of a variety of approaches to individualized outcome measures (Donnelly & Carswell, 2002), including goal attainment scaling (Kiresuk & Sherman, 1968), the Canadian Occupational Performance Measure (Law et al., 1990; Law et al.,1994) and in person-centered planning (Holburn & Vietze, 2002; Mount, Riggs, Brown, &Hibbard, 1997; Schalock & Alonso, 2002). Individualized measures comprise an excellent approach to empowering insiders in clinical contexts, as insiders and outsiders share control of measurement, and the measured insider is heard.

Within CI *research,* however, evidence of a thriving empowerment paradigm is scant. For example, PAR has not been as widely used in (physical) rehabilitation and CI research as in other fields (e.g., public health) (or perhaps it is just not used as frequently as discussed in published reports). In fact, a recent *PubMed* search for research publications on PAR resulted in 214 citations since 1981, only 4 of which were related to physical disability or rehabilitation.

EMPOWERMENT OF THE MEASURED INSIDER

As important as PAR may be in empowering those insiders directly involved in measurement decision making, PAR does not necessarily lead to the *measured* insider's having his/her perspective heard. Although PAR-led research may increase the likelihood that topics of importance to the measured insider are being addressed, the process does not guarantee the sensitivity of PAR-developed measures to the concerns and values of each person with a disability who is measured, or to the concerns of groups of individuals who are outside the direct decision-making circle.

Additional means are needed to optimize empowerment of *measured* insiders through tapping into the measured insider's perspective. Whether working within or without PAR, those who hold the reins of research decision making can optimize empowerment of measured insiders through two steps: (a) systematically *selecting and shaping measures* to include more of the measured insider's perspective (e.g., his/her evaluation of importance and satisfactoriness), and (b) then *empirically testing* the resulting measure in terms of its validity in tapping into the perspective of insiders. These steps are discussed in turn below.

In selecting and shaping measures, CI researchers must address a variety of research goals, in addition to expanded empowerment of the measured insider. At minimum, potential measurement approaches must adhere to concerns for quality in measurement, in the traditional psychometric sense, or in adhering to established principles of qualitative research. Within this real-world context, empowerment can be optimized when subjective/evaluative approaches are adopted.

The insider's perspective is maximally empowered in *qualitative* research, because the measured insider, while addressing the established purposes of the study, is much freer than in quantitative research to introduce a wide range of comments and thoughts, with few strictures placed by the outsider on the insider's evaluations. However, this approach does not address the typical need of outsiders/researchers to obtain systematic measures of variables of interest. Within *quantitative* research, measures that potentially maximize the insider's "voice" require that the insider himself/herself be asked to evaluate the satisfactoriness of variables that are of high importance (at minimum, of *known* importance) to the measured insider. This is also seen in adaptations of goal attainment scaling within research (e.g., Malec, Smigielski, DePompolo, & Thompson, 1991). Approaches that tap into the insider's perspective can be designed to augment or complement objective measures, to address varying mandates with two or more sets of related measures.

At our RTC, the insider's evaluation of the importance of measured elements, as well as his/her evaluation of the satisfactoriness of these elements in his/her life (Brown & Gordon, 1999) has been incorporated into a quantitative approach to empower insiders in the context of being measured. The "Participation Objective, Participation Subjective" instrument (POPS) (Brown, et al., 2004, Gordon, Brown, & Hibbard, 1998a; Gordon & Brown, 2003) is a dual-perspective measure of CI, that is, each item in the measure is scaled objectively and subjectively. For example, when asked about access to transportation in the POPS, the respondent reports objectively on the frequency of transportation used, and also subjectively on how well it meets his or her needs and how important this is to his or her satisfaction with life. Using this approach, an objective profile of the person's life in the community can be generated (i.e., a measure of CI from a normative perspective), as can a subjective profile, indicating points of satisfaction/dissatisfaction in areas that are important to the person's well-being.

In maximizing empowerment of the measured insider, once a set of measures has been selected to address a specific purpose, the next step is to test empirically the adequacy of the measure in reflecting the insider's perspective. To judge the relative validity of any set of measures as tools that reflect the measured insider's perspective, we suggest that a gold standard be established and used for this purpose (Brown & Gordon, 2004). What existing measure taps into the insider's voice, reflecting his/her perspective on what is important to his/her life? What is the gold standard for *this* validity issue?

Adhering to the definition of "perspective" suggested herein—in which the individual's evaluations of the importance and satisfactoriness of variables/constructs were emphasized—we suggest a gold standard that constitutes a summary of the insider's overall evaluation of all facets of life that he/she deems important. We believe that summary measures of subjective quality of life (SQOL), by definition, can serve as the gold standard for what we will term *insider perspective validity*. An example is Andrews and Withey's (1976) Delighted-Terrible (D-T) Scale, which asks respondents to provide ratings on a seven-point scale ranging from being delighted with life in general to viewing it as terrible. The Satisfaction with Life Scale (Diener, 1984; Pavot, Diener, Colvin, &Sandvik, 1991) is a second example. The suggestion that SQOL measures of this type summarize the valuations the person places on the elements in his/her life that he/she deems important is drawn from the model of SQOL developed by Flanagan (1978, 1982) and also by Ferrans and Powers (1985), who define the individual's evaluation of important life elements as underlying SQOL.

The selected SQOL gold standard is applied by using simple correlation or regression procedures to determine the degree to which any single measure or sets of measures correlate(s) with the SQOL standard. When using regression procedures, the appropriate statistic for comparing one set of measures with another, in terms of a measure's tapping into the insider's perspective, is adjusted R^2.

The discussion that follows illustrates how one can apply an SQOL gold standard in testing the capacity of candidate measures to reflect the insider's perspective. In this example, we sought to compare objective and subjective measures of the same variables. However, because no objective and subjective measures of CI on the same study participants were available to us at the time of writing, we chose to focus, instead, on measures of need (Brown, Gordon, & Haddad, 2000). In this example, four alternative, multi-item sets of measures were developed of the degree to which 11 types of needs are met, for example, needs for Material Comfort, Satisfying Work, Close Friends, Socializing, and the like (based upon the work of John Flanagan, 1978, 1982).[1] Each of the four sets of measures was developed by selecting variables from an existing database generated in an RTC study of 430 individuals with TBI living in the community. In testing each of the four sets of measures, two SQOL measures were used as the gold standard: D-T Scale ratings (Andrews & Withey, 1976) plus the General QOL Measure (Brown & Vandergoot, 1998).

The first set of measures tested for their validity in reflecting the insider's perspective consisted of *objective* measures of the 11 Flanagan need areas. For example, the need for Close Friends was measured objectively in terms of the number of friends the person had contacted in the past month. These 11 objective measures together accounted for 19%–22% of the variance in SQOL ratings. Thus, objective measures of how well needs are met correlated with overall well-being in the low-to-moderate range.

The remaining three sets used *subjective* measures of each need area. The first of these used items originally drawn from Bigelow, Gareau, and Young's (1992) Quality of Life Questionnaire (QOLQ). For example, the Material Comfort need area was represented by three QOLQ items: satisfaction with current residence, satisfaction with household income, and the degree to which the person worries about future income. This type of subjective measure of each of the 11 areas of need together accounted for 38%–47% of SQOL variance. A second approach to subjectively measuring the 11 need areas was also tested, consisting of a summation of the respondent's ratings of the importance of each need area multiplied by his/her rating of the degree to which his/her needs in the area were met. The third subjective approach was the same, but without the importance ratings. These latter two models accounted for 35%–45% of variance in SQOL ratings; the approach incorporating importance ratings accounted for 5% more variance than in the model in which only the degree to which needs are met was rated. Thus, in using an SQOL gold standard to test the degree to which alternative approaches to measurement of need attainment give greater or lesser "voice" to the measured insider, we found that each of the three sets of subjective measures of the construct performed better than the objective set of measures, accounting for approximately twice the SQOL variance.

When selecting measures to maximize the empowerment of the insider, the standard that the RTC has adopted for judging the validity of the measure in representing the insider's voice is subjective well-being (this is, of course, in addition to traditional standards of validity). In effect, this stance views the insider's subjective quality of life as the bottom line. Minnes and colleagues (2003), in validating the CIM, adopted a similar approach.

OPTIMIZING RESEARCH METHODS IN AN EMPOWERMENT PARADIGM

If the research goal is to empower insiders in reaching their full potential, whether using PAR or not, how does one choose and design studies that support this goal? We suggest three criteria: As discussed above, the focus of study should be on something that outsiders and insiders can *do* something about and should be important to *insiders*. We suggest a third criterion: that in designing the study, the complexities of living life after disablement should be acknowledged rather than ignored. In doing research outside the relatively simple medical model, researchers will contribute to insider empowerment only by undertaking research that is based on a model of life, not illness.

For example, the RTC conducted a study that explores personal and environmental factors that promote and hinder post-TBI social-recreational participation (Brown, Gordon, & Spielman, 2003). This study addresses the first two criteria, in that we included predictor variables that *are* open to intervention, and social-recreational activity *is* an area of study of known importance to insiders (Brown & Vandergoot, 1998). Further, the design acknowledged complexity of social-recreational life in at least two ways: it did not pretend that only a few factors affect social engagement; and 19 variables organized into 6 sets were entered into regression analyses. Further, the ordering of entry of predictor variables into the analyses was based on preliminary analyses that demonstrated that the order of depression's entry was critical, as it had large effects on how other variables contributed to explained variance.

If we gauge the importance of any potential focus of research by documenting its relationship with SQOL, undoubtedly mood disorders comprise a key area demanding study—within the world of stroke, spinal cord injury, and TBI (Dijkers, 1997; Granger, Divan, & Fiedler, 1995; Pyne et al., 1997) among others. We also know that prevalence of mood disorders is high within each of these impairment groups (Busch & Alpern, 1998; Elliott & Frank, 1996; Gordon & Hibbard, 1997; Gordon et al., 1991; Hibbard, Vysal, Kepler, Bogdany, & Silver, 1998b; Krause, Kemp, & Coker, 2000; Rosenthal, Christensen, & Ross, 1998). Given the clear importance of mood disorders, many intervention-relevant research questions arise, each suggesting the complexity of modeling and design that is called for: Are there disability-specific triggers of and risk factors for depression? What factors are protective in preventing the emergence of mood disorders? What is the time course of mood disorders, and are the triggers the same across time? And, what interventions are effective, with whom?

Many other foci for CI research need exploring and clearly pass the can-we-do-something-about-it and is-it-important criteria. For example, one of the questions that often is raised when we are in feedback sessions with people with TBI is, "What's going to happen to me as I age?" The fact that this question is constantly coming to the fore in diverse audiences suggests that this also is an area of importance to insiders. And, it's an area that has been inadequately studied, with too much reliance on cross-sectional designs. This also relates to broader questions: What are the disability-specific health issues affecting physical well-being over the life span? Is disability in general or any specific disability a risk factor for secondary conditions—age-related or non-age-related? In the world of TBI, how does cognitive impairment mediate the aging process? What kinds of supports are needed in the community to maintain individuals with disabilities in their environment?

SAMPLING/INCLUSION ISSUES

With respect to sampling within CI research, two challenges are relevant to insider empowerment, in the sense that to be empowered within research, one must be defined as part of the population from which study samples are drawn. When a study is community-based and all members of an impairment group living in the community comprise the study population, careful case finding may be essential in assuring that samples actually represent all parts of the population. For example, in a 1992 survey of students at Hunter College, NYC, the RTC administered a symptom checklist and asked about history of blows to the head (Gordon, 1992). About 8% of the sample evidenced symptoms similar to individuals with known TBI and also reported having experienced a blow to the head. A subsequent RTC study (Gordon et al., 1998b) and another reported by Silver, Kramer, Greenwald, and Weissman, (2001), in which they analyzed data from the New Haven National Institute of Mental Health (NIMH) catchment area study, suggest that about 7% of people in the community appear to have experienced a TBI. Although those within this 7% typically do not identify themselves as having a disability, Silver and colleagues found that their persisting symptoms interfere with daily functioning. For example, compared to individuals reporting no head injury, those who *did* experience such an injury were almost twice as likely to be on public assistance and were four times more likely to have attempted suicide.

Thus, in populations such as persons with traumatic brain injury, identification and screening to find members of the population who do not self-identify, but who could be helped to better function if they were known, is a largely unrecognized problem. Further, in terms of insider empowerment, if researchers fail to include this part of the population in a sampling plan, their voices are never heard.

A related problem in sampling is comorbidity. Too much research assumes (wrongly) that members of the population sampled represent a single impairment. However, comorbidity, at least in the area of TBI, is quite common and typically has strong implications for designing research, services, and accommodations. For example, Silver screened a large sample of people with schizophrenia for comorbid TBI; he found that more than 20% had experienced a brain injury and that those with comorbid TBI were more likely to be homeless (Silver et al., 2001). Dennis Moore and his colleagues have studied comorbidity of substance abuse and a variety of other impairments (Substance Abuse and Mental Health Services Administration, 1998). For example, Moore and Weber (2000) found that in substance abusers with one additional disability, in 28% of the cases the disability was mental illness; for those with two or more additional disabilities, this figure rose to 92%.

In the RTC's screening of new clients of the New York Office of Alcohol and Substance Abuse Services, 45% of their clients met criteria of having a comorbid TBI (Gordon, 2002). In individuals with more than one TBI, the average age of first injury was 14 and current age was 27. Thus, the average person screened was injured prior to becoming a substance abuser and was *un*identified as a person with a TBI for an average of 13 years in a variety of settings—school, work, and hospitals, as well as in public assistance and treatment programs. This is not just an academic issue, as comorbid TBI often has strong implications for individual functioning and for how community-based programs can best help insiders in reaching their full potential.

In terms of sampling and empowerment, it is clear that people with unidentified impairments rarely are included in sampling plans. We have inadequate data on hidden disabilities across the board. And, all too often in research within the world of disablement (and without), comorbidity found via screening is typically a reason to *ex*clude a person from study. In seeking so-called clean samples, researchers fail to document the complex situations of people with a variety of disabling conditions. We need to improve methods of identifying people with hidden disabilities and to include individuals with comorbid conditions, as part of engaging in research that acknowledges the complexity of living with disablement and certainly as a means of documenting unmet needs of these infrequently studied people.

In concluding this discussion, we would like to emphasize that we have much to do as a society and within our CI research community in living up to the charge given us in Dart's gentle but powerful words. We have suggested an empowerment paradigm for CI research in which insiders become part of the research process through PAR, the perspective of insiders to disability is sought within measurement, research that is action-oriented and of known importance to insiders is given priority, and all subgroups within the focal population of insiders are accessed into study samples.

AUTHOR NOTE

Wayne A. Gordon is the Jack Nach Professor of Rehabilitation Medicine, Mount Sinai School of Medicine, New York City; Margaret Brown is an adjunct assistant professor in the Department of Community and Preventive Medicine at Mount Sinai School of Medicine; Allan I. Bergman was executive director of the Brain Injury Association of America; Ralph William Shields is a consumer advocate from Albany, NY.

This activity is supported in part by Grant No. H133B30038, to the Department of Rehabilitation Medicine, the Mount Sinai School of Medicine, New York City, from the National Institute on Disability and Rehabilitation Research, United States Department of Education. The contents of this chapter do not necessarily represent the views of the U.S. Department of Education; readers should not assume endorsement by the U.S. government.

Correspondence concerning this chapter should be addressed to Wayne A. Gordon, Department of Rehabilitation Medicine, Mount Sinai School of Medicine.

QUESTIONS FOR DISCUSSION AND/OR FURTHER STUDY

Service Domain

1. How do the ideas that Gordon and colleagues advocate apply within a service context? Imagine yourself a top administrator who felt that insider empowerment was an important way to go (in an agency that you know)—what would you see as needing change, and how could such changes be effected?

2. If you were a person with a disability receiving services in a state vocational rehabilitation agency, what elements of this chapter do you think would ring true, and what might seem pie-in-the-sky?

Research Domain

3. Develop a brief proposal for a study evaluating a vocational needs assessment of people with recent spinal cord injuries that operates within an empowerment paradigm.
4. Provide examples from the research literature that illustrate the differences between research that focuses on reduction of disablement, and research that addresses the needs of people. What arguments can you muster to support research of each type? How would these arguments differ for insiders with a disability and researchers/outsiders?
5. How might researchers with a disability and those without a disability differ in their perspectives on the importance of research on environmental barriers, return to work after rehabilitation, independence in ADL, technological aids, and housing? What factors other than being an insider versus an outsider might affect these perspectives?

Policy Domain

6. What measures would you incorporate into the process of funding research—from writing requests for proposals to developing standards for evaluating applications—to further the growth of the empowerment paradigm? What types of priorities, policies, and guidelines hinder such growth?

NOTE

1. Flanagan's list refers to 15 need areas; but measures for only 11 need areas could be generated from items in our database to fit all four approaches adopted

REFERENCES

Andrews, F. M., & Withey, S. B. (1976). *Social indicators of well-being: Americans' perceptions of quality of life.* New York: Plenum.

Bigelow, D. A., Gareau, M. J., & Young, D. J. (1992). A quality of life interview. *Psychosocial Rehabilitation Journal, 14,* 94–98.

Brown, M., Dijkers, M.P.J.M., Gordon, W. A., Ashman, T. Charatz, H., & Cheng, Z. (2004). Participation objective, participation subjective: A measure of participation combining outsider and insider perspectives. *Journal of Head Trauma Rehabilitation, 19,* 459–481.

Brown, M., & Gordon, W. A. (2004). Empowerment in measurement: "muscle," "voice" and subjective quality of life as a gold standard. *Archives of Physical Medicine and Rehabilitation, 85*(4, Suppl 2), S13–S20.

Brown, M., & Gordon, W. A. (1999). Quality of life as a construct in health and disability research. *Mount Sinai Medical Journal, 66,* 160–169.

Brown, M., Gordon, W. A., & Haddad, L. (2000). Models for predicting subjective quality of life in individuals with traumatic brain injury. *Brain Injury, 14,* 5–19.

Brown, M., Gordon, W. A., & Spielman, L. (2003). Participation in social and recreational activity in the community by individuals with traumatic brain injury. *Rehabilitation Psychology, 48,* 266–274.

Brown, M., & Heinemann, A. (1999). NIDRR's New Paradigm: Opportunities and caveats. *Rehabilitation Outlook, 4*(3), 1, 6, 7, 9.

Brown, M., & Vandergoot, D. (1998). Quality of life of individuals with traumatic brain injury: Comparison with others living in the community. *Journal of Head Trauma Rehabilitation, 13*(4), 1–23.

Busch, C. R., & Alpern, H. P. (1998). Depression after mild traumatic brain injury: A review of current research. *Neuropsychological Review, 8*(2), 95–108.

Carling, P. J. (1990). Major mental illness, housing, and supports: The promise of community integration. *American Psychologist, 45,* 969–975.

Corrigan, J. D., Smith-Knapp, K., & Granger, C. (1998). Outcomes in the first 5 years after traumatic brain injury. *Archives of Physical Medicine and Rehabilitation, 79,* 298–305.

Dembo, T. (1964). Sensitivity of one person to another. *Rehabilitation Literature, 25,* 231–235.

Diener, E. (1984). Subjective well-being. *Psychological Bulletin, 95,* 542–575.

Dijkers, M. (1997). Quality of life after spinal cord injury: A meta analysis of the effects of disablement components. *Spinal Cord, 35,* 829–840.

Donnelly, C., & Carswell, A. (2002). Individualized outcome measures: A review of the literature. *Canadian Journal of Occupational Therapy, 69*(2), 84–94.

Elliott, T. R., & Frank, R. G. (1996). Depression following spinal cord injury. *Archives of Physical Medicine and Rehabilitation, 77,* 816–823.

Felce, D., & Emerson, E. (2001). Living with support in a home in the community: Predictors of behavioral development and household and community activity. *Mental Retardation and Developmental Disabilities Research Review, 7*(2), 75–83.

Felmingham, K. L., Baguley, I. J., & Crooks, J. (2001). A comparison of acute and postdischarge predictors of employment 2 years after traumatic brain injury. *Archives of Physical Medicine and Rehabilitation, 82,* 435–439.

Ferrans, C., & Powers, M. (1985). Quality of life index: Development and psychometric properties. *Advances in Nursing Science, 8,* 15–24.

Flanagan, J. C. (1978). A research approach to improving quality of life. *American Psychologist, 33,* 138–147.

Flanagan, J. C. (1982). Measurement of quality of life: Current state of the art. *Archives of Physical Medicine and Rehabilitation, 63,* 56–59.

Fuhrer, M. J., Rintala, D. H., Hart, K. A., Clearman, R., & Young, M. E. (1992). Relationship of life satisfaction to impairment, disability, and handicap among persons with spinal cord injury living in the community. *Archives of Physical Medicine and Rehabilitation, 73,* 552–557.

Gordon, E. W. (1971). Race, ethnicity, and social disadvantagement and rehabilitation. In W. S. Neff (Ed.) *Rehabilitation psychology* (pp. 201–214). Washington, DC: American Psychological Association.

Gordon, W. A. (1992). [Survey data, Hunter College students]. Unpublished data.

Gordon, W. A. (2002). [Self-reported history of injury to the brain in substance abusers]. Unpublished data.

Gordon, W. A., & Brown, M. (2003). *Participation, objective. Participation, subjective.* New York: Research and Training Center on Community Integration of Individuals with TBI, Mount Sinai School of Medicine.

Gordon, W. A., Brown, M., & Hibbard, M (1998a). *Living life after TBI.* New York: Research and Training Center on Community Integration of Individuals with TBI, Mount Sinai School of Medicine.

Gordon, W. A., Brown, M., Sliwinski, M., Hibbard, M., Patti, N., Weiss, M. J., Kalinsky, R., & Sheerer, M. (1998b). The enigma of "hidden" traumatic brain injury. *Journal of Head Trauma Rehabilitation, 13*(6), 17–33.

Gordon, W. A., & Hibbard, M. (1997). A review of post-stroke depression. *Archives of Physical Medicine and Rehabilitation, 78,* 658–663.

Gordon, W. A., Hibbard, M. R., Brown, M., Flanagan, S., & Campbell-Korves, M. (1999). Community integration of individuals with TBI. In M. Rosenthal, E. R. Griffith, J. S. Kreutzer, & B. Pentland (Eds.), *Rehabilitation of the adult and child with traumatic brain injury* (3rd ed.). Philadelphia: F. A. Davis.

Gordon, W. A., Hibbard, M. R., Egelko, S., Riley, E., Simon, D., Diller, L., & Ross, E. D. (1991). Issues in the diagnosis of post-stroke depression. *Rehabilitation Psychology, 36,* 71–88.

Granger, C. V., Divan, N., & Fiedler, R. C. (1995). Functional assessment scales. A study of persons after traumatic brain injury. *American Journal of Physical Medicine and Rehabilitation, 74,* 107–113.

Heinemann, A. W., & Whiteneck, G. G. (1995). Relationships among impairment, disability, handicap and life satisfaction in persons with traumatic brain injury. *Journal of Head Trauma Rehabilitation, 10*(4), 54–63.

Hibbard, M. R., Uysal, S., Sliwinski, M., & Gordon, W. A. (1998a). Undiagnosed health issues in individuals with traumatic brain injury living in the community. *Journal of Head Trauma Rehabilitation, 13*(4), 47–57.

Hibbard, M., Uysal, S., Kepler, K., Bogdany, J., & Silver, J. (1998b). Axis I psychopathology in individuals with TBI. *Journal of Head Trauma Rehabilitation, 13*(4), 24–39.

Holburn, S., & Vietze, P. (2002). *Person-centered planning: Research, practice and future directions.* Baltimore: Brookes.

Kiresuk, T. J., & Sherman, R. E. (1968). Goal attainment scaling: A general method for evaluating comprehensive community mental health programs. *Community Mental Health Journal, 4,* 443–453.

Krause, J. S., Kemp, B., & Coker, J. (2000). Depression after spinal cord injury: Relation to gender, ethnicity, aging and socioeconomic indicators. *Archives of Physical Medicine and Rehabilitation, 81,* 1099–1109.

Krogh, K. (Ed.) (1998). Community partnerships: Research and action on disability issues [special issue]. *Canadian Journal of Rehabilitation, 12*(2).

Kruzich, J. M. (1985). Community integration of the mentally ill in residential facilities. *American Journal of Community Psychology, 13,* 553–564.

Law, M., Baptiste, S., McColl, M. A., Opzoomer, A., Polatajko, H., & Pollock, N. (1990). The Canadian Occupational Performance Measure: An outcome measure for occupational therapy. *Canadian Journal of Occupational Therapy, 57,* 82–87.

Law, M., Polatajko, H., Pollock, N., McColl, M. A., Carswell, A., & Baptiste, S. (1994). Pilot testing of the Canadian Occupational Performance Measure: Clinical and measurement issues. *Canadian Journal of Occupational Therapy, 61,* 191–197.

Malec, J. F., Smigielski, J. S., DePompolo, R. W., & Thompson, J. M. (1991). Goal attainment scaling and outcome measurement in postacute brain injury rehabilitation. *Archives of Physical Medicine and Rehabilitation, 72,* 138–143.

McColl, M. A., Carlson, P., Johnston, J., Minnes, P., Shue, K., Davies, D., & Karlovits, T. (1998). The definition of community integration: Perspectives of people with brain injuries. *Brain Injury, 12,* 15–30.

McColl, M. A., Davies, D., Carlson, P., Johnston, J., & Minnes, P. (2001). The community integration measure: Development and preliminary validation. *Archives of Physical Medicine and Rehabilitation, 82,* 429–434.

Millis, S. R., Rosenthal, M., & Lourie, I. F. (1994). Predicting community integration after traumatic brain injury with neuropsychological measures. *International Journal of Neuroscience, 79* (3–4), 165–167.

Minnes, P., Carlson, P., McColl, M. A., Nolte, M. L., Johnston, J., & Buell, K. (2003). Community integration: A useful construct, but what does it really mean? *Brain Injury, 17,* 149–159.

Moore, D., & Weber, J. (2000, November). *An analysis of statewide substance use treatment episode data and persons with coexisting disabilities.* Paper presented at the meeting of the American Public Health Association, Boston, MA.

Mount, B., Riggs, D., Brown, M., & Hibbard, M. (1997). *Moving on: A personal futures planning workbook for individuals with brain injury.* New York: Research and Training Center on Community Integration of Individuals with TBI, Mount Sinai Medical Center.

National Institute on Disability and Rehabilitation Research. (1999a). *Long-Range Plan 1999–2003.* Retrieved from www.ed.gov/pubs/edpubs.html

National Institute on Disability and Rehabilitation Research. (1999b, December 7). *Correction for final long-range plan for fiscal years 1999–2003.* Department of Education. *Federal Register, 64*(234).

O'Neill, J., Brown, M., Gordon, W., & Schonhorn, R. (1985). The impact of deinstitutionalization on activities and skills of severely/profoundly mentally retarded multiply-handicapped adults. *Applied Research in Mental Retardation, 6,* 361–371.

O'Neill, J., Brown, M., Gordon, W., Schonhorn, R., & Greer, E. (1981). Activity patterns of mentally retarded adults in institutions and communities: A longitudinal study. *Applied Research in Mental Retardation, 2,* 367–379.

Pavot, W., Diener, E., Colvin, C. R., & Sandvik, E. (1991). Further validation of the Satisfaction with Life Scale: Evidence for the cross-method convergence of well-being measures. *Journal of Personality Assessment, 57*(1), 149–161.

Pyne, J. M., Patterson, T. L., Kaplan, R. M., Gillin, J. C., Koch, W. L., & Grant, I. (1997). Assessment of the quality of life of patients with major depression. *Psychiatric Services, 48,* 224–230.

Racino, J. A. (2002). Community integration and statewide systems change: Qualitative evaluation research in community life and disability. *Journal of Health and Social Policy, 14*(3), 1–25.

Rosenthal, M., Christensen, B. K., & Ross, T. P. (1998). Depression following traumatic brain injury. *Archives of Physical Medicine and Rehabilitation, 79,* 90–103.

Salzberg, C. L., & Langford, C. A. (1981). Community integration of mentally retarded adults through leisure activity. *Mental Retardation, 19*(3), 127–131.

Schalock, R. L., & Alonso, M.A.V. (2002). *Handbook on quality of life for human service practitioners.* Washington, DC: American Association on Mental Retardation.

Schalock, R. L., Harper, R. S., & Genung, T. (1981). Community integration of mentally retarded adults: Community placement and program success. *American Journal of Mental Deficiency, 85,* 478–488.

Seekins, T. (2003, October). *Testing threats to social validity in research.* Paper presented at the annual meeting of the American Congress of Rehabilitation Medicine, Tucson, AZ.

Silver, J. M., Kramer, R., Greenwald, S., & Weissman, M. (2001). The association between head injuries and psychiatric disorders: Findings from the New Haven NIMH Epidemiologic Catchment Area Study. *Brain Injury, 15,* 935–945.

Substance Abuse and Mental Health Services Administration. (1998). *Substance use disorder treatment for people with physical and cognitive disabilities: Treatment Improvement Protocol (TIP) Series 29* (DHHS Publication No. SMA 98–3249). Washington, DC: U.S. Government Printing Office.

Sullivan, W. P. (1992). Reclaiming the community: The strengths perspective and deinstitutionalization. *Social Work, 37,* 204–209.

Wherley, M., & Bisgaard, S. (1987). Beyond model programs: Evaluation of a countywide system of residential treatment programs. *Hospital and Community Psychiatry, 38,* 852–857.

White, G. W. (2002). Consumer participation in disability research: The Golden Rule as a guide for ethical practice. *Rehabilitation Psychology, 47,* 438–446.

Whyte, W. F. (Ed.) (1991). *Participatory action research.* Newbury Park, CA: Sage.

Willer, B., Rosenthal, M., Kreutzer, J., Gordon, W. A., & Rempel, R. (1993). Assessment of community integration following rehabilitation for traumatic brain injury. *Journal of Head Trauma Rehabilitation, 8*(2), 75–87.

CHAPTER TWO

Considering Class, Culture, and Access in Rehabilitation Intervention and Research

Catherine A. Marshall
Priscilla R. Sanderson
Sharon R. Johnson
Barbara Du Bois
Joseph C. Kvedar

Rehabilitation psychologists and educators have long advocated that culture, including behaviors, beliefs, and values associated with ethnicity and race, be recognized as *essential context* in rehabilitation research and service delivery.[1] For example, Leung stated in 1993 that our "changing demography and its implication for vocational rehabilitation must be met directly and forcefully" (p. 10). Twenty years ago Atkins (1982) linked the rehabilitation needs of women with their cultural characteristics. Cross-cultural lessons have been offered for rehabilitation educators and professionals (Lopez Levers & Maki, 1994), and concerns regarding culturally appropriate service delivery have been well documented (Leal, Leung, Martin, & Harrison, 1988; Wright & Leung, 1992). Special focus on the needs and concerns of specific cultural groups, particularly populations that are otherwise ignored and invisible to policy makers, is essential. However, cultural topics that relate to disability and rehabilitation can no longer be confined to the occasional special issue of a rehabilitation journal or a conference. It is crucial that cultural focus not only become a core component of rehabilitation education and service delivery (Marshall, Johnson, & Johnson, 1996), but that cultural context be viewed as an essential aspect of service and research planning (Marshall, Leung, Johnson, &Busby, 2003).

Rehabilitation professionals may feel overwhelmed at having to learn about the cultures of others because cultures are so numerous, diverse, and susceptible to stereotyping, and because it is hard to know where and how to begin in understanding the effects of culture in rehabilitation, including research. Specific suggestions on where to begin in terms of understanding the cultures of others have been documented elsewhere (Makas, Marshall, & Wehman, 1997; Marshall, Johnson, & Johnson, 1996; Marshall, Martin, Thomason, & Johnson, 1991). Most importantly, one must simply begin.

A postcard advertising a Peruvian foundation concerned with the cardiac health of children reads, "El mundo y nuestro país está lleno de gente de diferentes culturas, pero muchos de nuestros gentes tienen algo en común, un corazón" [The world and our country are full of people of different cultures, but many of the people have something in common, a heart]. The United States is a nation of immigrants in a world increasingly characterized by instantaneous worldwide communication and interpenetrating global economic, political, social, and intellectual networks. We can learn much from the many world cultures that are closely intertwined with the different cultures within our own borders. Leung (1993) wrote a decade ago that our new demography, including the impact of immigration, provides what should be seen as positive opportunities for change. In particular, he noted that the very need for "inclusion of differences provides the opportunity to develop responsive institutions that fit the needs of clients who have traditionally and historically not been served well" (p. 5). Thus culture must indeed be seen as the essential context within which rehabilitation programs of research and intervention are designed and implemented.

We affirm that the cultural context, with its myriad changing elements and dynamics that shape the attitudes and behaviors of individuals, families, and communities, is to be seen as *fully positive* and not framed as a potential barrier to standard, one-size-fits-all procedures in rehabilitation and research. In ensuring the participation of people with disabilities in our communities and in refining our rehabilitation research agenda, culture must be acknowledged, documented, and embraced (Marshall, Bruyère, Shern, & Jircitano, 1996).

We believe that class issues should be approached in the same manner. Although many Americans think of the United States as a classless society with equality of opportunity for all, one has only to be a person of color, a woman (particularly a single mother on public assistance), old, poor, or with a disability to understand that this perception does not reflect our present reality. Ensuring the full community participation of people with disabilities also means ensuring their full access to the disability and rehabilitation services that will make this possible. Because disability and poverty are so closely linked in our society (as we discuss in more detail below), class is in fact a critical factor in relation to rehabilitation access and community participation.

This chapter looks at class, culture, and disability at a crucial point where they intersect: in access to rehabilitation interventions, as understood through examples involving training, transportation, and independent living. A new rehabilitation model that can enhance access, telerehabilitation, is explored in relation to culturally appropriate rehabilitation intervention. Finally, proposals for a rehabilitation research agenda that addresses important issues of class, culture, and access are detailed in three areas: independent living, disability conditions, and research itself.

ACCESS: THE INTERSECTION OF CLASS AND CULTURE

It is important to address the intersection of class and culture, where persons of limited economic means seek access to quality rehabilitation intervention that is consonant with their cultural values and mores. While one could argue that persons with disabilities and of cultures other than the dominant culture face problems of access in the United States regardless of their socioeconomic status, rehabilitation researchers need to focus on the status of rehabilitation intervention for low-income Americans—Americans who even after rehabilitation services may find themselves among the working poor. The American promise is still that education and training will lead to successful employment outcomes— outcomes that will assure sufficient income for the necessities of life: a home, a car, store-bought clothes, groceries, utilities, and perhaps simple pleasures such as a good haircut. It becomes increasingly evident that the promise does not always include access to quality health care or to rehabilitation services that result in employment with a health insurance benefit (Lustig & Strauser, 2003).

Public vocational rehabilitation is not an entitlement program but an eligibility program, and is most often based on financial need for cost-based services or technology. Americans with disabilities who depend on public aid for their main source of income face incredibly intricate financial systems on a day-to-day basis, and frequently are living in or on the edge of poverty (Banks & Ackerman, 2003; Lustig & Strauser, 2003). Conflicting rules and regulations, communications confusions, reporting difficulties, transportation problems, callousness or insensitivity on the part of systems representatives, inability to self-advocate—these are just a few of the problems they experience daily. Choices become more and more limited; control is lost. For example, poor people with disabilities are at risk of losing their independence, especially when affordable housing is an issue. The needs of poor people with disabilities may be consistently ignored and overlooked, but if they attempt to assert themselves they risk sacrificing their dignity and receiving punitive reactions that further threaten their access to services. The problems intensify if they attempt to return to work, because additional income may jeopardize their eligibility for needed benefits and services and can make a fragile balance difficult to maintain.

The common denominator among people with disabilities is poverty. From our clinical experience and perspective based on 25 years of service in the public vocational rehabilitation system, we have found that poverty among people with disabilities is a problem that cuts across culture, race, ethnic group, or geographical area (see also Utter, 1993.) It can also cut across social class and educational levels, as acquired disability can plunge one precipitously into poverty. Some vocational rehabilitation programs may analyze a client's financial situation to see what effect competitive employment will have on an individual's financial status. Some who could work might not be able to afford to do so, as accepting even a low-wage job can result in loss of benefits such as Medicare or Medicaid coverage (Lustig & Strauser, 2003).

The intersection of class and culture makes clear that the proper focus of publicly funded vocational rehabilitation programs should be on providing culturally appropriate resources and services to those without the income or education that would enable them to gain access to those services. In the following section we examine three arenas—education and training, transportation, and independent living—in which access to rehabilitation services can ameliorate problems relating to class and culture.

Education and Training as a Path to Employment

People with disabilities who are having trouble securing or maintaining employment because of a disability or handicapping conditions of the environment may turn to state and, where available, tribal vocational rehabilitation programs for employment-related assistance. While a wide range of services is available through these programs, one service that needs to be scrutinized is training. People with disabilities can acquire training on their own, but counseling and guidance services, case planning, and client advocacy are often critical in helping people appreciate choices and make decisions. Clients have the right to set their sights high and aspire to both the best education available and to the widest possible array of fields of work. All too frequently, however, appropriate and viable plans are discouraged or dismissed by state agency personnel because of financial considerations or logistics, such as distances to training sites (Wright, 1993). Agency policies and practices do not provide unlimited access to training—and therefore to the kinds of occupations or professions that individuals with disabilities can pursue.

Class, racial, ethnic, and gender stereotyping can also limit choices; rehabilitation psychologists and counselors are not immune to stereotypes and prejudice. Tailoring outcome expectations and thus vocational or professional education and training to the existing "social context" of rehabilitation clients, as recommended by Thomas and Weinrach (2002), may risk countenancing lower expectations as both reasonable and desirable for lower social class and low-income rehabilitation clients, or even for clients of certain ethnic or racial groups. When the training, or the best-quality training, for the work the client desires is unavailable in the local setting, the state agency should assume the ethical responsibility of providing counseling and financial assistance for the best opportunity, no matter where that might be found.

Transportation

Transportation is often a major obstacle that limits access to rehabilitation services, medical management, and independent living, in both urban and rural areas. President Bush's New Freedom Initiative (2001) called transportation "a primary barrier to work for people with disabilities: one-third of people with disabilities report that inadequate transportation is a significant problem" (p. 10). Rural areas are notoriously difficult in terms of public transportation, the lack of which can create nearly insurmountable or even life-threatening conditions.

Most major cities have some type of public transportation available for people with disabilities (e.g., accessible "kneeling" buses, accessible vans with portal-to-portal service), but even there inclement weather, unsafe neighborhoods, infrequent schedules, limited routes, and poor funding can limit access to transport. Consequently, people with mobility impairments can become housebound and isolated, unable to use health care facilities and maintain community involvement. Some individual communities and states are addressing transportation issues through innovative rehabilitation programs such as New Mexico's "Whatever It Takes: Solutions in Transportation" program (Yvonne Hart, Project

Director, personal communication, January 29, 2003). We call for the success of these programs to be reported widely in professional research and service-oriented publications as well as in community media, and replicated, preferably in numerous and diverse contexts.

Independence and Control in Community Participation

The philosophy of the independent living movement emphasizes the rights of people with disabilities to determine their own futures through choice and control (Nosek, Roth, & Zhu, 1990; Shapiro, 1995; Smith, Smith, Richards, Frieden, & King, 1994). Both establishing and maintaining the basic human rights of people with disabilities and enhancing their status in their communities are on independent living agendas world-wide (Batavia, 2001; Leutz, 1998; Smith, 2001). Successful independent living programs can provide important community resources that fulfill the potential of rehabilitation services. They offer accessible services and counseling, support the goals of persons with disabilities, and provide opportunities for rehabilitation professionals and community members to resolve barriers resulting from disability, class, and culture. Independent living centers respond to federal mandates to provide information and referral, independent living skills training, advocacy and systems change, and peer counseling, yet chronic underfunding can severely limit their effectiveness (Starkloff, 1997).

Some groups are at particular risk of not receiving independent living services. Nosek, Roth, and Zhu (1990) found that outreach is needed to specific populations, including young children and the elderly. As individuals with one or more disabilities grow older (and perhaps poorer, if their retirement depends primarily on Social Security income), their disabilities and functional limitations may become more severe. Health care delivery stakeholders and those providing rehabilitation and independent living services can form partnerships to meet the needs of these underserved consumers (Batavia, 2001; Moore & Stephens, 1994). Moore and Stephens recommended the expansion of independent living services for older blind individuals in all 50 states and territories. Even though the 1992 amendment to the Rehabilitation Act of 1973 (Chapter 2, Title VII) authorizes training, including the use of specialized adaptive living skills for older blind individuals to live independently, many do not receive these services.

Provision of training requires qualified service providers. In addition to administrative, financial, and clinical skills, Wong and Millard (1992) found that independent living service providers need training and technical assistance on cross-cultural ethical standards to promote competence and enhance services available to marginalized and underserved populations. Wong and Millard discussed conflicts in service delivery that can create ethical dilemmas for independent living service providers, such as when a provider's perceptions of need are contradictory to consumer choices. They recommended ethics training that covers (a) identification of ethical dilemmas in case studies, (b) developing resolutions to ethical dilemmas, and (c) providing the opportunity to explore decision-making skills in role-play scenarios with consumers.

Ensuring Access for the Underserved

One underserved group that receives little attention is people living with and surviving cancer. Conti (1990) found that many independent living centers and state vocational rehabilitation service agencies are not serving cancer patients and may not be aware of several key issues. First, cancer patients' rates of survival have increased over the years, and many cancer patients can qualify for disability benefits. Cancer survivors are among the lowest in cost to serve, and many people in this group are able to work. The disability-poverty relationship is striking in this population; "poor Americans, irrespective of race, have a 10 to 15% decreased rate of survival from cancer compared to the general population" (American Cancer Society, 2003, p. 1).

Eliminating health and employment disparities by 2010 is a major goal of the U.S. Department of Health and Human Services (2000). Both independent living and vocational rehabilitation services will be required to assure that our nation achieves this goal and ensures access to culturally appropriate and high-quality services for all Americans, regardless of class, culture, or income level. A novel means of achieving this goal is through the widespread application of telerehabilitation, particularly as regards access to the cultural expertise that makes those services genuinely available to traditionally underreached and underserved people in our country.

TELEREHABILITATION: A NEW MODEL FOR ACCESS

We are at an auspicious historical moment to consider, imaginatively and boldly, what new forms of rehabilitation resources and services we might create to meet the needs of underserved people with disabilities, and to ameliorate barriers to access resulting from culture and class. Telerehabilitation is one such new form, possible only now because of recent advances in computer technology and worldwide telecommunications. Telerehabilitation programs are under development through the Rehabilitation Engineering Research Center on Telerehabilitation (http://www.telerehab-nrh.org), among others. These efforts focus primarily on bringing vocational rehabilitation counseling and resources, including assistive technology, to clients who are otherwise unable to receive these services because of distance or functional limitations. Telerehabilitation offers significant expansion and strengthening of rehabilitation's potential to serve all people with disabilities, regardless of location or condition.

Telemedicine provides an instructive model for telerehabilitation. Telemedicine offers to everyone the promise of enhanced access to a knowledgeable and qualified health care advocate, as well as timely access to specialized medical knowledge. Partners Telemedicine (http://telemedicine.partners.org) is an award-winning, internationally recognized program with the mission of extending expert health care knowledge to patients and physicians worldwide, using modern information and communications technologies as a conduit. Founded in 1995 by Dr. Joseph Kvedar, with the support of Massachusetts General Hospital (MGH), the program has become a channel for disseminating knowledge from Harvard's preeminent teaching hospitals, Brigham and Women's Hospital, Massachusetts General Hospital, and the Dana Farber Cancer Institute. Partners Telemedicine has four well-formed strategic and programmatic areas of focus:

1. Online consultation, performed with worldwide reach through Partners Online Specialty Consultations (http://www.partners.org/econsults). Through this secure website, patients, in conjunction with their health care providers, can obtain a consultation with one of the faculty affiliated with one of the sponsoring institutions. In one year alone, 1,300 consultations were provided in all specialties to patients and physicians in over 30 countries.
2. Medical education, delivered to clinicians worldwide using both videoconferencing technologies (1,200 programs in fiscal year 2001) and the World Wide Web (http://www.partners.org/conferences).
3. Outreach to underserved populations (for example, see http://www.villageleap.com).
4. Monitoring of people with chronic illness in their homes.

The Partners Telemedicine program serving Robib, Cambodia, illustrates the fact that

> "telemedicine involves the use of communications technology to move medical information rather than moving patients, so that anyone,

anytime, anywhere can benefit from the best health care available. Throughout history, medical experts have tended to congregate in large metropolitan areas, limiting access of those who live in remote regions of the world. Telemedicine is becoming a powerful tool to bridge this inequality of access to quality medical care" (Kvedar, n.d., p. 1).

Telerehabilitation can enhance access for people with disabilities. Just as improved medical access is now available to patients in Cambodia, rehabilitation clients in places like Pearl River, Mississippi; Douglas, Arizona; and Nett Lake, Minnesota can have access to high-quality rehabilitation services. Telerehabilitation (Lloyd, 2002) can provide clients and counselors with access to rehabilitation expertise that has been unavailable due to economic factors, geographic distance, or barriers resulting from culture or class (Marshall, Bruyère, Shern, & Jircitano, 1996).

A significant and powerful element of telerehabilitation is its potential to bring cultural expertise to rehabilitation counselors and their interventions. Should a Hmong client apply for services in Arizona, the expertise needed to develop an employment plan may be available in St. Paul rather than in Tucson. Determining eligibility for an older Navajo client recovering from cancer might be facilitated through consultation with a senior counselor in Seattle who has specialized in this area rather than with a rehabilitation counselor who is geographically close to the client. Physical restoration services might best be planned with experts not available in rural areas. Finally, the value and uses of traditional healing practices such as acupuncture, herbal remedies, and indigenous ceremonies not understood or available in all areas of our country could be explained by experts and consumers through telerehabilitation; some healing modalities might even be made available through telerehabilitation training and videoconferencing.

The current pace of discovery in computer technology and telecommunications may outstrip our imaginations, but even within the limits of current applications some important implications of these new technologies are clear. Telerehabilitation can allow rehabilitation counselors who are unfamiliar with the cultural background of a new client to draw on the expertise of culturally skilled counselors, as well as provide guidance through expert consultation in the full range of rehabilitation services to clients and counselors who are isolated by geography or economic circumstances. Some readers may be concerned that a "digital divide" will limit the expertise which could be available through telerehabilitation from reaching clients who need it most. However, data from a recent report, *A Nation Online: How Americans are Expanding their Use of the Internet,* suggest that this may not be a problem. Evans (2002) noted that all groups are using communication technologies in increasing numbers.

Rehabilitation must follow the model of medicine in ensuring community participation and access to the highest quality of rehabilitation services. Rehabilitation can go beyond current models of telemedicine to ensure not only that services are provided, but that they are provided in consultation with cultural specialists whenever necessary.

TOWARD A REHABILITATION RESEARCH AGENDA

Richard W. Riley, former U.S. Secretary of Education, stated that "research has the potential to reinvent the future for millions of people with disabilities and their families" (Riley, 1998, p. 57190). President Bush, in announcing the New Freedom Initiative of 2001, said that he is "committed to tearing down the remaining barriers to equality that face Americans with disabilities today" (p.1). While it should be the goal of both rehabilitation researchers and providers to ensure that individuals with disabilities from all classes and cultural groups of our society have the opportunity for full community participation, it should be the particular goal of *publicly* funded rehabilitation research and services to ensure that low-income and underserved individuals have full access to all needed information and services. Given the advances of technology and telecommunication, lack of access to high-quality training, education, and expert consultation due to barriers resulting from transportation, economic status, or cultural factors, is no longer unavoidable or justifiable.

We advocate the active involvement of vocational rehabilitation counselors and other service providers in identifying and seeking solutions to community needs and problems faced by their clients. Further, we encourage rehabilitation researchers to apply innovative research designs and methods to the pressing problems identified by people with disabilities. We have called for the active involvement of researchers in communities under study and in seeking solutions to concerns that have been documented through their investigations (Marshall, et al., 2002). In addition, with others we have advocated for participatory action research as means of assuring that research goals and methods are relevant to persons with disabilities (Blanck, Ritchie, Schmeling, & Klein, 2003; Bruyère, 1993; Davis & Keemer, 2002; Marshall, Johnson, Martin, Saravanabhavan & Bradford, 1992).

Full community participation is lacking for many Americans with disabilities. Improved independent living outreach and service delivery can contribute to solving this problem, as will improved transportation services in both urban and rural areas. It is also likely that important answers lie in new approaches entirely, such as telerehabilitation, that promote sharing of cultural expertise and bridging of gaps resulting from class and cultural differences. Such options, currently untested, may provide solutions allowing for the highest possible quality of community participation.

Rehabilitation research must be pursued with full commitment to culturally appropriate contexts, using culturally appropriate research designs and instrumentation, of course, but also drawing upon the cultural history, wisdom, and resources of communities and research participants. One example is provided by disability-related research with sovereign American Indian nations, as exemplified in a recent symposium and monograph of the Work Group on American Indian Research and Program Evaluation Methodology (AIRPEM). Based on the broad and multifaceted experience of researchers, program evaluators, health and human service professionals, policy makers, and private practitioners who work with American Indians who have disabilities, this work represents current thinking on culture and research that we believe should inform policy, planning, practice, research, training, and education in rehabilitation and related fields (Davis et al., 2002).

Rehabilitation research must also include research participants from geographically isolated areas of the United States and persons from low-income groups, including the working poor. This latter criterion is not difficult to fulfill given the poor economic situation of many people with disabilities. Research findings should be disseminated in culturally appropriate formats and in languages appreciated by the community members who would benefit from the information, both in terms of program development and local capacity-building efforts. Telerehabilitation can allow researchers to identify experts who are documenting problems and identifying solutions in one part of the country that could then be shared quickly with other parts of the country.

We offer the following recommendations for a rehabilitation research agenda that addresses gaps in current priorities and points to new directions for addressing the urgent concerns discussed in this chapter. These recommendations fall into three main categories: independent living, disability conditions, and research.

Independent Living

1. Independent living centers should develop working partnerships with local clinics to enhance access to services and to emphasize peer support and peer recreation for individuals with mild to severe spinal cord and head injuries (McAweeney, Forchheimer, &

Tate, 1996; Starkloff, 1997). Specifically, further investigation is needed regarding effective strategies for empowering individuals with spinal cord injuries and head injuries as well as on the current functional measurements of impairments that clinical services use.

2. Little is known regarding the specific needs of homeless HIV-infected adolescents. Research should count and describe this population, assess policies regarding their eligibility for and access to benefits and services, and recommend new research directions. Social policies should recognize the right to independent living services, as noted by Rotheram-Borus, Koopman, and Ehrhardt (1991).

3. Hanson (2000) examined six state health care programs from different states that have incorporated the independent living philosophy into their health care delivery and found few studies on managed health care and health care reform that utilize independent living philosophy. Batavia (2001) discussed consumer-directed personal assistance services under the independent living model of community-based long-term care at the residences of working-age consumers. This model needs longitudinal research to determine the outcomes and lasting effects of community-based long-term care. Research is needed on managed care delivery systems that utilize the principles of independent living in order to further understanding of consumer and other stakeholder participation and of collaborative efforts among service providers. Research is also needed on long-term medical-model care versus consumer-directed care.

4. Independent living centers should hire personnel of both sexes and from a variety of racial, ethnic, language, religious, and class backgrounds. They should also provide community outreach services to ethnically diverse populations (Flowers, Edwards, & Pusch, 1996; Sanderson, Schacht, & Clay, 1996a, 1996b; Sanderson & Yazzie-King, 2001; Wright, Martinez, & Dixon, 1999). Flowers and colleagues described the implications of Section 21 of the 1992 Rehabilitation Act amendments on the need to provide equitable vocational rehabilitation and independent living services for the growing population of ethnically diverse people with disabilities in both rural and urban settings, including Indian Country. Further research is needed to compose a demographic profile of independent living center personnel and the consumers they serve. Research is also needed to investigate whether consumers believe their needs are being met within a cultural context that they approve.

Research Related to Specific Disability Conditions

1. More research is needed to understand the transition from school to employment for deaf persons, particularly among different cultural groups and new immigrant populations. Bullis and Reiman (1992) described the need for an instrument to assess the skill levels of deaf adolescents and young adults in transition from school to work after high school, and validated the Transition Competence Battery for Deaf Adolescents and Young Adults.

2. Little is known about the prevalence of Down syndrome in American Indian populations (Rhoades, 2000; Ebbott, 1983). Perhaps the incidence among American Indians is low. If so, is this true across tribal groups or specific to certain tribes? Have individuals with Down syndrome been removed from their families at a young age? Are they hidden within family structures? Is there some type of early mortality of which we are unaware? What can research tell us about the incidence of Down syndrome and other developmental disabilities among other populations in the United States, including recent immigrant populations? What are the specific rehabilitation needs of these individuals and what are appropriate interventions within the cultural context of the family?

3. Rehabilitation counselors are seeing a higher incidence of ADD (attention deficit disorder) and ADHD (attention deficit hyperactivity disorder) among applicants for vocational rehabilitation services, including students in high school. Is this observation the result of easy diagnosis that will suffice to obtain services for individuals, or does it reflect an increase in the numbers of people affected? Could the apparent increase be due to better diagnostic instruments and more perceptive diagnosticians? Do these disabling conditions affect all age groups, or primarily children and young adults? Are there any identifiable class or environmental differences in incidence and prevalence? What are the causes as well as the effects? Do we know the long-term effects of Ritalin and newer stimulant drugs used to combat the problems? Is there any connection with FAS (fetal alcohol syndrome)? Are any prenatal preventive approaches effective?

4. Many women with disabilities, including developmental disabilities in all age ranges, are physically and mentally abused by their personal assistants, caregivers, family, and present or past spouses (Morris, 1995; Powers et al., 2002; Swedlund & Nosek, 2000). Researchers have cited several barriers to women's seeking assistance, including inaccessible women's shelters

and centers for independent living, and vocational rehabilitation services personnel not knowing how to ask questions about abuse. Additionally, information is lacking on women of ethnically diverse backgrounds in abusive situations. There is a need to expand research in this area to improve the quality of life for women with disabilities and their children. In particular, investigation of women with disabilities experiencing abuse must be inclusive and participatory, involving not only the women experiencing abuse but also other stakeholders.

5. Aging "baby boomers" with disabilities, including developmental disabilities, may find their community participation at risk due to secondary disabilities. Researchers have recommended that centers for independent living and community programs reduce the incidence of secondary disabilities through public education, including public education in remote rural areas and in Indian Country (DeJong, 1979; Seekins, Clay, & Ravesloot, 1994; White, Gutierrez, & Seekins, 1996). Further research is needed regarding the health care needs of our growing senior citizen population and the prevention of secondary disabilities in this group. Research is needed to document the demographic characteristics of older blind individuals who receive independent living services. Research is also needed to document the demographic characteristics of older individuals who need independent living services but who are not receiving them.

6. Data on cancer survival rates and on cancer survivors' needs for independent living and vocational rehabilitation services is needed. Cancer survivors and those living with cancer point to the persistence of debilitating, disfiguring, and disabling effects of both the disease and its treatments by noting wryly that "cancer is the gift that keeps on giving" (BDuB), but cancer has been described by one public vocational rehabilitation counselor (SRJ) as "a disability we just don't see"—observations that point to the need for better outreach to counter limited access for this large and often invisible population. A national dissemination conference on cancer rehabilitation is recommended, with the goal of improving practice, informing policy, and raising awareness (Conti, 1990).

Rehabilitation Research

1. Given our diverse population, we are concerned with developing rehabilitation research capacity (Marshall, Leung, Johnson, & Busby, 2003). At a recent rehabilitation educators' conference, a participant remarked to the first author, "I've been very aware

of your research and have always wanted to meet you. I was wondering if you were Indian." This comment raises the question of how the researcher's ethnic or cultural characteristics may influence the research process and the quality and validity of data gathered (Lomawaima & McCarty, 2002; Marshall, Sanders, & Hill, 2001). Who should conduct rehabilitation research focused on ethnically distinct populations? What is the meaning and significance of the researcher's racial, ethnic, or disability status in terms of conducting rigorous and relevant research? Given that extra points may be awarded to a research center's grant application by the National Institute on Disability and Rehabilitation Research for employing researchers with specific demographic characteristics, the influence of these characteristics on the quality and outcomes of research should be documented and understood through carefully planned investigation.

2. As the cultural characteristics of researchers are believed to influence the design and quality of research, so, too, will the cultural characteristics of research participants, especially where participatory research strategies are employed and where culture is recognized as an essential context for developing research methods. We need to understand and document the rehabilitation needs of all Americans, not just those who are willing to participate in English-language surveys or services or who happen to live near a university—always being inclusive of those whose class and culture might make them reticent to participate in rehabilitation. Evidence-based practice requires studies that include recipients from diverse backgrounds, yet we fail to see adequate representation of such individuals in research that provides data regarding the effectiveness of interventions.

SUMMARY

As a society we have made a commitment to ensuring that all citizens with disabilities have access to the best available rehabilitation services. Publicly funded rehabilitation programs must enhance access for low-income people with disabilities, and must be planned and provided in culturally appropriate ways to the many diverse groups that make up our society. Improved access requires that class and cultural needs be considered in the planning and provision of rehabilitation services and training. Many obstacles continue to frustrate our national policy commitment. It is at the intersection where class and culture meet that we can clearly see need and where we can clearly see the most promising directions for immediate and future efforts.

QUESTIONS FOR DISCUSSION AND/OR FURTHER STUDY

Service Domain

1. Describe the factors to be considered regarding class and culture, in regard to telerehabilitation access in a poor rural remote community with limited utilities and transportation.
2. Thomas and Weinrach (2002) offer a "social context" perspective to use in determining options for client vocational training. What arguments can you make for client vocational training using a social justice perspective?

Research Domain

3. Describe the benefits and weaknesses of participatory action rehabilitation research in rural remote communities.
4. How should study protocols consider class and culture when the research involves American Indians and Alaska Natives?
5. The authors argue that the vision of a classless society does not reflect our present reality. Develop a research study that would allow you to marshal arguments for or against this position.

Policy Domain

6. If you were a member of Congress, what policies would you develop to address the issue of people with disabilities who are at the poverty level?
7. Describe the challenges of developing a policy that will be accepted by the public and Congress.
8. The authors conclude, "As a society we have made a commitment to ensuring that all citizens with disabilities have access to the best available rehabilitation services." What points are made in the chapter that argue for or against the truth of this statement?

ACKNOWLEDGMENTS

The authors would like to acknowledge the valued comments and suggestions our colleague, Elizabeth Kendall, PhD, provided on an earlier version of this manuscript.

NOTE

1. The authors note the observation of Coe (2003) that "while anthropologists have had more than a century to reach a consensus on how the term *culture* should be defined, they have yet to do so" (p. 260). In regard to its use in this chapter, we ask the reader to consider a fairly narrow definition of culture, one that focuses on what Pedersen (2003) refers to as "ethnographic variables (nationality, ethnicity, language)." For the reader who would like to further explore definitions of culture and in regard to people with disabilities, we recommend the work of Loveland (1999), who offered that "culture refers to the learned behaviors, values, norms, and symbols that are passed from generation to generation within a society" (p. 18).

REFERENCES

American Cancer Society. (2003). Targeted grants for research directed at poor and underserved populations. Retrieved March 12, 2003, from http://www.cancer.org/docroot/RES/content/RES_5_2x_Targeted_Grants_for_Research_Directed_at_Poor_and_Underserved_Populations.asp?sitearea = RES

Atkins, B. J. (1982). Women as members of special populations in rehabilitation. In L. G. Perlman & K. C. Arneson (Eds.), *Women and rehabilitation of disabled persons* (pp. 38–46). Alexandria, VA: The National Rehabilitation Association.

Banks, M. E., & Ackerman, R. J. (2003). All things being unequal: Culturally relevant roads to employment. In F. E. Menz & D. F. Thomas (Eds.), *Bridging gaps: Refining the disability research agenda for rehabilitation and the social sciences. Conference Proceedings* (pp. 35–63). Menomonie: University of Wisconsin–Stout, Stout Vocational Rehabilitation Institute, Research and Training Center.

Batavia, A. I. (2001, Spring). A right to personal assistance services: "Most integrated setting appropriate" requirements and the independent living model of long-term care. *American Journal of Law and Medicine, 27*(1), 17–43.

Blanck, P., Ritchie, H., Schmeling, J., & Klein, D. (2003). Technology for independence: A community-based resource center. *Behavioral Sciences & the Law, 21*(1), 51–62.

Bruyère, S. M. (1993). Participatory action research: Overview and implications for family members of persons with disabilities. *Journal of Vocational Rehabilitation, 3*(2), 62–68.

Bullis, M., & Reiman, J. (1992, September). Development and preliminary psychometric properties of the Transition Competence Battery for Deaf Adolescents and Young Adults. *Exceptional Children, 59*(1), 12–26.

Coe, K. (2003). *The ancestress hypothesis: Visual art as adaptation.* New Brunswick: Rutgers University Press.

Conti, J. V. (1990, October–December). Cancer rehabilitation: Why can't we get out of first gear? *The Journal of Rehabilitation, 56*(4), 19–22.

Davis, J. D., Erickson, J. S., Johnson, S. R., Marshall, C. A., Running Wolf, P., & Santiago, R. L. (Eds.). (2002). *Work Group on American Indian Research and Program Evaluation Methodology (AIRPEM), Symposium on Research and Evaluation Methodology: Lifespan Issues Related to American Indians/Alaska Natives with Disabilities.* Flagstaff: Northern Arizona University, Institute for Human Development, Arizona University Center on Disabilities, American Indian Rehabilitation Research and Training Center.

Davis, J. D., & Keemer, K. (2002). A brief history of and future considerations for research in American Indian and Alaska Native communities. In J. D. Davis, J. S. Erickson,

S. R. Johnson, C. A. Marshall, P. Running Wolf, & R. L. Santiago (Eds.), *Work Group on American Indian Research and Program Evaluation Methodology (AIRPEM), Symposium on Research and Evaluation Methodology: Lifespan Issues Related to American Indians/Alaska Natives with Disabilities* (pp. 9–18). Flagstaff: Northern Arizona University, Institute for Human Development, Arizona University Center on Disabilities, American Indian Rehabilitation Research and Training Center.

DeJong, G. (1979). Independent living: From social movement to analytic paradigm. *Archives of Physical Medicine and Rehabilitation, 60,* 435–466.

Ebbott, E. (1983). *Indians in Minnesota* (4th ed.). (J. Rosenblatt, Ed.). Minneapolis: University of Minnesota Press.

Evans, D. L. (2002). Foreword. *A nation online: How Americans are expanding their use of the internet.* U.S. Department of Commerce, Economics and Statistical Administration, National Telecommunications and Information Administration. Retrieved April 19, 2002, from http://www.ntia.doc.gov/ntiahome/dn/anationonline2.pdf

Flowers, C. R., Edwards, D., & Pusch, B. (1996, July–September). Rehabilitation cultural diversity initiative: A regional survey of cultural diversity within CILs. *The Journal of Rehabilitation, 62*(3), 22–28.

Hanson, S. P. (2000, Winter). Applying independent living principles to state health-care programs for people with disabilities. *Journal of Disability Policy Studies, 11*(3), 161. Retrieved April 6, 2002, from http://web4.infotrac.galegroup.com/itw/infomark/0/1/1/purl = rc6_EAIM?sw_aep = nau_cline

Kvedar, J. C. (n.d.). *Robib and telemedicine.* Retrieved March 16, 2006, from http://www.camnet.com.kh/cambodiaschools/villageleap/telemedicine_robib.htm.

Leal, A., Leung, P., Martin, W. E., & Harrison, D. K. (1988). Multicultural aspects of rehabilitation counseling: Issues and challenges. *The Journal of Applied Rehabilitation Counseling, 19*(4), 3.

Leung, P. (1993). A changing demography and its challenge. *Journal of Vocational Rehabilitation, 3*(1), 3–11.

Leutz, W. (1998, Summer–Autumn). Home care benefits for persons with disabilities. *American Rehabilitation, 24*(3), 6–14.

Lloyd, M. (2002, May 3). Project lets village doctors in Mexico call on U. of Texas experts. *The Chronicle of Higher Education,* A34.

Lomawaima, K. T., & McCarty, T. L. (2002). Reliability, validity, and authenticity in American Indian and Alaska Native research. ERIC Digest. Retrieved March 16, 2006, from http://eric.ed.gov/ERICDocs/data/ericdocs2/content_storage_01/0000000b/80/2a/38/24.pdf.

Lopez Levers, L., & Maki, D. (1994). *An ethnographic analysis of traditional healing and rehabilitation services in southern Africa: Cross-cultural implications.* A report prepared for the World Rehabilitation Fund, National Institute on Disability and Rehabilitation Research, U.S. Department of Education.

Loveland, C. (1999). The concept of culture. In R. Leavitt (Ed.), *Cross-cultural rehabilitation: An international perspective* (pp. 15–24). London: WB Saunders LTD.

Lustig, D., & Strauser, D. (2003). *Fringe benefits for consumers with disabilities: Current research on VR performance.* Paper presented at the annual meeting of the National Council on Rehabilitation Education, Tucson, AZ.

Makas, E., Marshall, C. A., & Wehman, P. (1997). Cultural diversity and disability: Developing respect for differences. In P. Wehman (Ed.), *Exceptional individuals in school, community and work.* Austin, TX: Pro-Ed.

Marshall, C. A., Bruyère, S., Shern, D., & Jircitano, L. (1996). *An examination of the vocational rehabilitation needs of American Indians with behavioral heath diagnoses in New York State.* Final Report. Flagstaff: Northern Arizona University, Institute for Human Development, Arizona University Affiliated Program, American Indian

Rehabilitation Research and Training Center. (Available from the American Indian Rehabilitation Research and Training Center, Institute for Human Development, Northern Arizona University, PO Box 5630, Flagstaff, AZ 86011.)

Marshall, C. A., Johnson, M. J., & Johnson, S. R. (1996). Responding to the needs of American Indians with disabilities through rehabilitation counselor education. *Rehabilitation Education, 10* (2 & 3), 185–199.

Marshall, C. A., Johnson, M. J., Martin, W. E., Jr., Saravanabhavan, R. C., & Bradford, B. (1992). The rehabilitation needs of American Indians with disabilities in an urban setting. *Journal of Rehabilitation, 58*(2), 13–21.

Marshall, C. A., Johnson, S. R., Kendall, E., Busby, H., Schacht, R., & Hill, C. (2002). Community-based research and American Indians with disabilities: Learning together methods that work. In J. D. Davis, J. S. Erickson, S. R. Johnson, C. A. Marshall, P. Running Wolf, & R. L. Santiago (Eds.), *Work Group on American Indian Research and Program Evaluation Methodology (AIRPEM), Symposium on Research and Evaluation Methodology: Lifespan Issues Related to American Indians/Alaska Natives with Disabilities.* Flagstaff: Northern Arizona University, Institute for Human Development, Arizona University Center on Disabilities, American Indian Rehabilitation Research and Training Center.

Marshall, C. A., Leung, P., Johnson, S. R., & Busby, H. (2003). Ethical practice and cultural factors in rehabilitation. *Rehabilitation Education, 17*(1), 55–65.

Marshall, C. A., Martin, W. E., Jr., Thomason, T. C., & Johnson, M. J. (1991). Multiculturalism and rehabilitation counselor training: Recommendations for providing culturally appropriate counseling services to American Indians with disabilities. *Journal of Counseling and Development, 70,* 225–234.

Marshall, C. A., Sanders, J .E., & Hill, C. R. (2001). Family voices in rehabilitation research. In C. A. Marshall (Ed.), *Rehabilitation and American Indians with disabilities: A handbook for administrators, practitioners, and researchers* (pp. 219–234). Athens, GA: Elliott & Fitzpatrick, Inc.

McAweeney, M. J., Forchheimer, M., & Tate, D. G. (1996, July–September). Identifying the unmet independent living needs of persons with spinal cord injury. *Journal of Rehabilitation, 62*(3), 29–34.

Moore, J. E., & Stephens, B. C. (1994, Spring). Independent living services for older individuals who are blind: Issues and practices. *American Rehabilitation, 20*(1), 30–34.

Morris, J. (1995, Autumn). Creating a space for absent voices: Disabled women's experience of receiving assistance with daily living activities. *Feminist Review, 51,* 68–93.

New Freedom Initiative. (2001). Retrieved April 19, 2002, from http://www.whitehouse. gov/news/freedominitiative/html

Nosek, M. A., Roth, P. L., & Zhu, Y. (1990, October–December). Independent living programs: Impact of program age, consumer control, and budget on program operation. *Journal of Rehabilitation, 56*(4), 28–35.

Pedersen, P. (2003). Multicultural aspects of counseling: Sage series guidelines. Statement of purpose. Retrieved December 9, 2003, from http://soeweb.syr.edu/chs/pedersen/ SAGE.html

Powers, L. E., Curry, M. A., Oschwald, M., Maley, S., Saxton, M., & Eckels, K. (2002). Barriers and strategies in addressing abuse: A survey of disabled women's experiences. (PAS Abuse Survey). *Journal of Rehabilitation, 68*(l), 4–13.

Rhoades, E. R. (2000). *American Indian health: Innovations in health care, promotion, and policy.* Baltimore: Johns Hopkins University Press.

Riley, R. W. (1998, October 26). National institute on disability and rehabilitation research: Notice of proposed long-range plan for fiscal years 1999–2004. *Federal Register, 63*(206), 57190.

Rotheram-Borus, M. J., Koopman, C., & Ehrhardt, A. A. (1991, November). Homeless youth and HIV infection [Special Issue: Homelessness]. *American Psychologist, 46*(11), 1188–1197.

Sanderson, P. L., Schacht, R. M., & Clay, J. A. (1996a). *Independent living outcomes for American Indians with disabilities: A summary of American Indian independent living consumer data.* Flagstaff: Northern Arizona University, Institute for Human Development, University Affiliated Program, American Indian Rehabilitation Research and Training Center.

Sanderson, P. L., Schacht, R. M., & Clay, J. A. (1996b). *Independent living outcomes for American Indians with disabilities: A needs assessment of American Indians with disabilities in northwest New Mexico: Cibola and McKinley Counties.* Flagstaff: Northern Arizona University, Institute for Human Development, University Affiliated Program, American Indian Rehabilitation Research and Training Center.

Sanderson, P. L., & Yazzie-King, E. (2001). Access to independent living and assistive technology for American Indians with disabilities. In C. A. Marshall (Ed.), *Rehabilitation and American Indians with disabilities: A handbook for administrators, practitioners, and researchers* (pp. 73–82). Athens, GA: Elliott & Fitzpatrick, Inc.

Seekins, T., Clay, J., & Ravesloot, C. (1994, April–June). A descriptive study of secondary conditions reported by a population of adults with physical disabilities served by three independent living centers in a rural state. *Journal of Rehabilitation, 60*(2), 47–51.

Shapiro, J. P. (1995, March 27). Others saw a victim, but Ed Roberts didn't (quadriplegic who fought for rights of the disabled) [Obituary]. *U.S. News & World Report, 118*(12), 6–7.

Smith, S. R. (2001, October). Distorted ideals: The "problem of dependency" and the mythology of independent living. *Social Theory and Practice, 27*(4), 579–598.

Smith, L. W., Smith, Q. W., Richards, L., Frieden, L., & King, K. (1994, Spring). Independent living centers: Moving into the 21st century. *American Rehabilitation, 20*(1), 14–22.

Starkloff, M. J. (1997, Spring). Spinal cord injury and centers for independent living [Spinal Cord Injury, Part 3]. *American Rehabilitation, 23*(1), 7–10.

Swedlund, N. P., & Nosek, M. A. (2000, October–December). An exploratory study on the work of independent living centers to address abuse of women with disabilities. *Journal of Rehabilitation, 66*(4), 57–64.

Thomas, K. R., & Weinrach, S. G. (2002). Racial bias in rehabilitation: Multiple interpretations of the same data. *Rehabilitation Education, 16*(1), 81–90.

U.S. Department of Health and Human Services. (2000). *Healthy people 2010: Understanding and improving health.* Washington, DC: Government Printing Office.

Utter, J. (1993). *American Indians: Answers to today's questions.* Lake Ann, MI: National Woodlands Publishing Company.

White, G. W., Gutierrez, R. T., & Seekins, T. (1996, July–September). Preventing and managing secondary conditions: A proposed role for independent living centers. *Journal of Rehabilitation, 62*(3), 14–21.

Wong, H. D., & Millard, R. P. (1992, October–December). Ethical dilemmas encountered by independent living service providers. *Journal of Rehabilitation, 58*(4), 10–16.

Wright, T. J. (1993). African Americans and the public vocational rehabilitation system. *Journal of Vocational Rehabilitation, 3*(1), 20–26.

Wright, T. J., & Leung, P. (1992). *The unique needs of minorities with disabilities: Setting an agenda for the future.* Proceedings of a conference cosponsored by The National Council on Disability and Jackson State University, Jackson, Mississippi. (Available from the National Clearing House of Rehabilitation Training Materials, 5202 Richmond Hill Drive, OSU, Stillwater, OK 74078.)

Wright, T. J., Martinez, Y. G., & Dixon, C. G. (1999, April–June). Minority consumers of independent living services: A pilot investigation. *Journal of Rehabilitation, 65*(2), 20–25.

CHAPTER THREE

Health Disparities: Focus on Disability

Martha E. Banks
Rosalie J. Ackerman

WHICH PEOPLE HAVE DISABILITIES, EMPLOYMENT, AND/OR SERVICES?

Demographic Concerns

It is critical to evaluate the societal status of people to determine the probabilities of disablement and opportunities for employment (Fujiura, 2000; Menz, 1997; Sanderson, 1997). With increased accuracy in counting and improved estimation, the 2000 U.S. Census documented shifts in the demography of the United States. Patterns of race/ethnicity, sex/gender, socioeconomic status, age, and geographic location are more accurately described than they were in the past. Despite the improved counting, there is continued difficulty tracking certain demographic characteristics about which the public is concerned, such as rates of disability, sexual orientation, and employment.

There are many definitions of disability. As a result, it is difficult to relate findings from one piece of research to another. Similarly, it is difficult to determine accuracy of racial and ethnic terminology. Current preferred usage involves differentiating between race (social construct, based primarily on appearance, skin color, hair texture, and other physical characteristics) and ethnicity (cultural identity). It is seldom clear how racial/ethnic terms are used in research; terminology can reflect self-identity of an individual or casual identification by an observer. The terminology for racial/ethnic groups varies considerably in the literature. In order to provide consistency within this chapter, the authors use continent of ancestral origin in the names of American ethnic groups. Lack of hyphenation indicates U.S. birth, whereas hyphenation indicates immigration to the United States. The term *Latinas/os* refers to people whose ancestry is in Central America, northern South America, and/or Spanish-influenced islands of the Caribbean region (e.g., Cuba, Haiti, Puerto Rico).

People of Color refers to U.S. citizens or immigrants who are not primarily of European descent. Most of the research included in the literature review is based on data collected prior to the 2000 U.S. Census; as a result, biracial/biethnic and multiracial/multiethnic people were each identified by a single race/ethnicity. Future research should include disaggregation into various biracial/biethnic and multiracial/multiethnic groups.

Due to the overrepresentation of People of Color among the poor, race/ethnicity is often confused with SES (Manly & Jacobs, 2002). Furthermore, the variability within groups is often ignored. Research on Latinas/os now refers to countries of origin, but often ignores level of acculturation or even number of generations of U.S. residency. In examining people of African descent, little attention is paid to African or Caribbean immigrants.

The literature on the employment of People with Disabilities, including Web-based resources, lags behind much of the other information available from the 2000 U.S. Census. Updated information about ethnicity does not include disability rates (e.g., McKinnon, 2003). Much of the current knowledge about People with Disabilities is based on the 1991–1992 and 1997 Surveys of Income and Program Participation (SIPP). The rates of disability varied considerably by race/ethnicity (Table 3.1). Although the 1991–1992 rate of disability is very high among American Indians and Alaska Natives

TABLE 3.1   U.S. Disability: Race/Ethnicity

Group	1991–1992 (SIPP)	1997 (SIPP)
White	18.0%	20.4%
Black, African American	20.8%	21.3%
Hispanic, Latino (any race)	16.9%	13.8%
Asian, Pacific Islander	9.6%	13.0%
American Indian and Alaska Native	26.9%	No Report

Source: "*Disability among racial and ethnic groups* (Disability Statistics Abstract, Number 10) by J. E. Bradsher, 1996, Washington, DC: U.S. Department of Education, National Institute on Disability and Rehabilitation Research. Copyright by National Institute on Disability and Rehabilitation Research. Adapted with permission.

(Johnson & Marshall, 2001), this information was not disaggregated and published for the 1997 SIPP (Stoddard, Jans, Ripple, & Kraus, 1998).

The SIPP also indicated that there were gender differences in rates of disability in 1997, although gender differences were not observed in 1991–1992 (Table 3.2). In the later survey, women had significantly higher rates of disability than men (Bradsher, 1996; McNeil, 2001; U.S. Department of Commerce, Economics, and Statistics Administration, U.S. Census Bureau, 2001).

Employment rates differ by both gender and disability status (Figure 3.1). Men with and without disabilities had higher employment rates than women with and without disabilities, respectively. People of

TABLE 3.2   U.S. Disability: Gender

Group	1991–1992 (SIPP)	1997 (SIPP)
Female	17.9%	20.7%
Male	17.9%	18.6%

Source: "*Disability among racial and ethnic groups* (Disability Statistics Abstract, Number 10)" by J. E. Bradsher, 1996, Washington, DC: U.S. Department of Education, National Institute on Disability and Rehabilitation Research. "Americans with Disabilities: *Household Economic Studies,* 1997 (Current Population Reports)" by J. McNeil, 2001, Washington, DC: U.S. Department of Commerce, Economics, and Statistics Administration, U.S. Census Bureau. Adapted with permission.

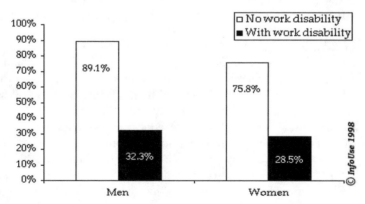

FIGURE 3.1   U.S. labor force participation: Men and women with or without work disabilities

Source: "*Chartbook on Work and Disability in the United States, 1998* (An InfoUse Report)" by S. Stoddard, L. Jans, J. Ripple, and L. Kraus, 1998, Washington, DC: U.S. National Institute on Disability and Rehabilitation Research. Copyright by National Institute on Disability and Rehabilitation Research. Reprinted with permission.

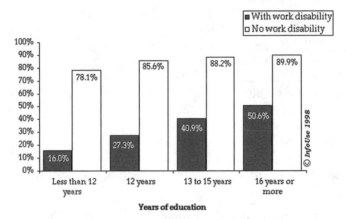

FIGURE 3.2   U.S. labor force participation: Education

Source: "*Chartbook on Work and Disability in the United States, 1998* (An InfoUse Report)" by S. Stoddard, L. Jans, J. Ripple, and L. Kraus, 1998, Washington, DC: U.S. National Institute on Disability and Rehabilitation Research. Copyright by National Institute on Disability and Rehabilitation Research.

both genders with disabilities had significantly lower rates of employment than those without disabilities (Stoddard et al., 1998).

Socioeconomic status (SES) is also difficult to define. SES can be used to reflect wealth (Brown, 1996; Myers & Chung, 1996), total current resources, past resources (e.g., family of origin resources), type of employment (e.g., professional, blue collar, clerical), and other access to financial resources. Educational attainment is often used as a substitute for SES. However, Manly and colleagues (1998) documented that the quality of education is often poorer for People of Color than for European Americans; therefore the same number of years of education is not comparable across groups. People with more education, regardless of disability status, are more likely to be employed (Stoddard et al, 1998). People with Disabilities, regardless of educational attainment, are less likely to be employed than people without disabilities (Figure 3.2).

Annual earnings are also used to estimate SES (McNeil, 2001). For People with Disabilities, annual earnings are a particularly inadequate way of illustrating SES. One concern is that there are limitations on jobs available to People with Disabilities, due to past and ongoing discrimination (Dunham et al., 1998; Fujiura, 2000; Wray, 1996). In addition, the medical expenses associated with disability (Olkin, 2003) more severely limit the financial resources for People with Disabilities as compared to those without disabilities, even when earned income is supplemented with disability insurance. As noted in Table 3.3, the earned income of

TABLE 3.3 Disability Status, Employment, and Annual Earnings (Ages 21–64 Years)

		Percent Employed	Median Earnings	Mean Earnings
Disability	Severe	31.4%	$13,272	$18,631
	Not Severe	82.0%	$20,457	$26,412
No Disability		84.4%	$23,654	$31,053

Source: "Americans with Disabilities: *Household Economic Studies,* 1997 (Current Population Reports)" by J. McNeil, 2001, Washington, DC: U.S. Department of Commerce, Economics and Statistics Administration, U.S. Census Bureau. Copyright by U.S. Census Bureau. Adapted with permission.

People with Disabilities is substantially less than that of people without disabilities.

Poverty status is another way to examine SES (McNeil, 2001). As Figure 3.3 illustrates, people with the most severe disabilities are more than three times as likely to be living in poverty than people without disabilities.

As People with Disabilities age, they are less likely to be gainfully employed (Figure 3.4); this pattern is different from those without dis-

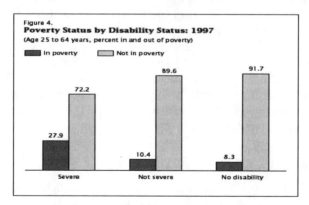

Figure 4.
Poverty Status by Disability Status: 1997
(Age 25 to 64 years, percent in and out of poverty)

■ In poverty   ▢ Not in poverty

	Severe	Not severe	No disability
In poverty	27.9	10.4	8.3
Not in poverty	72.2	89.6	91.7

FIGURE 3.3 People with disabilities: Poverty status

Source: "Americans with Disabilities: *Household Economic Studies,* 1997 (Current Population Reports)" by J. McNeil, 2001, Washington, DC: U.S. Department of Commerce, Economics and Statistics Administration, U.S. Census Bureau. Adapted with permission.

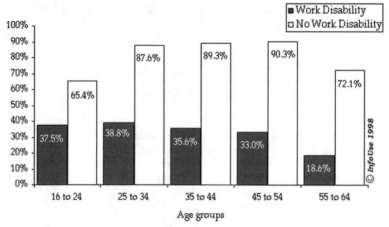

FIGURE 3.4   U.S. labor force participation: Age

Source: *"Chartbook on Work and Disability in the United States, 1998* (An InfoUse Report)" by S. Stoddard, L. Jans, J. Ripple, and L. Kraus, 1998, Washington, DC: U.S. National Institute on Disability and Rehabilitation Research. Copyright by National Institute on Disability and Rehabilitation Research. Reprinted with permission.

abilities (Stoddard et al., 1998). One of the concerns is that retirement literature does not address the needs of People with Disabilities who have reached traditional retirement age. There is a very sharp decline in the labor force participation of People with Disabilities who are 55 years old and older relative to their younger counterparts.

Szalda-Petree, Seekins, and Innes (1999) examined the rates of employment among people with and without disabilities living in rural and urban areas of the United States (Figure 3.5). People with Disabilities were far less likely to be gainfully employed than people without disabilities. Rural People with Disabilities were less likely to be employed than their urban counterparts.

Interactions Among Demographic Characteristics

It is important to note that people do not exist with single identities. Each person has at least one race and/or ethnicity, a sex/gender, sexual orientation, socioeconomic status, age, and geographic location. Therefore, it is critical, in examining employment patterns of People with Disabilities, not to assume unidimensionality. Majumder, Walls, Fullmer, and Misra (1997) provide a useful description of the competitive employment outcomes of people with different types of disabilities. Within those disability

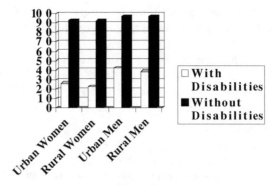

FIGURE 3.5   U.S. labor force participation:
Urban and rural

Adapted from "Women with Disabilities: Employment, income,
and health" by A. Szalda-Petree, T. Seekins, and B. Innes, 1999,
Missoula, MT: The University of Montana Rural Institute.
Copyright by The University of Montana Rural Institute.
Adapted with permission.

groups, demographic characteristics are examined. This research is a critical first step toward determining the impact of demographic characteristics on employment for People with Disabilities. This should be extended
to more closely examine the interactions among demographic characteristics. For example, it is likely that there are differences among employment experiences of people of various ages, education levels, geographic
locations, ethnicity, and gender. One would expect, for example, that
the vocational needs of a 35-year-old, PhD educated, rural heterosexual
African American woman, a 65-year-old high school dropout urban gay
European American man, a 51-year-old college educated urban Native
American lesbian, and a 28-year-old technical school educated rural heterosexual Asian American man, would differ considerably. What follows
are some examples of the interactions among demographic characteristics
to illustrate the need for disaggregation of demographic characteristics in
future research.

   In Figure 3.6, Jans and Stoddard (1999) demonstrated that, among
European Americans, African Americans, Asian Americans and Pacific
Islanders, and Latinas/os, women were more likely to report disabilities than men. For Native Americans, men were slightly more likely to
report disabilities than women (Bradsher, 1996). Among the racial/ethnic
groups, Asian Americans and Pacific Islanders were least likely to report
disabilities. Native Americans had the highest chances of reporting disabilities. Figure 3.6 can serve as a model for the kind of disaggregation

that is critical to our understanding of the status of various People with Disabilities; without gender disaggregation within ethnicity, the picture would be inaccurate.

Among women, rural women with disabilities are least likely to be employed from ages 16 to 64 years (Szalda-Petree et al., 1999) (Table 3.4). Rural women with disabilities who are 65 years old or older are four times more likely to be employed than their younger counterparts. This is clearly

TABLE 3.4   U.S. Labor Force Participation: Urban or Rural Location: Women and Age

	With Disability		Without Disability	
Age	Urban	Rural	Urban	Rural
16–64	7.5%	2.4%	71.2%	19.0%
65 +	27.4%	10.5%	46.9%	15.2%
Total	11.1%	3.8%	66.8%	18.3%

Adapted from "Women with Disabilities: Employment, Income, and Health" by A. Szalda-Petree, T. Seekins, and B. Innes, 1999, Missoula, MT: The University of Montana Rural Institute. Copyright by The University of Montana Rural Institute. Adapted with permission.

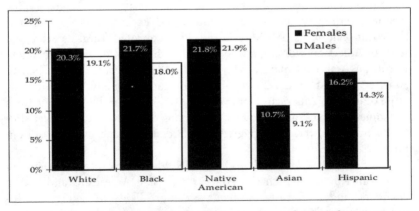

FIGURE 3.6   Percentage with disability gender and race/ethnicity

Source: "*Chartbook on women and disability in the United States. An InfoUse report*" by L. Jans, and S. Stoddard, 1999, Washington, DC: U.S. Department of Education, National Institute on Disability and Rehabilitation Research. Copyright by U.S. Department of Education. Reprinted with permission.

at odds with the overall trends illustrated in Figure 3.4; that figure is most likely reflective of rural and urban men who are employed at greater rates regardless of disability status.

As noted in Figure 3.5, there were significant gender differences in employment rates for rural and urban women and men. Men were far more likely to be employed than women. Table 3.5 illustrates gender discrepancy in annual earnings based on severity of disability (McNeil, 2001). Women earn less than men at all comparison levels. People with less severe disabilities earn significantly more (up to a third more) than their counterparts with more severe disabilities.

TABLE 3.5 U.S. Labor Force Participation: Annual Earnings: Gender

		Percent Employed	Median Earnings	Mean Earnings
Women	Severe	30.6%	$12,030	$16,333
	Not Severe	75.7%	$16,291	$20,921
Men	Severe	31.8%	$14,575	$21,048
	Not Severe	89.1%	$25,277	$31,809

Source: "Employment and Annual Rate of Earnings of Individuals 21 To 64 Years Old with A Disability" by U.S. Department of Commerce, Economics, and Statistics Administration, U.S. Census Bureau, 2001. Copyright by U.S. Census Bureau. Reprinted with permission.

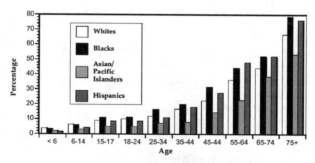

FIGURE 3.7 People with disabilities: Race/ethnicity and age

Source: "Disability among racial and ethnic groups (Disability Statistics Abstract, Number 10)" by J. E. Bradsher, 1996, Washington, DC: U.S. Department of Education, National Institute on Disability and Rehabilitation Research. Copyright by U.S. Department of Education. Adapted with permission.

From age 15 years, African Americans and Latinas/os have the highest rates of disability. They are followed by European Americans and Asian Americans/Pacific Islanders, respectively (Bradsher, 1996) (Figure 3.7).

Types and Rates of Disability

Figure 3.8 and Table 3.6 illustrate employment rates of people with different types of disability. It is clear that developing programs to improve the employment rates of People with Disabilities must be prepared to address a variety of physical and mental challenges. The people with mobility disabilities are least likely to be gainfully employed.

Difficulty in comparing the information in Figure 3.8 and Table 3.6 should also be noted. While the graph and the table both indicate a 41.3% employment rate for people with mental disabilities, the other categories do not match. This is one of the problems in disability research, as inconsistency in measurement makes it hard to document progress or to clearly identify areas that need particular attention. One of the issues raised by the data in Table 3.6 is a question about the impact of different types of disability on the accommodations required for employment. It is not clear, for example, if it is easier for employers to accommodate a person who is deaf or hard of hearing than a person with limited vision or blindness. Those are very different disabilities. In Figure 3.8, however, there

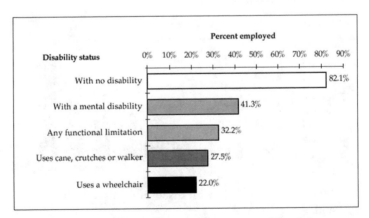

FIGURE 3.8   U.S. employment rates: Types of disability

Source: "*Chartbook on Work and Disability in the United States, 1998* (An InfoUse Report)" by S. Stoddard, L. Jans, J. Ripple, and L. Kraus, 1998, Washington, DC: U.S. National Institute on Disability and Rehabilitation Research. Copyright by National Institute on Disability and Rehabilitation Research. Reprinted with permission.

are two categories of mobility disabilities; comparison between them is relatively straightforward.

Stoddard and colleagues (1998) provided an overview of the employment rates, with inclusion of people in the U.S. labor force, but not employed (Table 3.7). It is useful to note that while most of the data available from the SIPP and the U.S. Census focus on the labor force only, the Current Population Survey (CPS) includes a comparison between people not working because they are not considered

TABLE 3.6   U.S. Labor Force Participation: Types of Disability

Disability[a]	Employed
Difficulty hearing	64.4%
Difficulty seeing	43.7%
Mental disability	41.3%
Difficulty walking	33.5%

Note. The participants surveyed were ages 21–64 years.

[a]Persons may have more than one type of disability.

Source: "Data on disability and employment: 1991/92, 1993/94, 1994/95, and 1997 (From the Survey of Income and Program Participation)" by U.S. Department of Commerce, Economics, and Statistics Administration, U.S. Census Bureau, 2001. Copyright by U.S. Census Bureau. Reprinted with permission.

TABLE 3.7   U.S. Employment Rates: Work Disability

		Work Disability		No Work Disability	
		Number	% of Total	Number	% of Total
Not in labor force		11,941,000	69.6%	27,490,000	17.7%
In labor force		5,216,000	30.4%	127,821,000	82.3%
	Employed	4,564,000	26.6%	121,764,000	78.4%
	Unemployed	652,000	5.8%	6,057,000	3.9%
Total		17,157,000	100.0%	155,311,000	100.0%
Unemployment rate			12.3%		4.8%

Adapted from "*Chartbook on Work and Disability in the United States, 1998* (An InfoUse Report)" by S. Stoddard, L. Jans, J. Ripple, and L. Kraus, 1998, Washington, DC: U.S. National Institute on Disability and Rehabilitation Research. Copyright by National Institute on Disability and Rehabilitation Research. Reprinted with permission.

to be in the labor force and contrasts them with people in the labor force who are not working. The 12.3% unemployment rate for People with Disabilities (and the 4.8% for people without work disabilities) reflects only people considered to be in the labor force; it excludes the 69.6% of People with Disabilities who are not in the labor force. The sobering bottom line is that 75.4% *of People with Disabilities are not employed,* more than three times the rate of people without work disabilities (21.6%).

Men are more likely to be employed regardless of disability status (Stoddard et al., 1998). Figure 3.9 illustrates the gender differences that are generally obscured when reporting aggregate data. This information would be even more useful with further disaggregation by ethnicity, age, and geographic location. Similarly, Table 3.8 would be more useful if the data were available disaggregated by gender and included a comparison with European Americans. Table 3.8 illustrates the differing employment rates by race/ethnicity, with Native Americans with severe disabilities being the least likely to be employed (U.S. Department of Labor, n.d.). Bradsher (1996) noted that "Native Americans have the highest rate of disability of any racial/ethnic group, while Blacks have the highest rate of severe disability" (p. 1). Bradsher's observations were based on the

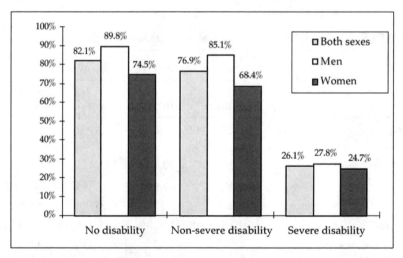

FIGURE 3.9   U.S. employment rates: Severity of disability

Source: *"Chartbook on Work and Disability in the United States, 1998* (An InfoUse Report)" by S. Stoddard, L. Jans, J. Ripple, and L. Kraus, 1998, Washington, DC: U.S. National Institute on Disability and Rehabilitation Research. Copyright by National Institute on Disability and Rehabilitation Research. Reprinted with permission.

1991–1992 SIPP, whereas the Department of Labor data appear to be based on an unspecified source.

Annual earnings information is not included for Asian Americans/ Pacific Islanders or American Indians and Alaska Natives in the SIPP (U.S. Department of Labor, n.d.) (Table 3.9). While it is clear that African Americans and Latinas/os with disabilities earn consistently less than their European American counterparts, without further disaggregation of the data, it is not possible to determine how other demographic characteristics impact the employment rates or the earnings.

TABLE 3.8 U.S. Employment Rates: People with Disabilities

	Total	Not Severe	Severe
African American	36.6%	69.0%	19.2%
Asian/Pacific Islander	48.1%	69.0%	23.1%
Native American	41.0%	66.2%	9.2%
Hispanic origin	44.8%	70.8%	21.1%

Source: "Cultural Diversity Initiative" by U.S. Department of Labor, n.d., Copyright by U.S. Department of Labor. Reprinted with permission.

TABLE 3.9 U.S. Labor Force Participation: Annual Earnings: Race/Ethnicity

		Percent Employed	Median Earnings	Mean Earnings
White, not of Hispanic origin	Severe	34.4%	$14,255	$19,801
Black	Not Severe	82.7%	$21,413	$27,721
	Severe	21.0%	$10,337	$15,195
Of Hispanic origin	Not Severe	80.2%	$17,371	$22,371
	Severe	26.5%	$11,487	$14,928
	Not Severe	78.9%	$13,904	$18,992

Source: "Data on disability and employment: 1991/92, 1993/94, 1994/95, and 1997 (From the Survey of Income and Program Participation)" by U.S. Department of Commerce, Economics, and Statistics Administration, U.S. Census Bureau, 2001. Copyright by U.S. Census Bureau. Reprinted with permission.

Cultural Differences and Cross-Cultural Concerns

Disability Identity

"The visible disability Community—disability advocates and scholars—in the United States is largely White, adult, educated, middle class, and empowered" (Devlieger & Albrecht, 2000, p. 51). As a result, the disability research is primarily focused on European American, adult, educated, middle class, and empowered People with Disabilities, with the goal of empowering similar people.

Gordon, Feldman, and Crose (1998) described some of the difficulties that arise for People with Disabilities who do not have disability incorporated into their identities. They interviewed women with a variety of chronic illnesses and found that many did not consider themselves to have disabilities, even when the illness had progressed to a point at which they were no longer able to continue gainful employment. Many of the women were clearly uncomfortable with the label of "disability"; this actually prevented some potential participants from becoming involved in the research. Gordon and colleagues noted that it is important for counselors to attend to the self-identity of clients with disabilities and to avoid stereotypical assumptions (see also Feldman & Tegart, 2003). In addition, some of the participants did not pursue personal care assistance or technological aids to which they were entitled.

Olkin (2002) addressed one of the possible underlying causes of the difference between the self-perception as a person without a disability and the perceptions of others. People in racial/ethnic minority groups usually develop in an environment that includes other people who face similar discrimination. There are obvious role models who demonstrate coping strategies and varying levels of pride in the racial/ethnic identity. The experience for People with Disabilities is different in that many who have early onset disabilities are unlikely to grow up with other people with similar disabilities, and those with late onset disabilities are very unlikely to have role models with whom they identify.

Another consideration involved in disability identity involves the cause of disability. Two specific issues are disabilities caused by the job and those caused by interpersonal violence (Ackerman & Banks, 2003). In the latter case, it can be expected that building disability into self-identity is a relatively minor consideration, due to the need to focus on immediate personal safety. Employment-caused disability is a critical issue for People of Color (Keppel, Pearcy, & Wagener, 2002). People of Color are employed in more physically dangerous jobs than European Americans. African Americans are overrepresented in jobs involving physically demanding work. As a result, African Americans are more apt to get injured than European Americans. However, African Americans are less likely than European Americans to get immediate medical treatment, thus increasing their chances of permanent, severe disabilities (Smart & Smart, 1997). In addition to physically demanding work, People of Color are disproportionately exposed to dangerous chemicals, including neurotoxins (LoSasso, Rapport, Axelrod, & Whitman, 2002), on the job and in the home environments, due to location of waste sites in poor neighborhoods (Reidy, Bowler, Rauch, & Pedroza, 1992; Valciukas, 1991).

Injuries sustained on the job are compounded by other health concerns, including health disparities between European Americans and People of Color (Keppel et al., 2002; U.S. Department of Health and Human Services, 2001). The combination of injury and ill health result in high levels of disability for People of Color (Bound, Schoenbaum, & Waidmann, 1996; Clark, Callahan, Mungai, & Wolinsky, 1996; Wray, 1996). It is also important to consider the impact of stress, both on the job (Botterbusch, 1999; Guyll, Matthews, & Bromberger, 2001) and outside of the work environment (Carels, Sherwood, Szcsepanski, & Blumenthal, 2000), on health. Poor health alone, as manifested by chronic illness, can lead to disability. Brown (1996) noted that lack of financial resources exacerbates this problem, as ill people do not receive adequate medical care (Santiago & Muschkin, 1996).

Services Provided to People of Color by European Americans

In an examination of satisfaction with community response to People with Disabilities, participants in one Midwestern American Indian tribe with strong American Indian identification were significantly less satisfied than those with bicultural or "anomic" (people who identify themselves as "human" without any specific ethnicity) identification (Pitchette, Berven, Menz, & La Fromboise, 1997). Some of the possible explanations for the dissatisfaction include service provider insensitivity to traditional Indian values and delivering culturally inappropriate service, or American Indian identified consumers might be likely to reject government and other organizations controlled by European Americans.

Ma, Coyle, Wares, and Cornell (1999) described the need for culturally appropriate services for Native Americans. These include incorporation of traditional healing into services for Native Americans with disabilities. Marshall, Johnson, and Johnson (2001) provide specific recommendations for effective cross-cultural vocational counseling with American Indians with disabilities.

Access to Services

Pitchette and colleagues (1997) observed that, although a multiplicity of employment and disability services were available through the Bureau of Indian Affairs, the Indian Health Service, the state-federal rehabilitation system, and local tribal agencies, because of the combination of economic dependence, depression, and poverty in their situations, many of the Native Americans eligible for these services were unaware of them. This could reflect a combination of lack of communication about the services or cultural interpretations of the meaning of disability, including the noninternalization of disability into self-identity (Gordon et al., 1998). Ma and colleagues (1999) documented some of the barriers that prevent Native Americans with disability from receiving available services.

Telehealth provides health care options for People with Disabilities. This could decrease the need for time away from the job for health care appointments. Telemetry can be used to monitor vital signs with asynchronous feedback from health professionals. Access to nurses by telephone can provide relatively quick response to health crises. Information on symptoms is more readily available to People with Disabilities in rural areas. It is critical to consider, however, that internet access is not affordable for poor people and that many health plans do not cover the expense.

Access to Employment Relevant Quality Education

People of Color generally have less formal education than European Americans (Smart & Smart, 1997). As noted earlier, the quality of that education also tends to be poorer for People of Color than for European Americans (Manly et al., 1998). Moore, Feist-Price, and Alston (2002) found that some People with Disabilities are unlikely to receive education that would provide them with the foundation for competitive employment.

Access to Financial Resources

Smart and Smart (1997) described racial/ethnic differences in access to various types of jobs (see also Dunham et al., 1998). These differences impose funding limitations on individuals pursuing education that could prepare them for better jobs.

An additional concern for older People with Disabilities is the need for employment in old age to cover the considerable medical expenses associated with disability. For older People of Color, there are seldom financial reserves, pensions, or spousal income available to meet those expenses (Holden & Kuo, 1996; Honig, 1996). As a result, as noted with older rural women with disabilities (Table 3.4), retirement is not an option.

Age Concerns

Upon attainment of adulthood, most young people actively pursue employment and/or continue education to improve their employment options. For young People with Disabilities, this can involve a complex move from dependence to independence. It is not clear if such a change is desired, and if desired, by whom. Little is known about the transition into adulthood for People with Disabilities; the difficulty in this transition is complicated by the varying ages considered for entry into the U.S. labor force. In addition, young people receiving Supplemental Security Income (SSI) were less likely to be admitted into rehabilitation programs than those without SSI (Berry, Price-Ellingstad, Halloran, & Finch, 2000). Clearly, the transition is defined in part by the nature and severity of the disability, as well as the cultural issues of ethnicity, gender, sexual orientation, socioeconomic status, and geography. For some disabilities, competence is an issue due to inadequate education and/or lack of preparation for making adult decisions. If a young person with a disability is not competent, then employment considerations need to involve a responsible adult. This is a critical area that needs much more detailed research.

As mentioned above, older People with Disabilities who have few resources remain in the labor force after traditional retirement age. Jackson, Lockery, and Juster (1996) note that, while disaggregated data reporting has improved in recent years, more information is needed about People of Color at retirement age (Hardy, 1996; Holden & Kuo, 1996; Honig, 1996).

Application of the Americans With Disabilities Act (ADA)

American Indian Tribal Law

Fowler and colleagues (2000) described the impact of self-government of American Indian tribes on implementation of the ADA for Native Americans. They found that one tribe had fully adopted the ADA, but that adoption was difficult and contentious due to inconsistencies with tribal traditions. Nineteen percent of tribes in the contiguous 48 states and 5% of tribes in Alaska provided employment services for People with Disabilities.

Ma et al. (1999) found that services for People with Disabilities were not reaching the Native American population. They noted lack of resources and service availability, lack of community awareness, and lack of specific agency responsibilities for services to American Indians with disabilities and confusion in implementation of federal, state laws, and tribal policies, which resulted in fragmented service delivery as well as the duplication of dispersed services; lack of acknowledgment of Indian cultural beliefs and practices in agency policies and operations, and time lag between referral and diagnosis. (p. 14)

Welfare-to-Work

The programs designed to decrease dependence on public assistance have disproportionately affected women, including those with disabilities. If people receiving welfare benefits are unable to become or remain gainfully employed, they lose welfare benefits. It is not clear what happens to People with Disabilities who are not considered qualified by disability programs or who have not met success through vocational rehabilitation. The latter is particularly an issue with respect to acceptance into vocational rehabilitation as "a woman was about seven times more likely to be working if she received job training and four times more likely to be working if she received job placement services" (Browne, Salomon, & Bassuk, 1999, pp. 421–422). There are several demographic questions remaining with respect to the impact of welfare reform on People with Disabilities (Pappas, 1998).

IDENTIFIED NEEDS FOR DISABILITY RESEARCH AGENDA FOR REHABILITATION AND THE SOCIAL SCIENCES

Information is definitely missing in several areas. In some cases, there is broad information available, but it has not been disaggregated to determine the best fit for members of specific populations. Other issues have not been adequately addressed.

The first task is to properly identify the population affected by disability. There are many definitions of disability. It would be useful if a limited set of definitions were made available to researchers in order to clarify the questions asked. Once the definitions are narrowed, it is necessary to disaggregate data. An analysis of the current disaggregation of U.S. disability data appears in Table 3.6. While there are several areas included in the research in the aggregate, it is clear that little has been disaggregated. Although there are check marks to the right of the Aggregate Data column, it should be noted that those marks seldom represent more than one study in the literature. Furthermore, for research indicated under Ethnicity, there is usually a focus on either a single ethnic minority group or on a comparison between one ethnic minority group and European Americans.

Second, there is a continued need for accurate documentation of the disability disparities among sociocultural groups. The disparities among sociocultural groups fall into several categories. By aggregating the information across diverse groups, information about people most in need of rehabilitation services is obscured. This was demonstrated in Figure 3.6, which clearly indicated that prevalence of disability varies not only by ethnicity, but also by gender within ethnicity. The concern about the joint impact of disability, gender, age, and geographic location was raised in Table 3.4: older women with disabilities were far more likely to be employed than their younger counterparts, with greater disparity among urban women than rural women.

There are many rehabilitation and employment strategies available. Most were developed for young European American men and have been modified as that group's needs have changed. Relatively few strategies have been documented that were specifically developed for other groups of

TABLE 3.10   Sociocultural Research on Disability

Demographics	Aggregate data	Gender	Ethnicity	Geographic location	Age	Sexual orientation	Gender & ethnicity	Gender & geographic location	Gender & age	Ethnicity & geographic location	Ethnicity & age	Geographic location & age	Gender, geographic location & age	Education
Prevalence of disability	☒	☒	☒				☒				☒			
Severity of disability	☒													
Types of disability	☒													
Onset type														
Onset age														
Socioeconomic status	☒													
Source of disability														
Poverty	☒													

(Continued)

TABLE 3.10 Continued

Demographics	Aggregate data	Gender	Ethnicity	Geographic location	Age	Sexual orientation	Gender & ethnicity	Gender & geographic location	Gender & age	Ethnicity & geographic location	Ethnicity & age	Geographic location & age	Gender geographic location & age	Education
Labor force participation	⊠	⊠	⊠	⊠	⊠								⊠	⊠
Annual earnings	⊠	⊠	⊠											
Disability identity	⊠	⊠												
Services provided	⊠													
Service providers														
Access to services	⊠		⊠											
Access to employment relevant quality education	⊠		⊠											
Access to financial resources			⊠		⊠							⊠		
Aging; human development across the lifespan														
Application of ADA	⊠		⊠											
Welfare-to-Work	⊠													
Inclusion of consumers in service development	⊠													

People with Disabilities. Specific information is needed with regard to how and why the existing strategies work for different groups of people. This necessitates inclusion of consumers in all stages of the research process.

RECOMMENDATIONS RESPECTIVE TO PUBLIC INTEREST RESEARCH

Which questions have not been answered for which segments of the population? Table 3.10 can serve as a general guide to indicate the gaps in those data.

- Employment levels and salaries do not show improvement from prior to ADA to 1997 (Kaye, 1998). What are the current rates?
- How have other countries addressed these concerns? Some of the research to review includes economic consequences of disability (Albers et al., 1999); geographic location (Bakheit and Shanmugalingam, 1997); sociodemographic predictors of treatment success and failure (Becker, Hojsted, Sjogren, & Eriksen, 1998; Bhandari, Louw, & Reddy, 1999; Frumkin, Walker, & Friedman-Jimenez, 1999; Mayer et al., 1998; Stronks, van de Mheen, van den Bos, & Mackenbach, 1995); and longitudinal studies (McDonough & Amick, 2001). Those studies provide models for the implementation of needed research examined in this chapter.

QUESTIONS FOR DISCUSSION AND/OR FURTHER STUDY

Service Domain

1. A client who is a member of a demographic group different from yours enters your office. You have read about members of the client's demographic group. How do you conduct an appropriate assessment without using inappropriate stereotypes?
2. Describe five types of disability and how a client with each type of disability can educate you about his or her disability.

Research Domain

3. Describe prevalence, severity, disability type, and geographic locations of six different groups of people throughout the world and disaggregate the findings by gender.

4. It is difficult to compare disability types, severity, and onset age. How might one develop standardized methods to account for the impact of SES status and chronicity across the lifespan on identity as a person with a disability?

Policy Domain

5. Describe six different groups of people who have unique assessment and treatment needs for access to service, ability to afford treatment, access and financial support for reeducation and training, and ability to return to the work force. Which government agencies should receive this information?

6. How can ADA laws be applied to reduce poverty, increase access to relevant quality education, and increase access to labor force participation? Select six different groups of people and describe the differences in adaptation of ADA laws for members of those groups.

REFERENCES

Ackerman, R. J., & Banks, M. E. (2003). Assessment, treatment, and rehabilitation for interpersonal violence victims: Women sustaining head injuries. *Women & Therapy*, 26(3/4), 343–363. [Simultaneously published in M. E. Banks & E. Kaschak (Eds.), *Women with visible and invisible disabilities: Multiple intersections, multiple issues, multiple therapies* (pp. 343–363). New York: Haworth Press.]

Albers, J. M., Kuper, H. H., van Riel, P. L., Prevoo, M. L., van Hof, M. A., van Gestel, A. M., et al. (1999). Socio-economic consequences of rheumatoid arthritis in the first years of the disease. *Rheumatology (Oxford), 38*, 423–430.

Bakheit, A. M., & Shanmugalingam, V. (1997). A study of the attitudes of a rural Indian community toward people with physical disabilities. *Clinical Rehabilitation, 11*, 329–334.

Becker, N., Hojsted, J., Sjogren, P., & Eriksen, J. (1998). Sociodemographic predictors of treatment outcome in chronic non-malignant pain patients. Do patients receiving or applying for disability pension benefit from multidisciplinary pain treatment? *Pain, 77*, 279–287.

Berry, H. G., Price-Ellingstad, D., Halloran, W., & Finch, T. (2000). Supplemental Security Income and vocational rehabilitation for transition-age individuals with disabilities. *Journal of Disability Policy Studies, 10*, 151–165.

Bhandari, M., Louw, D., & Reddy, K. (1999). Predictors of return to work after anterior cervical discectomy. *Journal of Spinal Disorders, 12*, 94–98.

Botterbusch, K. F. (1999). *Outcomes and career achievements of persons with professional qualifications who have severe psychiatric disabilities: The Minnesota experience.* Menomonie, WI: Rehabilitation Research and Training Center, Stout Vocational Rehabilitation Institute, University of Wisconsin–Stout.

Bound, J., Schoenbaum, M., & Waidmann, T. (1996). Race differences in labor force attachment and disability status. *Gerontologist, 36*, 311–321.

Bradsher, J. E. (1996, January). *Disability among racial and ethnic groups* (Disability Statistics Abstract, Number 10). Washington, DC: U.S. Department of Education, National Institute on Disability and Rehabilitation Research.

Brown, C. C. (1996). Symposium II: Income and wealth. *Gerontologist, 36,* 341.

Browne, A., Salomon, A., & Bassuk, S. S. (1999). The impact of recent partner violence on poor women's capacity to maintain work. *Violence Against Women, 5,* 393–462.

Carels, R. A., Sherwood, A., Szcsepanski, R., & Blumenthal, J. A. (2000). Ambulatory blood pressure and marital distress in employed women. *Behavioral Medicine, 26,* 80–89.

Clark, D. O., Callahan, C. M., Mungai, S. M., & Wolinsky, F. D. (1996). Physical function among retirement-aged African American men and women. *Gerontologist, 36,* 322–331.

Devlieger, P. J., & Albrecht, G. L. (2000). Your experience is not my experience: The concept and experience of disability on Chicago's Near West Side. *Journal of Disability Policy Studies, 11,* 51–60.

Dunham, M. D., Holliday, G. A., Douget, R. M., Koller, J. R., Presberry, R., & Wooderson, S. (1998). Vocational rehabilitation outcomes of African American adults with specific learning disabilities. *Journal of Rehabilitation, 64* (3), 36–41.

Feldman, S. I., & Tegart, G. (2003). Keep moving: Conceptions of illness and disability of middle-aged African-American women with arthritis. *Women & Therapy,* 26(1/2), 127–143. [Simultaneously published in M. E. Banks & E. Kaschak (Eds.), *Women with visible and invisible disabilities: Multiple intersections, multiple issues, multiple therapies* (pp. 127–143). New York: Haworth Press.]

Fowler, L., Seekins, T., Dwyer, K., Duffy, S. W., Brod, R. L., & Locust, C. (2000). American Indian Disability Legislation and Programs: Findings of the first national survey of tribal governments. *Journal of Disability Policy Studies, 10,* 166–185.

Frumkin, H., Walker, E. D., & Friedman-Jimenez, G. (1999). Minority workers and communities. *Occupational Medicine, 14,* 495–517.

Fujiura, G. T. (2000). The implications of emerging demographics: A commentary on the meaning of race and income inequity to disability policy. *Journal of Disability Policy Studies, 11,* 66–75.

Gordon, P. A., Feldman, D., & Crose, R. (1998). The meaning of disability: How women with chronic illness view their experiences. *Journal of Rehabilitation, 64*(3), 5–11.

Guyll, M., Matthews, K. A., & Bromberger, J. T. (2001). Discrimination and unfair treatment: Relationship to cardiovascular reactivity among African American and European American women. *Health Psychology, 20,* 315–325.

Hardy, M. A. (1996). Symposium III: Employment, economic status, and retirement. *Gerontologist, 36,* 361–362.

Holden, K. C., & Kuo, H.-H.F. (1996). Complex marital histories and economic well-being: The continuing legacy of divorce and widowhood as the Hrs cohort approaches retirement. *Gerontologist, 36,* 383–390.

Honig, M. (1996). Retirement expectations: Differences by race, ethnicity, and gender. *Gerontologist, 36,* 373–382.

Jackson, J. S., Lockery, S. A., & Juster, F. T. (1996). Minority perspectives from the health and retirement study: Introduction: Health and retirement among ethnic and racial minority groups. *Gerontologist, 36,* 282–284.

Jans, L., & Stoddard, S. (1999). *Chartbook on women and disability in the United States. An InfoUse report.* Washington, DC: U.S. Department of Education, National Institute on Disability and Rehabilitation Research. Retrieved June 30, 2005, from http://www.infouse.com/disabilitydata/.

Johnson, S. R., & Marshall, C. A. (2001). Best practices for serving American Indians in vocational rehabilitation. In C. A. Marshall (Ed.), *Rehabilitation and American Indians with disabilities: A handbook for administrators, practitioners, and researchers* (pp. 99–112). Athens, GA: Elliott & Fitzpatrick.

Kaye, H. S. (1998, May). *Is the status of People with Disabilities improving?* (Disability Statistics Abstract, Number 21). Washington, DC: U.S. Department of Education, National Institute on Disability and Rehabilitation Research.

Keppel, K. G., Pearcy, J. N., & Wagener, D. K. (2002, January). *Trends in racial and ethnic-specific rates for the health status indicators: United States, 1990–98* (Healthy people statistical notes, no 23). Hyattsville, MD: National Center for Health Statistics.

LoSasso, G. L., Rapport, L. J., Axelrod, B. N., & Whitman, R. D. (2002). Neurocognitive sequelae of exposure to organic solvents and (meth)acrylates among nail-studio technicians. *Neuropsychiatry, Neuropsychology, and Behavioral Neurology, 15,* 44–55.

Ma, G. X., Coyle, C., Wares, D., & Cornell, D. (1999). Assessment of services to American Indians with disabilities. *Journal of Rehabilitation, 65*(3), 11–16.

Majumder, R. K., Walls, R. T., Fullmer, S. L., & Misra, S. (1997). What works. In F. E. Menz, J. Eggers, P. Wehman, & V. Brooke (Eds.), *Lessons for improving employment of people with disabilities from vocational rehabilitation research* (pp. 263–282). Menomonie, WI: Rehabilitation Research and Training Center, Stout Vocational Rehabilitation Institute, University of Wisconsin–Stout.

Manly, J. J., & Jacobs, D. M. (2002). Future directions in neuropsychological assessment with African Americans. In F. R. Ferraro (Ed.), *Minority and Cross-Cultural Aspects of Neuropsychological Assessment* (pp. 79–96). Heereweg, Lisse, The Netherlands: Swets & Zeitlinger Publishers.

Manly, J. J., Miller, S. W., Heaton, R. K., Byrd, D., Reilly, J., Velásquez, R. J., et al. (1998). The effect of African-American acculturation on neuropsychological test performance in normal and HIV-positive individuals. *Journal of the International Neuropsychological Society, 4,* 291–302.

Marshall, C. A., Johnson, M. J., & Johnson, S. R. (2001). Responding to the needs of American Indians with disabilities through rehabilitation counselor education. In C. A. Marshall (Ed.), *Rehabilitation and American Indians with disabilities: A handbook for administrators, practitioners, and researchers* (pp. 115–131). Athens, GA: Elliott & Fitzpatrick, Inc.

Mayer, T., McMahon, M. J., Gatchel, R. J., Sparks, B., Wright, A., & Pegues, P. (1998, discussion 606). Socioeconomic outcomes of combined spine surgery and functional restoration in workers' compensation spinal disorders with matched controls. *Spine, 23,* 598–605.

McDonough, P., & Amick, B. C., III. (2001). The social context of health selection: A longitudinal study of health and employment. *Social Science and Medicine, 53,* 135–145.

McKinnon, J. (2003). *The Black population in the United States: March 2002.* Washington, DC: U.S. Census Bureau, Current Population Reports, Series P20–541.

McNeil, J. (2001, February). Americans with disabilities: *Household economic studies,* 1997 (Current Population Reports). Washington, DC: U.S. Department Of Commerce, Economics and Statistics Administration, U.S. Census Bureau.

Menz, F. E. (1997). Places: Being in context with people and strategies. In F. E. Menz, J. Eggers, P. Wehman, & V. Brooke (Eds.), *Lessons for improving employment of people with disabilities from vocational rehabilitation research* (pp. 49–85). Menomonie, WI: Rehabilitation Research and Training Center, Stout Vocational Rehabilitation Institute, University of Wisconsin–Stout.

Moore, C. L., Feist-Price, S., & Alston, R. J. (2002). Competitive employment and mental retardation: Interplay among gender, race, secondary psychiatric disability, and rehabilitation services. *Journal of Rehabilitation, 68,* 14–19.

Myers, Jr., S. L., & Chung, C. (1996). Racial differences in home ownership and home equity among preretirement-aged households. *Gerontologist, 36,* 350–360.

Olkin, R. (2002). Could you hold the door for me? Including disability in diversity. *Cultural Diversity & Ethnic Minority Psychology, 8,* 130–137.

Olkin, R. (2003). Women with physical disabilities who want to leave their partners: A feminist and disability-affirmative perspective. *Women & Therapy, 26*(3/4), 237–246. [Simultaneously published in M. E. Banks & E. Kaschak (Eds.), *Women with visible and invisible disabilities: Multiple intersections, multiple issues, multiple therapies* (pp. 237–246). New York: Haworth Press.]

Pappas, G. (1998). Monitoring the health consequences of welfare reform. *International Journal of Health Services, 28,* 703–713.

Pitchette, E. F., Berven, N. L., Menz, F. E., & La Fromboise, T. D. (1997). Effects of cultural identification and disability status on perceived community rehabilitation needs of American Indians. *Journal of Rehabilitation, 63*(3), 38–44.

Reidy, T. J., Bowler, R. M., Rauch, S. S., & Pedroza, G. I. (1992). Pesticide exposure and neuropsychological impairment in migrant farm workers. *Archives of Clinical Neuropsychology, 7,* 85–95.

Sanderson, P. L. (1997). People characteristics that affect employment outcomes. In F. E. Menz, J. Eggers, P. Wehman, & V. Brooke (Eds.), *Lessons for improving employment of people with disabilities from vocational rehabilitation research* (pp. 33–48). Menomonie, WI: Rehabilitation Research and Training Center, Stout Vocational Rehabilitation Institute, University of Wisconsin–Stout.

Santiago, A. M., & Muschkin, C. G. (1996). Disentangling the effects of disability status and gender on the labor supply of Anglo, Black, and Latino older workers. *Gerontologist, 36,* 299–310.

Smart, J. F., & Smart, D. W. (1997). The racial/ethnic demography of disability. *Journal of Rehabilitation, 63*(4), 9–15.

Stoddard, S., Jans, L., Ripple, J., & Kraus, L. (1998). *Chartbook on work and disability in the United States, 1998* (An InfoUse Report). Washington, DC: U.S. National Institute on Disability and Rehabilitation Research.

Stronks, K., van de Mheen, H., van den Bos, J., & Mackenbach, J. P. (1995). Smaller socioeconomic inequalities in health among women: The role of employment status. *International Journal of Epidemiology, 24,* 559–568.

Szalda-Petree, A., Seekins, T., & Innes, B. (1999, June). Women with disabilities: Employment, income, and health. Fact sheet. Retrieved March 14, 2006, from http://rtc.ruralinstitute.umt.edu/RuDis/DisWomenFact.htm.

U.S. Department of Commerce, Economics, and Statistics Administration, U.S. Census Bureau. (2001, May). *Profiles of general demographic characteristics: 2000 Census of Population and Housing: United States 2000.* Washington, DC: Author.

U.S. Department of Health and Human Services. (2001). *Mental health: Culture, race, and ethnicity—A supplement to mental health: A report of the surgeon general.* Rockville, MD: U.S. Department of Health and Human Services, Public Health Service, Office of the Surgeon General.

U.S. Department of Labor. (n.d.). *Cultural diversity initiative.* Retrieved March 15, 2006, from http://www.dol.gov/odep/archives/programs/cultural.htm.

Valciukas, J. A. (1991). *Foundations of environmental and occupational neurotoxicology.* New York: Van Nostrand Reinhold.

Wray, L. A. (1996). The role of ethnicity in the disability and work experience of preretirement-age Americans. *Gerontologist, 36,* 287–298.

SECTION II

Health, Function, and Well-Being

INTRODUCTION TO SECTION II: HEALTH, FUNCTION, AND WELL-BEING

Health, function, and well-being are among the outcomes most often studied among persons with disabilities, but may be the least understood. The dynamic nature of these outcomes and the sheer number and complexity of factors that influence them makes this domain of disability and rehabilitation challenging to psychologists. The three chapters that follow challenge the reader to think critically about traditional conceptualizations of disability and rehabilitation, current research paradigms, and the limits of psychology's understanding of contributors to desired and undesired outcomes.

Linda Mona and her coauthors explore how theorists and researchers have broadened psychological paradigms of disability within clinical arenas of the behavioral sciences. They provide a historical review by which disability, impairment, and rehabilitation are conceptualized with special consideration of the "New Paradigm of Disability" articulated by the National Institute for Disability and Rehabilitation Research (NIDRR) in its 1999 Long Range Plan. They contrast NIDRR's New Paradigm with medical, social, and rehabilitation paradigms that are distinguished by a varying focus on internal and external factors that influence the experience of disability. They also discuss adjustment and adaptation outcomes that have been used to assess the quality of life of people with disabilities. In so doing, they seek to enhance our appreciation of how disability paradigms affect the ways in which we measure life satisfaction. Drawing from Rhoda Olkin's therapy model that incorporates the perspective of a disability minority culture, Mona and her colleagues discuss an expanded repertoire of clinical interventions for persons with disabilities. They also call for an expanded view of rehabilitation research that integrates consumer agency and goals and considers environmental and policy variables. Their theoretical foundation promotes clinical research that is diverse in how we conceptualize disability, deliver services, and measure outcomes.

Seth Warschausky reviews recent literature on the social development and integration of children with acquired and congenital neurodevelopmental disorders. He emphasizes that the field of neuropsychology has over just a few years learned a tremendous amount about the cognitive and physiological consequences of disabilities among children. This rapid increase in knowledge, however, may have contributed to a benign neglect of psychological research among these children and a relative deficit in knowledge

73

about their social development and integration among peers. He calls on rehabilitation psychology and neuropsychology to improve the ecological validity of outcome measures, including social development. There exists great promise in socioenvironmentally based interventions to reduce the stigma and increase peer acceptance for children with neurodevelopmental disabilities, but this research also needs to be conducted.

Mary McAweeney and her coauthors address the psychosocial implications and consequences of co-occurring substance use disorders (SUD) for persons with disabilities. They highlight the "double negative" consequences of being stigmatized with a disability and a substance use disorder. This chapter provides a summary of the past 25 years of research on the prevalence of substance use disorders and disabilities, offers an overview of the unique psychosocial issues facing persons with disabilities who have coexisting substance use disorders, and illustrates the unique psychosocial issues encountered by a specific disability group, persons with spinal cord injury. The authors also discuss how the National Institute on Disability and Rehabilitation Research's Model Spinal Cord Injury Systems address this topic and reviews the lessons learned by the Rehabilitation Research and Training Center on Drugs and Disability funded by the National Institute on Disability and Rehabilitation Research. McAweeney and colleagues call for continued development of innovative treatment programs that acknowledge the complexity of challenges facing individuals with disabilities who have co-occurring SUD. These experts recommend continued research into the factors contributing to substance use disorders and poorer outcomes. A multidomain model that is similar to those presented in several chapters is recommended to guide research and interventions for persons with disabilities and co-occurring SUD. The model includes demographic variables, personal characteristics, medical variables, and environmental factors.

Together, these chapters underscore the importance of multifactorial models to understanding and studying disability and rehabilitation. Psychologists have begun to effectively integrate consumers' perspectives when defining research problems and identifying target outcome variables. They have also begun to incorporate environmental and policy variables into research, leading to a more comprehensive and ecologically valid understanding of the challenges of disability. Opportunities remain, however, for research programs that can tease apart the complex interactions among individual characteristics, interpersonal and social influences, environmental variables, and policies that promote or detract from full participation among persons with disabilities. Opportunities abound also in the development of empirically and ecologically valid curricula and therapeutic interventions. These chapters establish a foundation for consideration of these issues.

CHAPTER FOUR

Broadening Paradigms of Disability Research to Clinical Practice: Implications for Conceptualization and Application

Linda R. Mona
Rebecca P. Cameron
Amadee J. Fuentes

PARADIGM SHIFTING

Historically, psychological perspectives on disability have been characterized by a deficit model, in which disability is viewed as a medical problem that creates impairment for an individual. According to that perspective, the locus of the problem is within the disabled person and the goal of clinical intervention is to promote the disabled person's adjustment to this impairment and to the world. Over the past 30 years, alternate perspectives have emerged. A range of models have evolved in which disability is viewed as an interaction between biological or medical circumstances and multiple contexts (e.g., family, housing, transportation, social, etc.). These offer a more holistic, multilevel approach to working with individuals with disabilities in which issues of person-environment fit and multiple intervention strategies are highlighted. However, there is an additional frame of reference that is often still omitted. This perspective arises from the sociopolitical view and the emerging field of disability studies: that of disability as a minority cultural perspective. This cultural perspective addresses issues of identity that arise from environmental and social deficits that inappropriately limit full self-determination and participation by individuals with disabilities, while also recognizing the interplay between biological and social/environmental factors in creating the experience of disablement.

Despite the emergence of these alternate perspectives, clinical psychology has yet to embrace issues of cultural competence in working with individuals with disabilities. Disability has been identified as an important area of competence in the ethical code of the American Psychological Association (APA), but is still marginalized: few psychologists or trainees are members of the disability community and few graduate training programs incorporate disability into the curriculum. Issues related to disability are typically addressed within rehabilitation psychology, which has begun to expand beyond its historical roots in the medical model, but disability is generally not addressed in the mainstream of clinical psychology. As a field, clinical psychology lacks: meaningful conceptual models for understanding psychological well-being in the context of disability; adequate strategies for assessment of individuals with disabilities; and mainstream awareness of models for culturally competent psychotherapy with persons with disabilities (PWD). Research on well-being, assessment, and treatment that incorporates the minority viewpoint of disability is needed in order to move toward empirically grounded and culturally appropriate clinical work with PWD. This chapter will highlight the limitations that currently exist in the field and attempt to draw attention to directions of needed inquiry. The term *disability* is used to describe a range of conditions, including physical, sensory, psychological, addictive, cognitive, developmental, and other. Although the issues we will present are broadly applicable across the diversity that comprises disability, we have chosen to focus primarily on physical disabilities for illustrative purposes. We begin with a brief overview of the paradigms that have guided work in this area.

The predominant paradigm for studying disability within psychology has been the medical or impairment perspective, which gained influence in the mid-1800s as interest in medicine and biological systems increased. This represented something of an advance over the previous stigmatizing view that disability was the result of an individual's moral failings. The model provided a pathological system to explain disabilities and removed theological or mythical implications of disability (Olkin, 1999). However, the medical model suggests that any difficulty experienced by a person with a disability can be understood through comparison to nondisabled medical and functional norms, and hence, movement towards becoming as nondisabled as possible will assist with the presenting issue at hand. By viewing nondisabled persons rather than enabling environments as the standard for comparison, the medical model approaches disability as negative, deficient, and centered within the individual (Gill, 1995). Accordingly, the remedy for disability-related problems is a cure or normalization of the individual, and the agent of remedy is a professional. Despite its archaic view of disability, a tremendous amount of work has been done within the medical model framework that has vastly improved the lives of many disabled persons by providing biomedical and technological advances (Olkin, 1999) such as cochlear implants, genetic testing, and prosthetics.

Closely related to the medical model of disability is the rehabilitation model, which also locates the "problem" of disability within the individual possessing an impairment. The rehabilitation model was designed to move away from the hospital care model and to improve upon an acute care approach to disability. This approach represents an effort to transform PWD from passive recipients of health care procedures by viewing long-term and chronic illness as a handicap and PWD as playing an active role in their own rehabilitation. Although this, like the medical model, represented a significant improvement in the role assigned to PWD, the rehabilitation model still views disabilities as deficiencies to be fixed (DeJong, 1984) and PWD as having the responsibility to accommodate to the outside world (Wessen, 1965). It regards the person as an individual "with a disability" in need of services from a rehabilitation or other helping professional who can provide training, therapy, counseling, or other services to help the PWD make up for the deficiency caused by the disability. Olkin critiques both the medical and rehabilitation models as "static, viewing differences as equally deficit, pathology oriented, predominantly intra-psychic, guided mostly by psychodynamic theory, about but not by persons with disabilities, working toward or amelioration or prevention of problems, sees those with disabilities as 'high risk,' and relies on methodology based on we-they, using either the non-disabled as norms or other outcast groups (e.g., convicts) as norms" (Olkin, 1999, p. 314).

During the 1960s an effort to adopt more integrated views of disability spurred researchers to investigate the effects of the environment on persons with disabilities. The idea emerged that individual functioning could not solely be determined by the nature of the disability itself, but had to be approached from the perspective that the environment could either facilitate or limit function. Nagi (1969) was a leader in developing this viewpoint, in which the environment is seen as a critical component of the phenomenon of disability. Furthermore, disability is dependent on the nature of the environment from which the degree of functionality is evaluated (Nagi, 1969). For example, a veterinary technician who loses her thumb in an accident would be considered disabled at her work because she no longer has the ability to restrain animals properly. However, as a professional lecturer, her ability to function within the lecturing community is not limited and the question of disability is less of an issue. Although the interplay between PWD and the disabling features of their environments was finally beginning to receive attention, the medical/rehabilitation models continued to exert influence. For example, Nagi (1969) described disability within formalized definitions of the consequences of pathology on functioning. This model suggests that disability is pathological in nature and may have resulted from infection, metabolic imbalances, traumatic injury, or other etiological factors, which are commonly referred to as "active pathologies" (p. 101). Nagi (1969) suggested that the goal of disability rehabilitation is to remove or control the active pathology and attempt "to restore optimal functioning and reintegrate the disabled into society" (p. 104). Despite limitations, the focus on the association between functionality and environment spurred further research on this interactive process.

The World Health Organization (WHO) provides an example of the evolution over time toward a more integrative model of disability in the development and revision of the International Classification of Impairments, Disabilities and Handicap (ICIDH) (WHO, 1980) from its original publication in 1980 to its revision 20 years later as the ICIDH-2 (Üstün, Chatterji, Bickenbach, Trotter, & Saxena, 2001). The ICIDH was developed for international use, and included three levels at which to examine disability: impairment (medical abnormality of the body), disability (activity or behavioral dysfunction of the person), and handicap (disadvantage conferred at the social level; Üstün et al., 2001). This model was broader than a purely diagnosis-based approach, but was critiqued for not going far enough (Üstün et al., 2001). Specifically, the classification system still had disease-related terminology embedded within it, still conveyed that disability at person or social levels flowed from bodily condition, and still failed to recognize the role of environmental factors in creating disability. In failing to place adequate attention on the role of social or cultural factors (e.g., the role that ignorance and bias play in maintaining disabling environmental and social conditions), the original ICIDH failed to account for the societal and political ramifications of what it meant to have a disability.

Impairment-based models have been challenged by WHO over the past 30 years and revisions of the ICIDH have occurred in response to the criticisms listed above, leading to increased emphasis on the subjective component of the health experience (e.g., quality of life) and the overall social context (Üstün, et al., 2001). These changes reflected, in part, the realization that medical diagnosis is an inadequate tool for characterizing individuals' functional status and for planning the application of social resources to enhancing individual functioning. Instead, similar functional difficulties might arise from very different medical conditions (e.g., mobility impairments and psychiatric impairments might result in similar areas of dysfunction), whereas two individuals with the same diagnosis might be dissimilar in areas of functioning. In addition, the ICIDH-2 approaches disability as a "universal classification of human functionality itself, both positive and negative" (Üstün et al., 2001, p. 8). Thus, the experience of disability is seen to be on a continuum, with all of us experiencing some degree of disablement. Specific aspects of an individual's environmental, social, and cultural milieu play a powerful role in their experience of enablement-disablement.

Along with the broader conceptual focus, the ICIDH-2 adopted a classification language more neutrally and flexibly oriented, reducing the amount of negativity associated with its predecessor (Üstün et al., 2001). The terms *impairment, disability, and handicap* have given way to three new levels of function: Body Function and Structure, Activity, and Participation. According to this model, these three dimensions of disability are outcomes of interactions between the health conditions and other features of the individual as well as features of the social and physical environment. Philosophically, the three dimensions of disability are not perceived as links in a causal chain leading from the impaired body to social disadvantage, but as interactive but conceptually distinct aspects of the disablement process. This model suggests then that multiple interventions may be warranted when working with a person with a disability. That is, rehabilitative interventions and social or political efforts may be equally valid modalities for change (Üstün et al., 2001).

The WHO, collaborating with nongovernmental organizations, disability groups, and individual experts and key informants, continued to work on the ICIDH-2 classification system. Within this new draft, efforts were made to move beyond defining disability as a consequence of disease to highlighting functioning as a component of health. The newly proposed classification system was created in multiple languages to assist with culturally specific linguistic differences and was then placed on the Internet for comments from consumers and providers. In December 2000, the classification system was renamed International Classification of Functioning, Disability, and Health (ICF) (Üstün, Chatterji, Bickenbach, Kostanjsek, & Schneider, 2003). Overall, the ICF provides a framework for the description of health and health-related states from different perspectives: the perspective of the body (classification of body functions and of body structures) and the perspective of the individual and the society (classification of activities and participation) (de Kleijn-de Vrankrijker,

2003). Furthermore, "functioning" is the ICF umbrella term encompassing body functions, structures, activities, and participation. On the other hand, *disability* is the ICF broad term for impairments, activity limitations, and participation restrictions. A major change from the ICIDH-2 to the ICF system is that it takes into account environmental factors that interact with all of the dimensions listed above.

It is important to note that the ICIDH-2 and ICF processes incorporated the voices of PWD. However, despite the increased involvement of PWD and despite improvements in the models guiding health care policy and service delivery, there are still significant limitations that occur when nondisabled professionals set the parameters for understanding disability. For example, the view of PWD as service consumers and able-bodied professionals as service providers remains an implicit, widespread assumption in thinking about reducing disablement and enhancing participation. What about the notion of members of the disability community providing service to other members rather than remaining in their role as service consumers?

The latter concept is one of the core principles of the Independent Living movement. This important social movement was developed in the 1970s, around the same time of Nagi's (1969) work, but is often overlooked. A greater understanding of this movement within clinical psychology could lead to enriched conceptualizations and enhanced services to PWD. The Independent Living movement goes further than other models in empowering PWD through empowering the disability community to be self-determining. The tenets of this movement are: "that people with disabilities should be service providers for other people with disabilities; that persons with disabilities should retain self-determination; that independence is a goal, and assistance (both personal services and assistive devices) should be aimed at helping the person maximize independence and self-determination; that community integration is a goal; and that separate is not equal" (Olkin, 1999, p. 139). The main focus of this philosophy was to create a supportive community of individuals who faced the same social and political barriers. This resulted in the rapid growth of Independent Living Communities. The ideals embodied in this movement are a significant departure from the impairment-focused medical and rehabilitation models, but are more compatible with the newer direction of models such as the ICF classification system.

Among the newer models, the sociopolitical perspective represents a conceptual contribution from academic fields outside of psychology (i.e., anthropology, sociology, disability studies) that affords particular attention to the degree in which environmental, cultural, and political factors influence the life experiences of people with disabilities. Olkin (1999) indicates that this paradigm "shifts to a systemic perspective; views adaptation as a fluid process; inquires about health and resilience; considers disability as culture; views the major problems of disability as prejudice, discrimination, and denial of civil rights; looks for information and solutions in public policy and legislation; and tends to be not only about but by persons with disabilities" (p. 314). This systemic approach does not ignore the individual experience of disability but changes the nature of inquiry by shifting to a focus on strengths. There are many similarities between Olkin and the ICIDH-2's newest classification of the disability experience, yet Olkin's sociopolitical model (Olkin, 1999, p. 314) defines the individual experience of disability from a health perspective compared to a disorder or deficiency-based construct. This model also emphasizes that people with disabilities themselves often actively participate in important life decisions influenced by political and/or legislative barriers, therefore incorporating many of the independent living philosophy tenets.

The sociopolitical model may be critiqued for underplaying the importance of the impairment itself. Individuals with chronic or lifelong illnesses still need to live with the reality of their condition and continue to seek medical care. An individual with chronic fatigue syndrome does not evaluate his or her life solely on the basis of how the environment accommodates him or her, but also in terms of issues like varying levels of stiffness and fatigue, as well as the impact of medications on his or her physical and psychological well-being.

Compared to the sociopolitical model, the New Paradigm of Disability acknowledges disability as impairment and searches for the interplay between individual and environmental factors. Keeping in line with the importance of expanding the deeper understanding of the disability experience, the New Paradigm of Disability (National Institute on Disability and Rehabilitation Research [NIDRR], 1999) maintains that disability is a product of interaction between characteristics of the individual and characteristics of the natural, built, cultural, and social environments. This approach argues that past conceptualizations of disability ascribe disability to the individual and underplay the interaction that occurs between various environments and the individual. Furthermore, according to this paradigm, disability is located on a continuum between the ability to perform and not perform in a given environmental condition or situation (Pledger, 2003). This paradigm further suggests an applied social model that interrelates the impact of environmental factors (e.g., families, immediate environments, various systems, public policies, culture, and society) on participation, productivity, involvement, quality of life, and psychological adjustment of those affected by disability.

As we have reviewed, the available models for classifying and characterizing the disability experience have increased dramatically in sophistication and complexity as they have expanded beyond the medical or rehabilitation perspectives with their focus on impairment, diagnosis, and one-way accommodation of the PWD to the nondisabled world. The environmental aspects and social experiences of disablement have begun to be seen as truly equivalent in importance to the medical and person-based aspects of disablement, yielding the possibility of integrated views of multiple aspects of disability. Each approach we have described has a particular focus that adds to the richness of our conceptualizations (e.g., empowerment of PWD as service providers); the relationships among different disability domains (NIDRR, 1999); or disability as a universal life experience (Olkin & Pledger, 2003). The field of disability studies adds to this richness by fully articulating the phenomenon of disability as a minority group perspective relevant within the universal human experience of enablement-disablement.

Disability studies is only beginning to inform the field of psychology, following other fields of interdisciplinary study such as African American and gender studies, which took approximately 30 years to develop before beginning to be incorporated into the discourse within psychology. Like other minority-group studies, disability studies approaches disability by developing "a definition of self (i.e., who are we?), preferred language (i.e., what do we call ourselves?), and the training and research agenda for the field" (Olkin & Pledger, 2003, p. 297). Furthermore, according to Olkin and Pledger (2003), disability studies attempts to track societal, political, historical, cultural, empowerment, stigma, and marginalization issues. In comparing the theories presented here, one major distinction is that disability per se is not viewed as impairment or disorder in either the sociopolitical or disability studies model.

With this expansion of theoretical arguments demanding larger and more precise examination of the disability experience, how have the interrelated views of health, impairment, social and environmental factors, and participation in life been employed in our direct service work with people with disabilities? This is a two-part question: (a) How have we defined satisfactory quality of life or treatment advancement when working with this population? (b) What models or treatment approaches have we used to work with the disability community? Both of these areas will be explored, with hopes of further refining what is known and not known about the current state of psychology's efforts in working clinically with people with disabilities.

PSYCHOLOGICAL VIEWS OF
DISABILITY AND QUALITY OF LIFE

Psychotherapy is an enterprise that arises from diverse philosophies and theoretical models, most of which are pathology-focused. There has been an increased focus on health and well-being in recent years, but the field of psychotherapy is not guided by a particular view of what it means to be healthy. Psychotherapy has been conducted with either broad goals in mind that may not be well-articulated or with well-defined and operationalized goals, depending in part on the theoretical orientation of the therapist and on the role of third-party payers, which often require the identification of a list of problems to be corrected during the course of psychotherapy. And as clinicians more routinely than in the past accept the need to set goals, they are perhaps increasingly mindful of the desired end-state of psychotherapy (defined by the removal or reduction of negative symptoms and/or by an increase in social or occupational functioning and resources like social support, coping strengths, etc.). Thus, at some level, psychotherapy is conducted in the context of a more- or less-articulated image of health. Yet, models of health are still far less salient in psychotherapy than are models of psychopathology.

In particular, when it comes to PWD, clinicians are poorly trained in conceptualizing health, and thus have difficulty moving beyond impairment models in organizing psychotherapy. Few clinicians have a sense of how to define psychological health or quality of life in the context of long-term physical differences; instead they utilize problematic constructs such as adjustment and adaptation. Thus therapists who recognize the limitations of impairment models may be unclear of their role in trying to expand the conceptual basis of their work with PWD to include newer models. Just as therapists lack training in a conceptualization of health in the context of disability, they lack assessment strategies for working with PWD that are flexibly able to provide meaningful feedback regardless of the nature of a client's disability. Traditional assessment methodologies compare disabled individuals to standardized ideals of normality, resulting in pathologic views of PWD. And psychology has yet to develop or really even to consider assessment strategies that would provide feedback on minority identity among PWD. Finally, locating problems in the environment is less a central part of assessment than is describing the individual's role in their difficulties. Thus, case conceptualizations remain focused on impairment rather than health, and on individual-level factors rather than external environmental or political factors. Clinicians will be unable to provide coherent services to PWD until progress is made in these areas, and until therapists are well-trained to consider these conceptual issues.

ADJUSTMENT

Adjustment is generally associated with arranging matters in the correct order. Of course, this assumes that there is one "right" way to become well adjusted. One of the staples of rehabilitation psychological research and practice has been of adjustment to disability. There has been an associated assumption that disability causes distress, depression, and maladjustment. In fact, NIDRR's New Paradigm of Disability (1999) continues to employ this word usage when the model is discussed in terms of evaluating the influence of the individual and environment on psychological adjustment. What is adjustment? How do we measure it among people with disabilities? How is it different among those with lifelong disabilities versus those with acquired disabilities? Psychological adjustment to stress has been defined in a variety of ways, including a persons' ability to decrease physiological arousal (e.g., heart rate and pulse) when coping with a stressful event; measure levels of psychological distress during difficult times; and examine the length of time it takes people to return to their prestress activities (Taylor &Aspinwall, 1996). However, with regard to this latter definition, "there is an implicit bias in this criterion to the effect that a person's prior living situation was in some sense an ideal one" (Taylor & Aspinwall, 1996, p. 41).

Clinicians typically use assessment tools to measure an individual's psychological adjustment to stressful events. For the disability population, adjustment to a new way of experiencing life or facing chronic life obstacles can have a variety of different meanings. Psychology should not assume that the disability, per se, is always the presenting issue in clinical treatment. It may be that monetary barriers or social prejudice prevent attainment of life's goals. It may be that disability, in and of itself, is a part of who the person is and treatment is sought for a reason unrelated to it. How is psychological distress unrelated to disability teased out from the disability status itself? With regard to returning to prestress activities (applicable only to those who have acquired disabilities later in life), some persons with disabilities may report that there are activities in which they cannot participate, whereas others may report alternative ways of accomplishing the same prestress activities. How do these issues relate to the experience of adjustment?

In the world of rehabilitation there are various measures utilized to assess adjustment, including measures of personality psychopathology, depression, and normative personality characteristics. These include measures such as the Minnesota Multiphasic Personality Inventory (MMPI and MMPI-2; Hathaway &McKinley, 1989), the Millon Clinical Multiaxial Inventories (MCMI through MCMI-III; Millon, 1982; Millon, Millon, & Davis, 1994), the Symptom Checklist 90-Revised (SCL-90R; Derogatis, 1977), and The Center for Epidemiological Studies—Depression Scale (CES-D); (Radloff, 1977). Each has a large body of literature associated with it, but each also has significant limitations with respect to use with PWD. Elliott and Umlauf (1995) provide a review of many of these. There are several issues that may affect generalizability: differences in physical functioning that may result in either inability to complete certain measures validly (e.g., those available only in paper and pencil might not be usable by someone with certain motor limitations; the comparability of the measure if administered in a nonstandardized format may be unknown); differences in normative responses for a particular group (e.g., PWD may score higher on scales assessing somatic concerns); and differences in the implication of scores (e.g., perhaps high scores on somatic preoccupation signal better functioning among those for whom vigilant self-monitoring is a key to maintaining health). The role of environmental circumstances in producing responses is not well understood, and may lead to misinterpretation (for example, a PWD might respond affirmatively to questions assessing the fairness of their life circumstances; this would not necessarily indicate entitlement, but might simply be a factual observation). Finally, most of these scales are designed to aid in the detection of psychological problems, not psychological strengths, and thus they contribute to an imbalanced perspective on the mental health functioning of PWD.

Disabilities come in all forms, including sensory, physical, neurological, and developmental. Given that tools such as the MMPI and MCMI are designed to be administered in a standardized manner, can we clearly conclude that evaluation is not a function of how the test is administered? Elliot and Umlauf (1995) explain that the paper-and-pencil version of the MMPI may not be entirely appropriate for inpatient rehabilitation patients because the measure itself is very long and if an individual is presenting fatigue or difficulty sitting up, responses may elevate somatic descriptor items on the MMPI. Additionally, Olkin (1999) argues that although many assessment measures are becoming more adapted to PWDs we cannot conclude that these measures are conveying valid results because modifications to these measures may not be appropriate for any given PWD. For example, assessing the adjustment achieved by a visually impaired individual would require a reader to be present during administration of the test. The presence of this reader may result in the individual feeling more anxiety and responses could report elevated subscales scores; or, the individual may fear disclosure issues and falsely answer certain questions. These are certainly considerations to take into account when assessing adjustment in individuals with disabilities.

Data that would guide interpretations and allow for meaningful interpretations of assessment instruments are typically quite limited. First, most instruments have been normed on nondisabled populations and have little or no normative information for PWD, or only for one subpopulation of PWD. What literature there is suggests that there may be differences in how PWD respond to these instruments, which suggests caution in interpretation. One obvious area in which existing norms may not apply has to do with items assessing somatic symptoms. The endorsement of these may lead to an interpretation that psychopathology or a particular style of managing stress and anxiety is present, when in fact these items may simply reflect realities of the person's health. Clinicians, despite being aware of the need to interpret all assessment data in light of individual circumstances, may have little training or practical frame of reference to guide these interpretations. Some work has been done to examine responses of PWD with acquired disabilities, such as spinal cord injuries (SCI) in certain instruments. Elliott and Umlauf (1995) cite work by Taylor (1970) and Kendall, Edinger, and Eberly (1978) showing differences in how PWD responded to 12 items. However, the MMPI-2 has not been similarly evaluated, and much work remains to be done in this area.

An important area for careful assessment is mood; depressive disorders can significantly affect health management and quality of life. Yet, this issue is complicated among individuals with health concerns. Depression may be over-diagnosed when somatic symptoms are viewed as arising from depression rather than physical health factors. It can be difficult for clinicians to tease apart the role of health factors from that of depressive symptoms as these may overlap (e.g., symptoms of fatigue, digestive problems, reduced appetite, aches and pains). The bias inherent in conceptualizations of disability that nondisabled practitioners are subject to complicates this issue as well; health professionals expect PWD to experience depression (i.e., "Who wouldn't feel depressed with that problem?"), but attribute this to an inevitable aspect of lost physical functioning and not to social and environmental injustices that are demoralizing. Thus, depression may be under-diagnosed as well; when acceptance of depressive symptoms as an inevitable part of the phenomenology of disability results in failure to recognize actual, treatable cases of depression, leading in turn to prolonged and less effective treatments. Lichtenberg (1997; in Olkin, 1999) found that major medical conditions of depression were overlooked and resulted in 50% or less of people with major conditions being diagnosed. Clearly, a more nuanced and sophisticated approach to the assessment of depression among PWD is needed.

Interpretive approaches to psychological assessment instruments often neglect to account for the environmental and societal/economic barriers experienced by PWDs. Olkin (1999) provides an example of this point in her description of a study conducted by Dorman, Hurley, and Laatsch, (1984) which reported that adolescents with cerebral palsy had a mean IQ of 86. Olkin argues that the researchers did not take into consideration that these adolescents "were not in mainstream classrooms . . . and mainly lived in residential homes with other children with disabilities" (p. 211). Their restricted participation in mainstream environments may have served to artificially lower their assessed intelligence. These are fine points that diagnostic tools are unable to resolve. Instead, use of assessment instruments needs to be guided by the contextual information gleaned from careful and thorough interviewing, as well as enough cross-cultural insight that the clinician can anticipate and avoid biased interpretations of assessment data.

Along these lines, assessment measures fail to account for the cross-cultural nature of the experience of disability as well as cultural variability due to factors such as ethnicity. Thus, PWD may be members of more than one minority group (Elliot, 1993: Olkin, 1999; Pledger, 2003), resulting in even more questionable application of assessment instruments generally accepted as reliable and valid for able-bodied dominant cultural groups (Padilla, 2001). The MMPI and the MCMI are instruments most commonly used to assess ethnic minority groups (Nagayama Hall & Phung, 2001) and the authors state that although studies indicate that these measures "show limited differences between European Americans and ethnic minority groups," cultural sensitivity should be practiced and that "expertise . . . in assessment and in ethnic minority groups" be acquired before applying these measures (p. 324). Without clarification of the norms for disabled individuals on these same instruments there is no clear way to determine the extent of misinterpretation that may occur with ethnic minority PWDs. However, the concept of cultural sensitivity and the need for special expertise should be similarly understood to apply to the disability minority group. These issues are particularly controversial as they relate to measures of quality of life and subjective well-being. These measures are fraught with validity and reliability questions when used among ethnic minority groups because they are developed using Western ideology and language (Utsey, Bolden, Brown, & Chae, 2001). Given our lack of clarity about psychological health among PWD, it is likely that these measures suffer from nondisabled biases as well. Research is needed in this area to inform both assessments of psychopathology as well as healthy adjustment. With the new focus on disability as a minority cultural experience, it would be informative to devise or adapt assessment instruments in order to measure cultural identification of PWD with nondisabled and disability cultural norms.

Psychological adjustment to acquired disabilities has been viewed historically in the literature as a sequential process involving three to five naturally occurring stages (Bracken, Shepard, & Webb, 1981; Hohmann, 1975; Siller, 1963; Stewart, 1977). Stage theories often suggest that psychological difficulties are a natural response that should be expected when persons undergo grieving processes. For example, Stewart (1977) proposed a three-stage model of coping and adaptation that included (a) denial, (b) depression, and (c) moratorium/restitution (a stage typically marked by some form of acceptance of the disability). Yet, stage theories like Stewart's do not discuss the degree to which psychological factors such as denial, depression, and moratorium are not sequential, but may be present at multiple stages in the grieving process, and in turn, how they affect adjustment over time. Stage models assume a linear process following a discrete event; however, disability is an experience that may be lifelong, that may have a gradual onset, that may wax and wane, or that may gradually intensify. In addition, moving between different environments and social milieu may create a nonlinear experience of disablement, in which disability may become more or less salient, anger or feelings of helplessness may vary as a function of external circumstances, and social relationships may be more or less of a resource. These are among the reasons that linear models are not adequate to capture the experience of maintaining or improving well-being in the face of difficult circumstances that the term *adjustment* implies. More holistic approaches would be helpful, as are models that place a decreased emphasis on the assumption of the necessity of grief and depression as *the* critical psychological phenomena that define well-being in disability. Finally, as long as *adjustment* to the disability remains the focus of this area of work, it may be difficult to shift from a preoccupation with PWD as differing from and therefore worse off than nondisabled persons, but actively seeking to reapproach their predisablement functioning. Models of *thriving* are more elusive but would afford a fresh perspective on the generativity and well-being that are as much the birthright of PWD as they are of nondisabled individuals. From the perspective of PWD as thriving individuals, it would be easier to shift to an understanding of the limiting and burdensome nature of the environment as a cause of distress.

In summary, psychological adjustment to disability has been examined in a variety of contexts and with numerous definitions of adjustment, most based upon impairment-based models. That is, the impairment itself, or the loss of functionality as a result of the specified impairment, are the factors deemed to be pivotal in evaluating the adjustment process. According to the literature, persons with acquired disabilities who report better adjustment seem to maintain better health practices (Macleod, 1988), live longer (Krause & Crewe, 1987; Krause, 1991), report higher levels of life satisfaction (Shulz & Decker, 1985), and have more social support (Dunn, 1977; Romano, 1976; Shulz & Decker, 1985). These findings make sense, yet they perpetuate an imbalanced view of problems as existing within the individual and available for correction at the individual level. However, the degree to which adjustment rests upon environmental factors (e.g., access to monetary resources, living in an architecturally and attitudinally accessible environment, knowledge about how to advocate for rights) remains unexamined from a psychological perspective. Furthermore, what is known about how people with lifelong disabilities adjust to their disability status is much less clear, as the acute onset of loss and grief no longer applies, and the concept of stages loses relevance.

ADAPTATION

Adaptation is typically used to describe an individual modification to new conditions. This term actually seems more fluid than that of adjustment and has been used frequently in the rehabilitation literature. However, the questions of environmental adaptation to the needs of PWD and social adaptation to the diversity that disability engenders still remain at the periphery of discussions of adaptation. Adjustment processes in persons with acquired disabilities have been examined in terms of individuals' level of comfort with experienced physical losses (Bracken et al., 1981; Hohmann, 1975; Siller, 1963; Stewart, 1977), but they are rarely explored within the context of adaptation to ways of viewing the self and/or behavior. Given that most research on disability and chronic health conditions relies upon the view that the loss of functionality and the lack of independent living skills are foremost for individuals, assessing adaptation based upon satisfaction with life, having adequate resources, and the current experience of self are often left unstudied. This manner of understanding adaptation is quite different from examining the adjustment process as a function of losses associated with a past way of viewing the self and evaluating one's life.

Traditional adaptation models have come from the health psychology field. Taylor's (1983) well-known theory of cognitive adaptation, developed while working with breast cancer patients, offers a model that takes into consideration psychological factors associated with adaptation to threatening events. Each construct, including personal control, meaning, self-esteem, and unrealistic optimism, was introduced as being responsible for the promotion of better psychological adaptation to a sudden, life-changing event. This model seeks explanations for adaptation based upon the individual's psychological processes instead of looking at environmental and social structure constraints as potential reasons behind lack of adaptation. Taylor's (1983) theory is applicable to those with acquired conditions if, in fact, acquiring the disability is perceived as a threatening event. Similar to the criticism of theoretical ideas within adjustment, Taylor's (1983) adaptation views may be difficult if not impossible to expand to those individuals who have lived with lifelong disabilities.

Yet neither of these approaches addresses how environmental and societal adaptation to disabilities impacts the PWD. If a person with cerebral palsy has every resource available to get to school, take exams, and has complete wheelchair access, is this person truly adapting? We are only assuming that this person's situation is ideal because there is a lack of research in the direction of how changes to the environment and society affect individuals with disabilities. We cannot be certain that these environmental changes ensure that adaptation is really taking place. We will always need nomothetic perspectives provided by empirical research within the disability community, coupled with idiographic assessment within clinical situations, rather than a priori assumptions to ascertain how best to foster quality of life and enhance adaptation.

Assessing the intricacies among the definitions of adjustment and adaptation is important if in fact psychology is committed to enhance its measurement of quality of life within the disability community. Some theorists would state that we need to look at how people with disabilities adapt to their life situation while others would argue that we need to examine the degree to which the environment and social world adapt to include the disability community. According to one disability studies theorist,

> "The positive news is that we all adjust and adapt to different environments for our emotional, psychological, and social health and survival. A certain amount of this is obviously healthy. The negative news is that in terms of people with disabilities and the social model on another level, both terms may imply adjusting to a constructed sociocultural environment that is normative. In this case, perhaps it would be best not to adjust or adapt to values and attitudes that have a norm at their center and to try to expand the center to accept more diversity. It is a matter of sorting out the types of society's attitudes, values, and orientations that would be psychologically and emotionally healthy to adapt or adjust to"
> (R. Shuttleworth, personal communication, July 18, 2000).

These are important questions to ask when exploring approaches to service with people with disabilities. These issues are complex in a society that struggles with monocultural versus pluralistic values. Yet, for PWD, true equality and dignity and thus a society that truly fosters psychological health seem inextricably bound to environmental and sociopolitical adaptations to the needs of PWD. In order to achieve greater parity of access, the disability community will need to be willing to show health by refusing to conform, by *not* "adjusting" to the nondisabled environment, perhaps by staying angry and rejecting a conformity that doesn't fit, despite the way this stance will lend itself to marginalization and pathological interpretation.

To recap, psychologists working in clinical areas can't always assume that disability experience is a fundamental part of the individual's presenting issue but should maintain that it is always an important part of the individual. With social and environmental models of disability now available, it is imperative that psychologists examine society's role in embracing people with disability in their complexity rather than being quick to focus upon an individual's need to change to fit existing standards of being.

Bearing in mind Shuttleworth's important argument (R. Shuttleworth, personal communication, July 18, 2000), psychologists are charged with challenging traditional beliefs of adjustment and adaptation in their work with people with disabilities. It may be true that individuals with acquired disabilities go through many of the typical grieving processes hypothesized by stage theories and examined within rehabilitation models. However, to understand issues only at this level would be to minimize or ignore a large part of the disability experience. If instead psychologists explore disability as they would any other sociodemographic factor, they can begin to tease out the importance of the disability experience to any given clinical situation.

TREATMENT ISSUES

Paradigms guiding the field of psychology are beginning to embrace:

- Perspectives on disability that integrate biological, environmental, and sociocultural factors that create the experience of disablement
- Views of PWD as resilient, self-determining agents in their own lives and communities
- Expectations of the world in which environments change to create enablement
- Visions of relationships in which nondisabled individuals do not set the agenda for the emotional lives of PWD
- Recognition that disability is a minority identity

Are clinicians prepared to work with clients in ways that enact these new perspectives and engender these views within their clients? The mainstream literature on clinical interventions rarely addresses the applicability of treatment models and strategies to clients with disabilities, and few disability-specific treatments have been developed. Although it is reasonable to assume that certain treatment strategies (e.g., empirically validated therapies for depression and anxiety) may be helpful, the nuances brought about by the social experience of disability call for strategies and therapists that explicitly incorporate disability-relevant factors and consciousness.

Therapy with PWD cannot be assumed to be limited to the standard focus on ameliorating psychological distress. Instead, therapists must be able to assist clients with an ongoing process of reevaluating their perception of their disability, values, future, relationships with others and the community, and state of independence (Olkin, 1999). Older, impairment-based views of disability carry implications for clinical work that are inadequate in numerous ways. For example, nondisabled norms will guide the goals of treatment, leading to an implicit message that, although the PWD may do his or her best to "adjust," he or she will be simply making the best of a bad situation or "overcoming" something, rather than being as fully him- or herself as any other client. There will be an expectation that grief is essential to adjustment, that anger is pathological and indicates unrealistic entitlement or other failure to accept the world as it is, and that the therapist is more of a provider and less of a facilitator (Olkin, 1999). In addition, outsiders will be looked to for definition of the task at hand, as the agency of the client will be minimized. Identifying and treating problems will take precedence over identifying strengths and considering how to enhance them; true fulfillment and psychological prosperity will not be considered as a goal. The environment and society will be seen as static, a given, rather than a source of disablement and oppression to be challenged. Civil rights will not enter the discourse, and abusive relationships will be less likely to be challenged. To conduct clinically rich therapy with PWD essentially requires an orientation in which therapists view PWD as equal in agency, worth, and potential to nondisabled clients, while not failing to appreciate the myriad ways in which the experience of disability is different from that of being nondisabled.

Disability Affirmative Therapy (DAT) (Olkin, 1999) reflects a predominantly sociocultural, but also very integrative conceptual stance. Thus, it encompasses factors of empowerment, social marginalization, and environmental barriers relevant to PWD, while not discounting medical realities and personal coping strategies. This model provides a framework and therapeutic techniques that incorporate the many loci in which disability is created (from individual to societal levels), but also acknowledges issues of time, both in the relationship between daily realities and longer-term experiences, and in recognition of the fact that the disability experience is not static, and there is no final plateau of adjustment beyond which disability becomes a moot area of one's psychological life. Keeping all of these perspectives in mind, Olkin (1999) provides six main goals for DAT.

The first goal is to gain insight into how the client perceives his or her disability. This goal requires that clinicians be familiar with a range of disability/rehabilitation models such as those overviewed above. Olkin (1999) focuses primarily on three models of disability that shape clients' self-views and conceptualization of the goals of treatment (i.e., the moral, medical, and minority models). For example, a client who has recently been diagnosed with rheumatoid arthritis may believe that medication is the answer to her difficulties, and invest psychic energy in hoping for an eventual cure. Or she may berate herself on days on which the pain is particularly pronounced, thinking that she "should" be able to prevent or manage her symptoms better, given that she is highly educated and has access to health care. Finally, she may be aware of her supervisor's failure to appreciate her need for a flexible work schedule, and find herself wishing she could work for a boss who also possessed a disability. These interpretations of her situation (medical, moral, and minority, respectively) may or may not coexist in the same individual and may change over time. Becoming aware of the assumptions implicit in these interpretations can aid the therapist and eventually the client in identifying underlying sources of distress as well as areas available for therapeutic change (What if no cure is found? How are you a bad person for having symptoms? How can we prepare you to assert your need for reasonable accommodations in the workplace?) The goal is not to convert clients to a minority perspective on disability; however, developing support in the disability community is often tremendously helpful.

A second goal centers around empowering clients with disabilities through recognition of their unique relationships to power, choice, independence, interdependence, assistance, and control. Olkin (1999) states that when individuals with disabilities lose the ability to make decisions concerning their own needs and priorities, "resulting disempowerment can lead to depression, rage, anxiety, passivity, and hopelessness" (p. 174). The goal is for clients to be truly in charge of their own lives, with power to make decisions, access needed resources, and determine the course of their health care, relationships, and other important areas of life, in as direct a sense as possible. Furthermore the goal of the therapy is to help clients with disabilities find an interdependent approach, representing equilibrium between independence and dependence. Thus, clients can accept assistance from friends, family, and coworkers without rescinding agency.

Often times, individuals' culturally sanctioned or preexisting value systems do not interact well with disability to enhance adjustment or adaptation. Olkin (1999) includes value changes as the third goal of DAT. Individuals need to essentially reprioritize their values such that identity and well-being are not tied to values that may have become a source of distress and loss rather than affirmation and growth. Values that are not likely to suffer from disability-related factors need to be moved to or maintained at higher positions within a hierarchy of values; in contrast, values that are deeply affected by disability need to be lowered in importance. A primary example is that for many PWD, placing a high value on physique and certain types of physical activities is no longer particularly functional; thus subordinating the physique within the value system can be beneficial. In order to maintain unaffected values at previously high levels of importance, one cannot allow them to be inappropriately associated with the disability. For example, for a client who values dressing in the latest styles, the experience of disability accompanied by physical changes that are not consistent with society's beauty ideals should not automatically indicate renunciation of fashion sense. For a person who is accustomed to leading neighborhood cleanup efforts, does the loss of physical mobility for bending over to pick up litter necessarily result in the loss of leadership skills or the abandonment of values of service to his or her community? Finally, resources and values need to be considered according to their inherent worth or utility rather than as they compare to other resources and values. For example, a person who loves to sit outside and read might prefer a large backyard to a neighborhood park. However, if disability leads to the decision to live in a condominium or apartment to eliminate certain kinds of maintenance chores or expenses, the utility of the neighborhood park might include more time to read. But if the decision is solely evaluated according to "less desirable than my old backyard," this comparison reduces the ability to take pleasure in the resource.

A fourth goal, "containing spread effects" (Olkin, 1999, p. 177), addresses the extent to which disability displaces other aspects of the person to whom it belongs. Often, disability becomes the central defining feature of a person, at least in the eyes of others; other aspects of identity are presented as existing *despite* the disability. Although disability may engender reevaluation and reprioritizing of values and interests, it does not replace the person. It is a possession with specific areas of impact rather than a personality characteristic that renders the person knowable in a simplified or stereotyped fashion. This goal reminds therapists to help clients discuss disability *as needed,* particularly with employers and romantic partners. Instead of "I have a disability, but . . ." clients can learn to discuss the nature of their disability, its effects, the accommodations that it calls for, and so forth, in a matter-of-fact way. This discourages others from dismissing the client's worth, skills, or actual personality characteristics as secondary to the central identity of disabled person.

A large part of moving forward and living with a disability is finding ways to manage the ongoing demands created by the disability. Some aspects of disability experience are repetitive, like managing a medication regimen or getting up early enough to get ready for work on time. Many can be punishing, like shopping or dining out and finding that bathrooms are not accessible or that shopkeepers, waiters, and other service persons talk down to you. These types of disability experiences can be demoralizing and even depressing over time, and, although some call for environmental or social change, there is also often a need to cope effectively at the individual level as well. One approach is reframing: "getting up early to get ready for work isn't so bad; I enjoy the birds singing in the early morning and seeing the sunshine gradually creep in the window." Another is to attend to the need for reinforcers, sources of pleasure and anticipation that need to be scheduled daily, weekly, monthly, and annually, if they do not occur naturally ("every Friday I have lunch with a friend at a restaurant we know is accessible"; "next fall we will go on a 2-week vacation") (Olkin, 1999).

Finally, a sixth goal is to help a client develop a supportive social group. All families have to adapt to changing developmental needs of family members, but families in which a member has a disability often struggle more than usual with developmentally necessary role shifts (especially the shift involving a child with a disability becoming a self-determining adult). The usual dance of give-and-take within friendships can be complicated by the meaning associated with asking for and receiving help for the PWD, who may avoid being on the receiving end even when it is appropriate and would enhance intimacy and mutuality. However, PWD, so often the subject of outsiders' curiosity, prejudice, and assumptions, need relationships within which they feel safe, understood, and unselfconscious. Therapists need to foster clients' social embeddedness among others who truly do not view the client as a diminished person (Olkin, 1999).

Olkin (1999) suggested that Disability Affirmative Therapy affords a coherent framework for approaching therapeutic work with clients with disabilities, despite differences in types of disabilities, presenting problems, psychological makeup, and levels of development. It is based in a conceptual foundation of sociocultural and integrative theory of disability, and it is cognizant of minority group status. If it were more widely taught, this model would provide clinical psychologists and trainees with a valuable tool for working with PWD in therapy. In order for this approach to become a long-term and authentic part of the scientist-practitioner's therapeutic mindset, research is needed to establish efficacy, limitations, and areas for improvement.

Further investigation of Disability Affirmative Therapy would be helpful to evaluate it as a treatment approach and to facilitate a broader conceptual approach to treatment of disabled people. This research process could also lay a foundation for integrating clinical information from rehabilitation, private practice, and community-based settings that provide services to individuals with a wide range of disabilities.

RECOMMENDED RESEARCH DIRECTIONS

By redefining paradigms of disability and seeking new understanding in research methodologies and design, psychology can begin to better acknowledge the disability experience at both research and practice levels. NIDRR (1999) proposes that one of the goals under the New Paradigm of Disability is "to change the focus of research such as studies of the dynamic interplay between an individual and the environment and of the adapting process by the society and the individual." Following are suggested ideas to fuel clinically relevant research reflective of the issues raised by Olkin (1999), NIDRR (1999), and Olkin and Pledger (2003) in expanding the research agenda on disability. These proposed ideas have the underlying goal of systematically exploring the rich life experiences of people with disabilities based upon relationships among individual, interpersonal, social, cultural, and political interactions. Research is needed in all the areas addressed above: conceptualizing quality of life, refining assessment tools, clarifying cultural aspects of disability, and developing intervention strategies.

Specifically, research is needed that investigates quality of life for PWD beyond adjustment, grief, and individual-level adaptation. This research agenda would be based in a resilience perspective in which the focus would be on well-being rather than deficits; outcome variables would include intimacy, happiness, creativity, leadership, spirituality, and so forth, rather than being limited to psychopathology and its exacerbation or reduction. Variables of interest would include environmental factors, both enabling and disabling, social policies, diversity awareness among the nondisabled community, diversity activism, and level of acculturation to, or identification with, the disability community, in addition to intrapsychic variables. As mentioned previously, the assumption of any particular approach to reducing disablement and enhancing quality of life would be avoided in favor of quantitative and qualitative research demonstrating an effect. Examples of topics of interest include the relationship between personal assistance services (PAS) and well-being, and the topic of sexual health.

To elaborate, PAS is defined as "involving a person assisting someone with a disability to perform tasks aimed at maintaining well-being, personal appearance, comfort, safety, and interaction with the community and society as a whole" (World Institute on Disability, 1999). More information is needed on the degree to which ideas of disability, independence, interdependence, and PAS are embraced among people with disabilities. Qualitative methods (e.g., structured interviews and focus groups) would be useful in exploring personal perspectives on the power of PAS, or lack thereof, to enhance fulfillment. Social policy issues (such as type of PAS program available based upon geographical region, amount of funding available, amount of out-of-pocket pay, and availability of qualified people) and individual-level issues (such as the nature of PAS experiences, including exposure to physical, emotional, or monetary abuse) could be examined to better capture the interplay among these factors, as the New Paradigm would suggest.

Another area of quality-of-life research that would benefit from exploration under the New Paradigm is access to intimate relationships and the expression of sexuality (Shuttleworth & Mona, 2002). Such research would go beyond a medical model focus on the sexual functioning of persons with spinal cord injuries (Baxter, 1978; Becker, 1978; Charlifue, Gerhart, Menter, Whiteneck, & Manley, 1992; Comarr, 1970; Griffith & Trieschmann, 1975; Leyson, 1979; Sipski, 1991; Tsuji, Nakajima, Morimoto, & Nounata, 1961; Yalla, 1982) and the psychological distress attendant on loss of certain sexual functions. Instead, sociopolitical issues such as constrained notions of beauty, attractiveness, suitability as a partner, and/or lack of services to assist with relationship development and sexual expression could be examined. Sexual relationships among PWD can depend upon the availability of assistance with communication, transportation to social meetings, PAS for activities of daily living (ADLs, e.g., eating, grooming), and access to relationships that support individual sexual and emotional intimacy. Because sexuality among PWD has been either ignored or examined primarily from the medical model perspective, our understanding of it as a psychosocial phenomenon subject to multiple influences is limited. In addition, assessment tools developed for use with nondisabled populations focus excessively on physiological aspects of sexuality, rendering them inappropriate for use with PWD. Societal attitudes of asexuality and the desexualizing of the disability community by these standards have had a great impact on the sexual self-beliefs of some people with disabilities. Further investigation is warranted (Mona, Gardos, & Brown, 1994; Mona et al., 2000).

Under the New Paradigm, research on traditional clinical topics such as the training of practitioners, the process of assessment, and the efficacy of therapy would incorporate the voices, needs, and experiences of PWD along with disability-specific models such as DAT. DAT as a treatment model aims to work toward goals common to the social experiences of people with disabilities. Research examining the interplay among psychological factors, presenting problems, environmental resources and constraints, support networks, social policies, and specific types of disabilities possessed by clients, along with issues such as therapeutic alliance and cultural competence of the therapist would be useful. This would include therapy process and outcome trials, as well as qualitative research with disabled individuals and trainees.

Finally, an area of relevance to quality of life and therapy research is the effect of dual minority status among ethnic minority PWDs. It is important to remember that the interpretation of the disability experience depends upon context but also on cultural values unrelated to disability per se. For example, moral and medical models of disability are employed by some cultural groups. To not accept these notions may be similar to denying one's heritage. Thus, Olkin's (1999) strategy is ideal in that it promotes discussion of and awareness of sociocultural notions but notes that interpretation of these constructs may vary depending upon the multiple identities that are held by all individuals. Quantitative measures aimed at measuring racial discrimination (see Utsey, 1998, for a review) could be reviewed and subsequently efforts made to develop instrumentation applicable to investigating the stressful effects of ableism on disability community members. When assessing levels of social alienation, which may vary by ethnocultural group and type of disability, it is imperative to understanding the social and environmental experiences of disability.

SUMMARY AND CONCLUSIONS

Psychology has been slow in embracing wider theoretical approaches to studying disability. However, given current trends in disability research funding suggested by the New Paradigm of Disability (NIDRR, 1999) and broader social models of disability (Olkin, 1999), behavioral sciences theorists and researchers have begun to examine shifting perspectives. This emerging paradigm shift is necessary to establishing new directions for research and practice. By embracing and applying the environmental, social, political, and cultural components of disability suggested by Olkin (1999) and NIDRR (1999), psychologists actually start to understand the breadth of the disability experience more accurately. The limitations of older, impairment-focused models are a failure to recognize the role of policy, laws, social institutions, and societal attitudes on well-being and intervention among PWDs. Along with eliciting a broader understanding of the experiences of this community, seeking a new disability research agenda in psychology provides the structure for deepening our understanding of the disability experience and begins to move toward forging stronger relationships with other disciplines studying disability (e.g., disability studies, medical anthropology, history, and sociology). With this unification, psychology's power as a behavioral science that researches disability can be improved along with increasing knowledge in clinical treatment adequacy and efficacy for the disability community.

QUESTIONS FOR DISCUSSION
AND/OR FURTHER STUDY

Service Domain

1. How do society, culture, politics, and history influence people's beliefs and views toward persons with disabilities? What models presented seemed to fit with society's perspective about persons with disabilities? How does each model expand or restrict conceptualizations of persons with disabilities?

2. Disability Affirmative Therapy (DAT) addresses factors that are associated with the complex and multilayered experience of disability. In what ways does this model take into account disability from a wide range of perspectives? How might this treatment model be applicable to other diverse individuals seeking psychotherapy?

3. How might society and culture influence the degree to which clinicians assist clients to move towards the six goals of DAT?

Research Domain

4. It often appears that research is driven by the power of culture and structured society. For example, research funding and interest on spinal cord injury (SCI) increased significantly when an actor with an SCI began advocating about the importance of this topic. What changes in cultural ideals and beliefs might it take to create a broader interest in other underrepresented research topics (e.g., sexuality, PAS) that affect the disability community?

5. Given the social constraints and environmental barriers faced by persons with disabilities, how might current research approaches and methodology prevent full participation of this community in research projects?

Policy Domain

6. How might the lack of funding for personal assistance services affect the quality of life of persons with disabilities? How might quality of life be different if there was a nationally based personal assistance program program that had sufficient funding and resources?

7. The degree to which people live fulfilling lives can be affected by how quality of life is defined within the context of chronic health issues and disability. How do current models of adjustment and adaptation to disability and chronic health problems address quality of life for persons with disabilities?

REFERENCES

Baxter, R. T. (1978). Sex counseling and the SCI patient. *Nursing, 78*(8), 46–52.

Becker, E. F. (1978). *Female sexuality following spinal cord injury.* Bloomington, IL: Cheever.

Bracken, M. B., Shepard, M. J., & Webb, S. B., Jr. (1981). Psychological response to acute spinal cord injury: An epidemiological study. *Paraplegia, 19,* 271–283.

Charlifue, S. W., Gerhart, K. A., Menter, R. R., Whiteneck, G. G., & Manley, M. S. (1992). Sexual issues of women with spinal cord injuries. *Paraplegia, 30,* 192–199.

Comarr, A. E. (1970). Sexual function among patients with spinal cord injury. *Urology International, 25,* 134–168.

DeJong, G. (1984). Independent living: From social movement to analytic paradigm. In R. P. Marinelli & A. E. Dell Orto (Eds.), *The psychological & social impact of physical disability.* New York: Springer Publishing Company.

De Kleijn-De Vrankrijker, M. W. (2003). The long way from the International Classification of Impairments, Disabilities, and Handicaps (ICIDH) to the International Classification of Functioning, Disability, and Health (ICF). *Disability and Rehabilitation, 25,* 561–564.

Derogatis, L. R. (1977). *Symptom Checklist-90R Administration, Scoring, and Procedures Manual.* Towson, MD: Clinical and Psychometric Research.

Dunn, M. (1977). Social discomfort in the patient with spinal cord injury. *Archives of Physical Medicine and Rehabilitation, 58,* 257–260.

Elliot, T. M. (1993). Training psychology graduate students in assessment for rehabilitation settings. In R. L. Glueckauf, L. B. Sechrest, G. R. Bond, & E. C. McDonel (Eds.), *Improving assessment in rehabilitation and health* (pp. 196–211). Newbury Park, CA: Sage.

Elliot, T. M., & Umlauf, R. L. (1995). Measurement of personality and psychopathology following acquired physical disability. In L. A. Cushman & M. J. Scherer (Eds.), *Psychological assessment in medical rehabilitation: Measurements and instruments in psychology* (pp. 325–358). Washington, DC: American Psychological Association.

Gill, C. J. (1995, July). *Disability and the responsive campus.* Paper presented at the national meeting of the Association on Higher Education and Disability, San Jose, CA.

Griffith, E. R., & Treischmann, R. B. (1975). Sexual functioning in women with spinal cord injury. *Archives of Physical and Medical Rehabilitation, 56,* 18–21.

Hathaway, S. R., & McKinley, J. C. (1989). *MMPI-2.* Minneapolis: University of Minnesota Press.

Hohmann, G. (1975). Psychological aspects of treatment and rehabilitation of the spinal cord injured person. *Clinical Orthopedics, 112,* 81–88.

Krause, J. S. (1991). Survival following spinal cord injury: A fifteen-year prospective study. *Rehabilitation Psychology, 36*(2), 89–98.

Krause, J. S., & Crewe, N. M. (1987). Prediction of long-term survival of persons with spinal cord injury: An 11-year prospective study. *Rehabilitation Psychology, 32,* 205–213.

Leyson, J.F.J. (1979). Counseling the female spinal cord injured patient. *Medical aspects of human sexual response, 13,* 59–60.

Macleod, A. D. (1988). Self-neglect of spinal cord injured patients. *Paraplegia, 26,* 340–349.

Millon, T. (1982). *Millon Clinical Multiaxial Inventory manual.* Minneapolis: Interpretive Scoring Systems.

Millon, T., Millon, C., & Davis, R. (1994). *Manual for the MCMI-III.* Minneapolis: NCS Assessments.

Mona, L. R., Gardos, P. S., & Brown, R. C. (1994). Sexual self-views of women with disabilities: The relationship among age-of-onset, nature of disability, and sexual self-esteem. *Sexuality and Disability, 12*(4), 261–277.

Mona, L. R., Krause, J. S., Norris, F. H., Cameron, R. C., Kalichman, S. C., & Lesondak, L. M. (2000). Sexual expression following spinal cord injury. *NeuroRehabilitation, 15*(2), 121–131.

National Institute on Disability and Rehabilitation Research. (1999). *NIDRR long-range plan.* Washington, DC: Office of Special Education and Rehabilitative Services.

Nagayama Hall, G. C., & Phung, A. H. (2001). Minnesota Multiphasic Personality Inventory and Millon Clinical Multiaxial Inventory. In L. A. Suzuki, J. G. Ponterotto, & P. J. Meller (Eds.), *Handbook of multicultural assessment: Clinical, psychological and educational applications* (2nd ed., pp. 309–330). San Francisco, CA: Wiley.

Nagi, S. Z. (1969). *Disability and rehabilitation: Legal, clinical, and self-concepts and measurement.* Columbus: Ohio State University Press.

Olkin, R. (1999). *What psychotherapists should know about disability.* New York: Guilford.

Olkin, R., & Pledger, C. (2003). Can disability studies and psychology join hands? *American Psychologist, 58*(4), 296–304.

Padilla, A. M. (2001). Issues in culturally appropriate assessment. In L. A. Suzuki, J. G. Ponterotto, & P. J. Meller (Eds.), *Handbook of multicultural assessment: Clinical, psychological and educational applications* (2nd ed., pp. 5–27). San Francisco, CA: Wiley.

Pledger, C. (2003). Discourse on disability and rehabilitation issues: Opportunities for psychology. *American Psychologist, 58*(4), 279–284.

Radloff, L. S. (1977). The CES-D Scale: A self-report depression scale for research in the general population. *Applied Psychological Measurement, 1,* 385–401.

Romano, M. (1976). Social skills training with the newly handicapped. *Archives of Physical Medicine and Rehabilitation, 57,* 302–303.

Shulz, R., & Decker, S. (1985). Long-term adjustment to physical disability: The role of social support, perceived control, and self-blame. *Journal of Personality and Social Psychology, 48,* 1162–1172.

Shuttleworth, R., & Mona, L. R. (2002). Disability and sexuality: Toward a focus on sexual access. *Disability Studies Quarterly, 22*(4), 2–3.

Siller, J. (1963). Reactions to physical disability. *Rehabilitation Counseling Bulletin, 7*(1), 12–16.

Sipski, M. L. (1991). Spinal cord injury: What is the effect on sexual response? *Journal of the American Paraplegia Society, 14*(2), 40–43.

Stewart, T. D. (1977). Coping behavior and the moratorium following spinal cord injury. *Paraplegia, 15,* 338–342.

Taylor, S. E. (1983). Adjustment to threatening events: A theory of cognitive adaptation. *American Psychologist, 38,* 1161–1173.

Taylor, S. E., & Aspinwall, L. G. (1996). Psychosocial aspects of chronic illness. In G. R. Vandenbos & P. T. Costa, Jr., (Eds.), *Psychosocial aspects of serious illness: Chronic conditions, fatal diseases, and clinical care* (pp. 7–60). Washington, DC: American Psychological Association.

Tsuji, I., Nakajima, S., Morimoto, J., & Nounata, Y. (1961). The sexual function in patients with spinal cord injury. *Urology International, 12,* 270–280.

Üstün, T. B., Chatterji, S., Bickenbach, J. E., Trotter, II, R. T., & Saxena, S. (2001). Disability and cultural variation: The ICIDH-2 cross-cultural applicability research study. In T. B. Üstün, S. Chatterji, J. E. Bickenbach, R. T. Trotter, II, R. Room, J. Rehm, & S. Saxena (Eds.), *Disability and culture: Universalism and diversity.* Seattle: Hogrefe & Huber Publishers.

Üstün, T. B., Chatterji, S., Bickenbach, J., Kostanjsek, N., & Schneider, M. (2003). The International Classification of Functioning, Disability, and Health: A new tool for understanding disability and health. *Disability and Rehabilitation, 25,* 565–571.

Utsey, S. O. (1998). Assessing the stressful effects of racism: A review of instrumentation. *Journal of Black Psychology, 24*(3), 269–288.

Utsey, S. O., Bolden, M. A., Brown, C. F., & Chae, M. H. (2001). Assessing quality of life in the context of culture. In L. A. Suzuki, J. G. Ponterotto, & P. J. Meller (Eds.), *Handbook of multicultural assessment: Clinical, psychological and educational applications* (2nd ed., pp. 191–212). San Francisco, CA: Wiley.

Wessen, A. F. (1965). Some conceptual issues in disability and rehabilitation. In M. B. Sussman (Ed.), *Sociology and rehabilitation.* Washington, DC: American Sociological Association.

World Health Organization. (1980). *International classification of impairments, disabilities, and handicaps* (rev. ed.). Geneva, Switzerland: Author.

World Institute on Disability. (1999). *Personal Assistance Services 101: Structure, utilization, and adequacy of existing PAS Programs.* Oakland, CA: Author.

Yalla, S. V. (1982). Sexual dysfunction in the paraplegic and quadriplegic. In A. H. Bennett (Ed.), *Management of male impotence* (pp. 182–191). Baltimore: Williams & Wilkins.

CHAPTER FIVE

Social Development and Adjustment of Children With Neurodevelopmental Conditions

Seth Warschausky

INTRODUCTION

Neurodevelopmental conditions place children at risk for truncated social development, limited social contact, and negative social experiences. Among children with cerebral palsy (CP), the leading cause of physical disability in children, research indicates risk for social rejection or neglect, in part associated with factors such as mental retardation, behavioral difficulties, and the social stigma of physical disability (Kokkonen, Suakkonen, Timonen, Selo, & Kinnunen, 1991; McDermott et al., 1996; Yude, Goodman, & McConachie, 1998). McDermott and colleagues (McDermott et al., 1996), in a rare population-based survey of the behavioral risks of children with CP, found high risk for peer difficulties. Studies have shown that children with CP have specific difficulty initiating social interactions (Dallas, Stevenson, & McGurk, 1993). Children with spina bifida reportedly have similar risk profiles, including a high rate of social isolation (Dorner, 1977; McAndrew, 1976, 1979).

Children with a history of traumatic brain injury (TBI) also are at significant social risk (Bohnert, Parker, & Warschausky, 1997; Yeates et al., 2004). Interestingly, when children and their parents independently rank the importance of life domains a year after surviving a TBI, children place friendships at the top of the hierarchy while parents put health and school functioning above their child's social adjustment (Bohnert et al., 1997). Regarding quality of life, the children's rankings probably are a more accurate reflection of the key issues in long-term outcomes following TBI.

It is difficult to compare social risks of children with congenital and acquired neurodevelopmental conditions, in part because there is tremendous heterogeneity in the cognitive and physical profiles within these sets of conditions. Those with congenital neurodevelopmental conditions, however, are more likely to exhibit physical impairments than those with TBI. Thus, stigma and access to activities may have a greater influence on the social development of this population. Among those with a history of TBI, age at onset is a critical predictor of outcomes, with greater neuropsychological and behavioral risks for those injured earlier in life. Surprisingly little is known, however, about specific risk for social maladjustment associated with age at onset. In what has been termed a "magnification phenomenon" (Woodhead & Murph, 1985), early impairments lead to a presumed negative developmental cascade in which the compromise of prerequisite skills adversely affects the development of higher level functions. For example, there have been specific discussions of potential cognitive precursors in infancy that foreshadow development of "Theory of Mind" (Baron-Cohen, 2000). At the behavioral level, early social play may be conceptualized, in part, as scaffolding for the development of mature social behavior (Bateson, 1976). To the extent that the young child's social play is restricted (e.g., by lack of access or stigmatization), social development could be truncated.

GENDER DIFFERENCES

Studies of typically developing (TD) children reveal gender differences in friendship characteristics (Maccoby, 1998). As gender identity emerges around age 3, children show preference for same-sex playmates (Maccoby & Jacklin, 1987). In the TD population, girls tend to exhibit more prosocial behavior and have fewer but stronger relationships (Eisenberg & Fabes, 1998; Schraf & Hertz-Lazarowitz, 2003). Boys value competition and independence in their friendships (Caldwell & Peplau, 1982). Given these gender differences in the TD population, it would not be surprising to find important gender differences in the peer relations of children with disabilities, yet surprisingly few studies with these populations have examined gender effects. In addition, there are intriguing findings that suggest that girls may be less vulnerable to certain types of brain injury or perinatal risk (Donders & Woodward, 2003; Hindmarsh, O'Callaghan, Mohay, & Rogers, 2000) leading to the possibility of less vulnerability to social impairments in girls with specific conditions. If indeed there is relative preservation of memory functions in girls with specific neurodevelopmental conditions (Donders & Woodward, 2003), it is conceivable that they would develop richer social schemata databases, leading to more flexible and effective social problem solving.

Bohnert et al. (1997) found interesting gender differences in a study of the friendships in 8- to 15-year-old children who were at least 10 months post-TBI. Whereas all of the girls with TBI reported that their best friendships predated the injury, only 29% of the boys had maintained their premorbid best friendships. Children with more recent injuries tended to have more opposite-sex friends, primarily reflecting greater numbers of girls in the boys' social networks. A critical consideration in the future study of gender effects on the peer relations of children with disabilities would be the interaction between gender and period of development, both from the standpoint of the child with a disability and those of peers.

SOCIAL INFORMATION PROCESSING

In the TD population, children's social information processing (SIP) predicts social behavior. Some of the most robust evidence has been in the associations between the tendency to generate aggressive solutions to social problems and actual aggressive behavior (Dodge, Laird, Lochman, & Zelli, 2002). There are an increasing number of studies that examine social cognition in children with neurodevelopmental conditions. These lines of research were stimulated by the increasing emphasis in SIP models on underlying neuropsychological factors such as processing speed, attention, and memory on SIP functions (Crick & Dodge, 1994). Investigators began to test hypotheses that the different components of SIP would be differentially affected by cognitive impairments.

In an initial study of the SIP profiles of children who had sustained TBI, we examined children's ability to generate a maximum number of responses to hypothetical social situations (Warschausky, Cohen, Parker, Levendosky, & Okun, 1997). Children ages 7–13 who had either a history of TBI, or were typically developing and were matched on multiple demographic factors, viewed pictures of problematic situations and scenarios that involved either peer-entry (e.g., joining a group of peers who were engaged in a game) or provocation (e.g., getting pushed out of line) (Dodge, Pettit, & Bates, 1994; Pettit, Dodge, & Brown, 1988). Solution types were coded as assertive, aggressive, passive, involving authority intervention, or irrelevant. The TBI group generated fewer total solutions and, specifically, fewer positive assertive solutions to peer-entry situations. The group differences in solutions to peer provocation situations were not significant.

In one of the first studies to examine the associations between SIP and social functioning, Janusz, Kirkwood, Yeates, and Taylor (2002) evaluated the developmental level of social problem-solving solutions and response evaluation. They demonstrated that children with histories of TBI tended to generate solutions at similar developmental levels to those of matched peers but selected lower developmental level responses as optimal solutions and that these lower-level response choices were associated with poorer social functioning.

When we compared the SIP skills of children who sustained TBI to those of children with congenital neurodevelopmental conditions, the groups exhibited similar profiles (Warschausky, Argento, & Hurvitz, 2003). Both groups generated a relatively low total number of solutions and fewer specifically to peer-entry situations. Perhaps of greater interest, findings suggested that the neuropsychological correlates of SIP solutions types differ by group. In both groups, level of intellect was associated with frequency of solution type, but aspects of executive functioning were more strongly associated with SIP in the congenital group. In particular, children who exhibited more perseverative errors on the Wisconsin Card Sorting Test (Heaton, Chelune, Talley, Kay, & Curtiss, 1993) generated fewer assertive social solutions. It is possible that there are differences in the salience of types of neuropsychological influences on development and manifestation of SIP skills.

In the most rigorous study to date of neuropsychological function and SIP as predictors of social functioning of children with neurodevelopmental conditions, Yeates and colleagues (2004) tested the hypothesis that SIP skills mediated the relations between neuropsychological status and global social outcomes in children with moderate to severe TBI. There was evidence that aspects of executive functions, pragmatic language, and social problem-solving predicted social functioning, but the results did not support the hypothesized mediational model. Similar to the findings of Warschausky and colleagues (2003), executive functions were not strong predictors of SIP in the TBI sample. Pragmatic language, however, was an important predictor, both of SIP and global social outcomes.

Dodge and colleagues (2002) have provided evidence of the validity of distinct SIP constructs including emotion understanding, intent attributions, social response generation, and response evaluation. In addition, they provide evidence of the situation specificity of SIP, though cross-situational attributional biases are noted, as well. Recent studies of SIP risks associated with neurodevelopmental conditions have drawn upon these types of theoretical and empirical developments, but there remains a lack of situational specificity in the study of SIP. As importantly, we continue to struggle to define exactly what we are trying to predict. The global social competence or adjustment scores obtained from screening instruments such as the Personality Inventory for Children–2 (Wirt, Lachar, Klinedinst, & Seat, 1990), Child Behavior Checklist (Achenbach, 1991), or Vineland Adaptive Behavior Scales (Sparrow, Balla, & Cicchetti, 1984) will not capture the situation specificity of children's social difficulties. To an extent, investigators appear to have approached the study of social risks in neurodevelopmental conditions backwards, with greater initial enthusiasm for predictors than for defining the nature of the problem itself. Largely, this stems from the tremendous growth in neuropsychological understandings of neurodevelopmental conditions, particularly TBI. Fortunately, there does appear to be an effort to put psychology back into neuropsychology, as once again neuropsychologists struggle with the lack of ecological validity of traditional assessment instruments. For example, ecologically valid measures of executive functions, such as the BRIEF (Gioia, Isquith, Guy, & Kenworthy, 2000) may be more highly correlated with aspects of social behavior than the Wisconsin Card Sorting Test (Heaton et al., 1993). That said, Taylor (2004) has argued that an instrument such as the BRIEF, with its high test construct verisimilitude (Gioia & Isquith, 2004), is itself a measure of behavior outcome rather than basic processing deficits, per se.

Consistent with this need for research that utilizes more proximal, ecologically valid predictors, some of the most promising and perhaps interesting lines of research on social outcomes have focused on semantic-pragmatic language and pragmatic communication. These studies largely examine the effects of TBI, with very few studies of children with congenital conditions (Simpson, Mohr, & Redman, 2000; Udwin & Yule, 1991). Dennis and colleagues (Dennis, Barnes, Wilkinson, & Humphreys, 1998; Dennis, Purvis, Barnes, Wilkinson, & Winner, 2001) have conducted a series of studies that demonstrate the effects of pediatric brain injury on nonliteral language comprehension. These studies have revealed impairments in comprehension of intentionality with preservation of literal language comprehension. Surprisingly, these deficits were noted in those who sustained mild and severe TBI. In related studies of pragmatic competence, Turkstra, McDonald, & DePompei (2001) have also shown difficulties with nonliteral language comprehension, including ability to detect sarcasm in adolescents who sustained TBI. Particularly in light of the recent Yeates (2004) evidence of the importance of pragmatic language in predicting social adjustment, as well as the relatively weak findings regarding associations of SIP with social outcomes in this population, further study of the predictive value of comprehension of intentionality and pragmatic communication is much needed.

STIGMATIZATION

Stigmatization typically is defined as overgeneralizing the influence of a perceived negative characteristic of a person. There is an extensive literature on the stigmatization of children with physical disabilities that largely focuses on the population with congenital conditions. This focus has largely been on TD children's social reactions to children with disabilities. There is some evidence that parents' reactions and concerns regarding stigma may adversely affect the amount of peer contact of their children with disabilities (Green, 2003). Limited research has focused on the effects of self-stigmatization in children with disabilities and very little research has examined the processes of stigmatization in persons who sustain TBI (Simpson, Mohr, & Redman, 2000; Stambrook, Moore, & Peters, 1990).

FAMILY CONTRIBUTIONS

Yeates and colleagues (2004) noted that while distal family factors such as global family functioning and resources moderate the process of recovery of social functioning of children who sustain TBI, there is substantial residual variance. At this point, there is a need to examine proximal factors such as parenting and direct efforts to facilitate social development. In the typically developing population, there are strong associations between parenting characteristics, including permissive and authoritative styles and child outcomes (Baumrind & Black, 1967; Querido, Warner, & Eyberg, 2002).

An intriguing set of findings in families of children with congenital neurodevelopmental conditions has shown complex family influences on the children's social functioning and specifically their risk for social passivity. Holmbeck, Coakley, Hommeyer, Shapera, and Westhoven (2002) found that children's verbal intellect mediated the greater passivity in family interactions noted in children with spina bifida. They also showed that the child's verbal intellect partially mediated the parental overprotectiveness (Holmbeck et al., 2002). This was particularly important because, among preadolescents, overprotectiveness was associated with lower levels of autonomous decision making. Clearly, this line of research is of tremendous value in increasing our understanding of the dynamics of specific social risks and suggesting important avenues for intervention. At this point, similar studies have not been conducted with families of children who sustained TBI. Taylor and colleagues (2001) in an elegant prospective study of parent and child psychological status after pediatric TBI showed bidirectional influences on behavior. This type of design may offer a productive model for the study of the bidirectional effects of parenting and children's social adjustment after TBI.

EFFICACY OF SOCIAL INTERVENTIONS

A 1999 review of empirical support for the efficacy of social interventions for children who sustained TBI concluded that while there was evidence to support targeted behavioral interventions, there was a paucity of studies that provided empirical support for social skills group interventions (Warschausky, Kewman, & Kay, 1999). In general, there is not a strong literature to support the use of social skills groups. In addition, most social intervention programs may be inappropriate for children with neurodevelopmental conditions because these interventions tend to either be designed for children with intact cognition or for those with significant cognitive impairment such as mental retardation, neither of which fits a significant portion of the population with neurodevelopmental conditions (Dixon & Warschausky, 2006). Meta-analysis of social skills intervention outcomes for typically developing children have shown that programs are moderately effective in improving outcomes such as social competence (Moote, Smyth, & Wodarski, 1999; Schneider, 1992). However, particularly for children with neurodevelopmental conditions, these intervention effects are not accompanied by maintenance and generalization of skills (Lloyd & Cuvo, 1994; Warschausky et al., 1999).

Given the concerns with generalization, there have been attempts to develop effective classroom-based interventions. There is some evidence that such interventions can affect typically developing peers' acceptance of children with disabilities (Favazza, Phillipsen, & Kumar, 2000). Programs that promote inclusion, including peer tutoring and teacher modeling, have been shown to be effective (Hunt, Alwell, Farron-Davis, & Goetz, 1996; Salisbury, Galluccu, Palombaro, & Peck, 1995). Apart from formal interventions, there is long-standing evidence that providing typically developing children with contact with and education about peers with disabilities or illness increases acceptance (Chekryn, Deegan, & Reid, 1986; Morgan, Bieberich, Walker, & Schwerdtfeger, 1998). The efficacy of these efforts has been demonstrated at the preschool level, highlighting the importance of promoting inclusive early intervention/preprimary impaired programs. A primary caution, however, is that inclusion is not integration; acceptance in interactions is not synonymous with reciprocity. Hunt and colleagues (1996) obtained success in increasing reciprocal interactions between children with and without interventions. There have been outcome studies of interventions that target the development of friendships, but initial gains typically are not maintained over time (Glang, Todis, Cooley, Wells, & Voss, 1997; Van Horn, Levine, & Curtis, 1992).

CONCLUSIONS AND FUTURE DIRECTIONS

There is long-standing interest in the social development and integration of children with neurodevelopmental conditions. The empirical research has included increasingly sophisticated examination of socioenvironmental influences, including seminal research on parent-child interactions (Holmbeck et al., 2003). However, neuropsychological influences on social development remain largely unexplored in this population. In part, this is related to the relative lack of focus on the neuropsychology of conditions such as cerebral palsy. The irony of traditional neuropsychological assessment instruments is that, typically, these instruments are not accessible to children with significant communicative or motoric impairments (Warschausky, 2006). In contrast, the literature on social outcomes for children with acquired conditions, such as TBI, has placed significant emphasis on neuropsychological factors and much less so on socioenvironmental influences. Regarding the study of neuropsychological influences, there is increasing interest in the use of ecologically valid measures and it is anticipated that this will lead to a refined model of the key predictors of social adjustment and integration in these populations, including the identification of critical functional skill mediators of outcomes.

There is tremendous heterogeneity in the status of children with congenital and acquired neurodevelopmental conditions. At this point, little is known about the differences in social risks of the two populations. Children with TBI who sustain injury early in life appear to be at greater neuropsychological and social risk than those with injuries later in childhood (Anderson et al., 1997; Ewing-Cobbs et al., 1997). Initial findings suggest that children with congenital and acquired conditions exhibit similar SIP profiles, though subtle differences are suggested (Warschausky et al., 2003). Little is known about the relative social developmental risks in these two populations, including how those risks change with age.

Much of the rigorous SIP and childhood social adjustment literature has focused on externalizing disorders such as aggression, or internalizing disorders including depression and anxiety. For children with neurodevelopmental conditions, however, there is a critical need for greater emphasis on studies of dependency and prosocial or assertive behavior. Unfortunately, the most common psychopathology screening instruments used in child assessments do not typically include dependency scales. Clearly, there have been important developments in our understanding of the social adjustment of children with neurodevelopmental conditions and we are at the stage in which there is an empirical basis to support multivariate prospective studies of social development. However, in what could be termed the neglect of passivity, there remains a need to address essential measurement gaps for these populations.

QUESTIONS FOR DISCUSSION AND/OR FURTHER STUDY

Service Domain

1. How should the magnification phenomenon be considered when rehabilitation interventions for children are designed?
2. Why is it important to assess pragmatic communication skills in children who sustain significant brain injury?
3. Describe family influences on the social development of children with spina bifida.
4. If you were developing a social skills intervention for children with neurodevelopmental conditions, what would be critical components of the intervention?

Research Domain

5. What is the evidence regarding gender differences in the social adjustment of children with disabilities?

Policy Domain

6. Considering the empirical literature on social development of children with neurodevelopmental conditions, what are the implications for policies regarding inclusion of children in regular classroom settings?

ACKNOWLEDGMENTS

Completion of this chapter was supported by U.S. Department of Education grants including an Office of Special Education Programs (OSEP) model demonstration project (H324M020077), a field-initiated project (H324C0020026), and an Office of Special Education and Rehabilitative Services (OSERS), National Institute on Disability and Rehabilitation Research, SCI Model Systems grant (H13300009).

REFERENCES

Achenbach, T. M. (1991). *Manual for the Child Behavior Checklist and 1991 Profile.* Burlington, VT: University Associates in Psychiatry.

Anderson, V. A., Morse, S. A., Klug, G., Catroppa, C., Haritou, F., Rosenfeld, J., et al. (1997). Predicting recovery from head injury in young children: A prospective analysis. *Journal of International Neuropsychological Society, 3,* 568–580.

Baron-Cohen, S. (2000). The cognitive neuroscience of autism: Evolutionary approaches. In M. S. Gazzaniga (Ed.), *The new cognitive neurosciences* (2nd ed., pp. 1249–1257). Cambridge, MA: The MIT Press.

Bateson, P. P. G. (1976). Rules and reciprocity in behavioural development. In P. P. G. Bateson & R. A. Hinde (Eds.), *Growing points in ethology* (pp. 401–421). Cambridge, UK: Cambridge University Press.

Baumrind, D., & Black, A. E. (1967). Socialization practices associated with dimensions of competence in preschool boys and girls. *Child: Care, Health and Development, 38,* 291–327.

Bohnert, A. M., Parker, J. G., & Warschausky, S. A. (1997). Friendship and social adjustment of children following a traumatic brain injury: An exploratory investigation. *Developmental Neuropsychology, 13*(4), 477–486.

Caldwell, M. A., & Peplau, L. A. (1982). Sex differences in same-sex friendship. *Sex Roles, 8,* 721–732.

Chekryn, J., Deegan, M., & Reid, J. (1986). Normalizing the return to school of the child with cancer. *Journal of the Association of Pediatric Oncology Nurses, 3,* 20–24, 34.

Crick, N. R., & Dodge, K. A. (1994). A review and reformulation of social information-processing mechanisms in children's social adjustment. *Psychological Bulletin, 115,* 74–101.

Dallas, E., Stevenson, J., & McGurk, H. (1993). Cerebral-palsied children's interactions with siblings. II. Interactional structure. *Journal of Child Psychology and Psychiatry, 34,* 649–671.

Dennis, M., Barnes, M. A., Wilkinson, M., & Humphreys, R. P. (1998). How children with head injury represent real and deceptive emotion in short narratives. *Brain and Language, 61,* 450–483.

Dennis, M., Purvis, K., Barnes, M. A., Wilkinson, M., & Winner, E. (2001). Understanding literal truth, ironic criticism and deceptive praise following childhood head injury. *Brain and Language, 78,* 1–16.

Dixon, P., & Warschausky, S. (2006). Social integration. In J. Farmer, J. Donders, & S. Warschausky (Eds.), *Neurodevelopmental disorders.* New York: Guilford.

Dodge, K. A., Laird, R., Lochman, J. E., & Zelli, A. (2002). Multidimensional latent- construct analysis of children's social information processing patterns: Correlations with aggressive behavior problems. *Psychological Assessment, 14*(1), 60–73.

Dodge, K. A., Pettit, G. S., & Bates, J. E. (1994). Socialization mediators of the relation between socioeconomic status and child conduct problems. *Child Development, 65,* 649–665.

Donders, J., & Woodward, H. R. (2003). Gender as a moderator of memory after traumatic brain injury in children. *Journal of Head Trauma Rehabilitation, 18,* 106–115.

Dorner, S. (1977). Sexual interest and activity in adolescents with spina bifida. *Journal of Child Psychology & Psychiatry & Allied Disciplines, 18*(3), 229–237.

Eisenberg, N., & Fabes, R. A. (1998). Prosocial development. In W. Damon & N. Eisenberg (Eds.), *Handbook of child psychology: Social, emotional and personality development* (5th ed., Vol. 3). New York, NY: John Wiley.

Ewing-Cobbs, L., Fletcher, J. M., Levin, H. S., Francis, D. J., Davidson, K., & Miner, M. E. (1997). Longitudinal neuropsychological outcome in infants and preschoolers with traumatic brain injury. *Journal of International Neuropsychological Society, 3,* 581–589.

Favazza, P. C., Phillipsen, L., & Kumar, P. (2000). Measuring and promoting acceptance of young children with disabilities. *Exceptional Children, 66*(4), 491–508.

Gioia, G. A., & Isquith, P. K. (2004). Ecological assessment of executive function in traumatic brain injury. *Developmental Neuropsychology, 25,* 135–158.

Gioia, G. A., Isquith, P. K., Guy, S. C., & Kenworthy, L. (2000). *The behavior rating of executive functions.* Odessa, FL: PAR.

Glang, A., Todis, B., Cooley, E., Wells, J., & Voss, J. (1997). Building social networks for children and adolescents with traumatic brain injury: A school based intervention. *Journal of Head Trauma Rehabilitation, 12*(2), 32–47.

Green, S. E. (2003). "What do you mean 'what's wrong with her?' Stigma and the lives of families of children with disabilities." *Social Science and Medicine, 57,* 1361–1374.

Heaton, R. K., Chelune, G. J., Talley, J. L., Kay, G. G., & Curtiss, G. (1993). *Wisconsin card sorting test manual: Revised and expanded.* Los Angeles, CA: Western Psychological Services.

Hindmarsh, G. J., O'Callaghan, M. J., Mohay, H. A., & Rogers, Y. M. (2000). Gender differences in cognitive abilities at 2 years in ELBW infants. *Early Human Development, 60,* 115–122.

Holmbeck, G. N., Coakley, R. M., Hommeyer, J. S., Shapera, W. E., & Westhoven, V. C. (2002). Observed and perceived dyadic and systemic functioning in families of preadolescents with spina bifida. *Journal of Pediatric Psychology, 27,* 177–189.

Holmbeck, G. N., Johnson, S. Z., Wills, K. E., McKernon, W., Rose, B., Erklin, S., et al. (2002). Observed and perceived parental overprotection in relation to psychosocial adjustment in preadolescents with a physical disability: The mediational role of behavioral autonomy. *Journal of Consulting and Clinical Psychology, 70,* 96–110.

Holmbeck, G. N., Westhoven, V. C., Phillips, W. S., Bowers, R., Gruse, C., Nikolopoulos, T., et al. (2003). A multimethod, multi-informant, and multidimensional perspective on psychosocial adjustment in preadolescents with spina bifida. *Journal of Consulting and Clinical Psychology, 71,* 782–796.

Hunt, P., Alwell, M., Farron-Davis, F., & Goetz, L. (1996). Creating socially supportive environments for fully included students who experience multiple disabilities. *Journal of the Association for Persons with Severe Handicaps, 21*(2), 53–71.

Janusz, J. A., Kirkwood, M. W., Yeates, K. O., & Taylor, H. G. (2002). Social problem-solving skills in children with traumatic brain injury: Long-term outcomes and prediction of social competence. *Child Neuropsychology, 8*(3), 170–194.

Kokkonen, J., Suakkonen, A. L., Timonen, E., Selo, W., & Kinnunen, P. (1991). Social outcomes of handicapped children as adults. *Developmental Medicine and Child Neurology, 33,* 1095–1100.

Lloyd, L. F., & Cuvo, A. J. (1994). Maintenance and generalization of behaviours after treatment of persons with traumatic brain injury. *Brain Injury, 8,* 529–540.

Maccoby, E. E. (1998). *The two sexes: Growing up apart, coming together.* Cambridge, MA: Belknap Press/Harvard University Press.

Maccoby, E. E., & Jacklin, C. N. (1987). Gender segregation in childhood. In H. W. Reese (Ed.), *Advances in child development and behavior* (Vol. 20, pp. 239–287). San Diego, CA: Academic Press, Inc.

McAndrew, I. (1976). Children with a handicap and their families. *Child Care, Health, and Development, 2*(4), 213–237.

McAndrew, I. (1979). Adolescents and young people with spina bifida. *Developmental Medicine and Child Neurology, 21,* 619–621.

McDermott, S., Coker, A., Mani, S., Krishnaswami, S., Nagle, R., Barnett-Queen, L., et al. (1996). A population-based analysis of behavior problems in children with cerebral palsy. *Journal of Pediatric Psychology, 21*(3), 447–463.

Moote, G. T., Smyth, N. J., & Wodarski, J. S. (1999). Special skills training with youth in school settings: A review. *Research on Social Work Practice, 9*(4), 427–465.

Morgan, S. B., Bieberich, A. A., Walker, M., & Schwerdtfeger, H. (1998). Children's willingness to share activities with a physically handicapped peer: Am I more willing than my classmate? *Journal of Pediatric Psychology, 23*(6), 367–375.

Pettit, G. S., Dodge, K. A., & Brown, M. M. (1988). Early family experience, social problem-solving patterns, and children's social competence. *Child Development, 59,* 107–120.

Querido, J. G., Warner, T. D., & Eyberg, S. M. (2002). Parenting styles and child behavior in African American families of preschool children. *Journal of Clinical Child and Adolescent Psychology, 31*(2), 272–277.

Salisbury, C. L., Galluccu, C., Palombaro, M. M., & Peck, C. A. (1995). Strategies that promote social relations among elementary students with and without severe disabilities in inclusive schools. *Exceptional Children, 62*(2), 125–137.

Schneider, B. (1992). Didactic methods for enhancing children's peer relations: A quantitative review. *Clinical Psychology Review, 12,* 363–382.

Schraf, M., & Hertz-Lazarowitz, R. (2003). Social networks in the school context: Effects of culture and gender. *Journal of Social & Personal Relationships, 20,* 843–858.

Simpson, G., Mohr, R., & Redman, A. (2000). Cultural variations in the understanding of traumatic brain injury and brain injury rehabilitation. *Brain Injury, 14*(2), 125–140.

Sparrow, S. S., Balla, D. A., & Cicchetti, D. V. (1984). *Vineland Adaptive Behavior Scales: Interview edition.* American Guidance Service: Circle Pines, MN.

Stambrook, M., Moore, A., & Peters, L. (1990). Social behaviour and adjustment to moderate and severe traumatic brain injury: Comparison to normative and psychiatric samples. *Cognitive Rehabilitation, 8,* 26–30.

Taylor, H. G. (2004). Research on outcomes of pediatric traumatic brain injury. *Developmental Neuropsychology, 25,* 199–225.

Taylor, H. G., Yeates, K. O., Wade, S. L., Drotar, D., Stancin, T., & Burant, C. (2001). Bidirectional child-family influences on outcomes of traumatic brain injury in children. *Journal of the International Neuropsychological Society, 7*(6), 755–767.

Turkstra, L. S., McDonald, S., & DePompei, R. (2001). Social information processing in adolescents: Data from normally developing adolescents and preliminary data from their peers with traumatic brain injury. *Journal of Head Trauma Rehabilitation, 16*(5), 469–483.

Udwin, O., & Yule, W. (1991). Augmentative communication systems taught to cerebral-palsied children—a longitudinal study. II. Pragmatic features of sign and symbol use. *British Journal of Disorders of Communication, 26*(2), 137–148.

Van Horn, K. R., Levine, M. J., & Curtis, C. L. (1992). Developmental levels of social cognition in head injured patients. *Brain Injury, 6*(1), 15–28.

Warschausky, S., Argento, A. G., & Hurvitz, E.B.M. (2003). Neuropsychological status and social problem-solving in children with congenital or acquired brain dysfunction. *Rehabilitation Psychology, 48*(4), 250–254.

Warschausky, S., Cohen, E., Parker, J. G., Levendosky, A., & Okun, A. (1997). Social problem solving skills of children with traumatic brain injury. *Pediatric Rehabilitation, 1*(2), 77–81.

Warschausky, S., Kewman, D., & Kay, J. (1999). Empirically supported psychological and behavioral therapies in pediatric rehabilitation of TBI. *Journal of Head Trauma Rehabilitation, 14*(4), 373–383.

Warschausky S. (2006). Physical impairments and disability. In J. Farmer, J. Donders, & S. Warschausky (Eds.), *Neurodevelopmental disabilities: Clinical research and practice* (pp. 81–97). New York: Guilford Press.

Wirt, R. D., Lachar, D., Klinedinst, J. K., & Seat, P. D. (1990). *Multidimensional description of child personality: A manual for the personality inventory for children.* Los Angeles, CA: Western Psychological Services.

Woodhead, J. C., & Murph, J. R. (1985). Influence of chronic illness and disability on adolescent sexual development. *Seminars in Adolescent Medicine, 1*(3), 171–176.

Yeates, K. O., Swift, E., Taylor, H. G., Wade, S. L., Drotar, D., Stancin, T., et al. (2004). Short- and long-term social outcomes following pediatric traumatic brain injury. *Journal of the International Neuropsychological Society, 10,* 412–426.

Yude, C., Goodman, R., & McConachie, H. (1998). Peer problems of children with hemiplegia in mainstream primary schools. *Journal of Child Psychology and Psychiatry, 39*(4), 533–541.

CHAPTER SIX

Psychosocial Aspects Related to Dual Diagnosis of Substance Use Disorder and Disability

Mary McAweeney
Martin Forchheimer
Dennis Moore
Denise Tate

The costs to society of substance abuse are staggering. In 1995, the national costs of alcohol and drug abuse were estimated to be $176 billion and $114 billion respectively (Rice, 1995), unemployment rates are higher among problem drinkers (Mullahy & Sinelar, 1996), and both men and women who are heavy drinkers are less likely to utilize basic preventative health care services (Kunz, 1997). Zucker and colleagues (1996) developed a risk aggregation model focusing on the development of alcohol abuse, dependence, and other drug involvement. The most salient risk factors included age, gender, education, socioeconomic status, marital status and a family history of the disease. Many of these factors are disproportionately common among persons with disabilities (DeVivo, Go, & Jackson, 2002; DiNitto & Webb, 1998; Moore & Li, 1998).

Estimates of the prevalence and incidence of substance use disorders (SUD), including both alcohol and other drugs, among persons with disabilities are difficult to determine. These estimates vary depending on data source, disability type, and definitions of *disability, substances, abuse,* and *dependence* (DiNitto & Webb, 1998; Kessler et al., 1996; Li & Moore, 1998, 2001; Moore & Li, 1994a; Substance Abuse and Mental Health Services Administration/Office of Applied Studies [SAMHSA/OAS], 2002). Regardless of the actual estimates of the occurrences, research has clearly shown that a *substantial* number of persons with disabilities experience SUD at some point in their lives (Groah, Goodall, Kreutzer, Sherron, & Wehman, 1990; Heinemann, Mamott, & Schnoll, 1990; Helwig & Holicky, 1994; Moore & Li, 1994b; Moore & Li, 1998; Tate, Forchheimer, Krause, Meade, & Bombardier, 2004). It has been estimated that as many as 5 to 10 million individuals have both a disability and co-occurring SUD (Ford, 2001; Mullahy & Sinelar, 1996; NAADD, 1999). In turn, most psychosocial domains in their lives including their health, well-being, community integration and employment are negatively affected by the abuse of substances (Brodwin, Tellez, & Brodwin, 2002; Marinelli & Dell Orto, 1999; Smart, 2001).

This chapter focuses on the psychosocial implications and/or consequences for persons with disabilities who have coexisting SUD. This dual diagnosis is often referred to as the "double negative" that is being socially stigmatized with both disability and SUD (Li & Moore, 2001; Moore & Siegal, 1989). We divide this chapter into five sections: (a) a summary of the past 25 years of research which has reported on the prevalence of SUD and disabilities; (b) an overview of the unique psychosocial issues facing persons with disabilities who have coexisting SUD; (c) an example of psychosocial issues encountered by a specific disability group, spinal cord injury (SCI), an incorporation of the alcohol and drug data collected by the Model Spinal Cord Injury Systems (MSCIS) project; (d) a discussion of the lessons learned at the Rehabilitation Research and Training Center on Drugs and Disability (RRTC), funded by the National Institute on Disability and Rehabilitation Research (NIDRR); and finally, (e) future directions for practice and research.

To clarify our terminology, when we discuss SUD we are including all psychoactive substances including alcohol, illicit drugs, and prescription medications. We include both abuse and dependence diagnoses when discussing SUD. We use the term alcohol use disorders (AUD) when referring to persons who have only alcohol dependence. We use the Americans with Disabilities Act (ADA, 1990) definition of disabilities. The ADA has a three-part definition of disability that is based on the definition under the Rehabilitation Act. Under the ADA, an individual with a disability is a person who has a physical or mental impairment that substantially limits one or more major life activities, has a record of such impairment or is regarded as having such impairment.

RESEARCH ON DISABILITY
AND SUD OVER THE LAST 25 YEARS

During the 1980s, there was an increasing awareness by the American pub-lic of the particular or unusual risks for abuse of substances by subgroups such as minorities and women (DiNitto & Webb, 1998; Moore, Greer, & Li, 1994). A benchmark for attention to the issues of SUD among persons with disabilities was the 1980 special issue of *Alcohol Health and Research World* (Hindman & Widem, 1980). In one of the first studies that quantified the rates for groups with physical disabilities, Greer, Roberts, and Jenkins (1990) found that the prevalence rates ranged from 62% for a sample of subjects with spinal cord injury (SCI) to 25% for subjects who were blind or severely mobility impaired and living in centers for independent living. Later in this chapter a review of the prevalence of persons with SCI and SUD will be presented.

Interest in the co-occurrence of mental illness and SUD has also surged in recent years (DiNitto & Webb, 1998). Using data from the Epidemiologic Catchment Area (ECA) study, Regier and colleagues (1990) reported that among those with a lifetime mental disorder, 22% also had a diagnosis of alcohol abuse or dependence and 15% had drug abuse or dependence. In 1996, Kessler and colleagues (1996) identified even higher rates with the National Comorbidity Survey. Over 50% of persons with a lifetime SUD also had a lifetime mental disorder.

Rates of SUD vary for different disability groups (Moore, Greer & Li, 1994) and different types of onsets or etiologies. Moore and col-leagues (1994) surveyed eight different disability categories: (a) quad-riplegia, (b) visual impairments or blindness, (c) arthritis, (d) hearing impairment or deafness, (e) learning disability, (f) traumatic brain injury (TBI), (g) mental illness, and (h) cerebral palsy. Those with quadriplegia reported the highest incidence for prescription medication use, current alcohol and cannabis use. Those with mental illness reported the high-est use of cigarette smoking. As Moore and colleagues (1994) pointed out, the lowest incidence of prescribed medication was by people with hearing impairment, and respondents with cerebral palsy reported the lowest alcohol and tobacco use. The findings suggest patterns of alcohol and other drug use appear to vary widely by disability type. People who experience a later onset or traumatic origin represent the heaviest users in most cases (Moore et al., 1994). The disabilities of quadriplegia, trau-matic brain injury, and mental illness had significantly higher alcohol abuse scores than did the other groups.

Further, Moore and colleagues (1994) found that people experienc-ing onset after 19 years of age had significantly more symptoms of alcohol abuse than did people who had a congenital or early childhood disability onset. Kolakowsky-Hayner and colleagues. (1999) and others (Heinemann & Hawkins, 1995; Heinemann, Keen, Donahue, & Schnoll, 1988) reported similar findings in the TBI and SCI fields. Heinemann and his colleagues speculated that "premorbid" lifestyles including alcohol abuse may have contributed to the onset of their disability. Other studies investigating illicit drug use at the time of the injury reported that over 30% of people admitted to hospitals with a diagnosis of SCI tested positively for illicit drugs (Kolakowsky-Hayner et al., 1999).

Another unique way of examining the prevalence of SUD among persons with disabilities is through the State-Federal Vocational Rehabilitation (VR) System. The Rehabilitation Research and Training Center on Drugs and Disability (RRTC) at Wright State University (WSU) reported that incidence of SUD among persons with disabilities within the VR system was greater than it was for the general population. Table 6.1 highlights the comparison between VR consumers and the general population (RRTC, 1999). As a group VR System consumers are dependent upon or abuse illicit drugs and illicit drugs coupled with alcohol at substantially higher rates than the general population. These estimates are supported directly by the results of several epidemiology studies reported recently by the RRTC on Drugs and Disability (Hollar & Moore, 2004; Moore & Weber, 2000; RRTC, 2002), which showed a similar pattern of comparative prevalence rates for alcohol and illicit drug use over the years 1995 to 2000.

Treatment settings also shed light on the co-occurrence of SUD and disabilities. It has been estimated that as many as 25% to 30% of the 1,600,000 persons served by the nation's SUD Treatment System have a co-occurring disability (Moore & Weber, 2000; SAMHSA, 1999). In other

TABLE 6.1   Comparative Rates of Substance Abuse/Dependence: Individuals Served by VR vs. General Population

VR consumers* (FY 2000 RSA 911 Database)	Type of substance	General population (National Household Survey, 2000)
13.9%	Either Alcohol or Illicit Drugs	6.5% (14.5 million)
2.1%	Both Alcohol and Illicit Drugs	0.9% (1.9 million)
7.0%	Illicit Drugs, but Not Alcohol	1.1% (2.4 million)
4.8%	Alcohol, but Not Illicit Drugs	4.6% (10.2 million)

*Percentage of persons who have SUD as primary or secondary diagnosis.

mental health settings similar estimates are reported (Mowbray et al., 1995; Mueser, Drake, & Miles, 1997; RRTC, 1999).

In spite of increased public awareness and published research, SUD among people with disabilities frequently goes unrecognized and the needs of those who need treatment are not met. There are a number of reasons for this problem. First, individuals with disabilities themselves are likely to deny, hide, or discount SUD in order to escape the "double negative" of being socially stigmatized with both disability and SUD (Li & Moore, 2001; Moore & Seigal, 1989). Additionally, poor self-concept and low self-esteem may keep a person with a disability from seeking help or from recognizing the potential for recovery. From the practical perspective, SUD is unrecognized when it goes untreated. Since most people with disabilities do not have the ability to pay for treatment and are unaware of the alternative options for having these treatments paid for, many simply do not seek treatment (SAMHSA, 1998). Finally, mental health professionals may overlook SUD with the misperception that "they are just self-medicating" (DiNitto & Webb, 1998).

PSYCHOSOCIAL ISSUES FACING PERSONS WITH DISABILITIES AND SUD

In this section, we present a broad overview of psychosocial issues and societal trends facing people with disabilities who have SUD. A common set of four bio-psychosocial domains affecting the lives of persons with disabilities include demographic, personal/psychological, medical/disability related, and environmental (Table 6.2) (Brodwin, Tellez, & Brodwin, 2002; Marinelli & Dell Orto, 1999; Smart, 2001). There are dynamic interrelationship among these domains: a change in one domain often influencing the others. For example, employment has been shown to influence self-esteem, which in turn affects acceptance of disability further reinforcing continuous employment (Drake, Becker, Bond, & Mueser, 2003; Mueser, Becker, & Wolfe, 2001). These results underscore the potential benefits of employment for persons with disabilities who also have SUD. A supported employment intervention specific to this population will be discussed later in this chapter.

Frequently cited risk factors for substance abuse include adjustment to disability, onset of disability, chronic pain, recurring medical problems, isolation, attention difficulties, availability of prescription medications, societal entitlement to use, pervasive poverty, high unemployment, and the inaccessibility of appropriate drug education (DiNitto, & Webb, 1998; Ford, 2001; Moore, Greer, & Li, 1994; Moore & Polsgrove, 1991; RRTC, 1999).

TABLE 6.2 Bio-Psychosocial Domains

Demographic	Personal	Medical	Environmental
Age	Acceptance of Disability	Diagnosis	Social support
Race	Pre-disability self-concept	Prognosis	Accessibility of health care
Culture	Locus of control	Severity of impairment	Societal attitudes
Gender	Spirituality	Functional limitations	Societal myths
Education	Intelligence	Pain	Architectural barriers
Occupation	Adaptability	Visibility of the disability	Access to resources
Social class		Presence of multiple disabilities	Physical accessibility
		Duration of the disability	Discrimination

There is some question as to what the concept of "acceptance of disability" means, although there has been research on this topic spanning several decades. The classic definition of disability acceptance comes from Wright (1983), who defined it as a process by which a person comes to view his or her disability as nondevaluing. For several years, researchers from WSU, home to the Substance Abuse Resources and Disability Issues (SARDI) program, have investigated the relationship between acceptance of disability and substance use patterns. They measured disability acceptance utilizing an abbreviated version of the Acceptance of Disability Scale, which was developed by Linkowski (1971).

Results from the use of this scale have been consistent in studies both among vocational rehabilitation consumers and also among persons with disabilities who were attending SUD treatment. In both cases, lower acceptance of disability scores tends to correlate with higher substance abuse levels or more severe SUD diagnoses (Moore & Li, 1998; Li & Moore, 1998; RRTC, 1999). The cross- sectional nature of the studies conducted to date has not permitted conclusions to be drawn about the causal nature of this relationship (e.g., does lower acceptance of disability increase risk for SUD, does preexisting substance abuse increase the risk for low acceptance of one's disability, or do both co-vary with a third factor?). Regardless of which comes first, it is clear that the combination of having a disability with the addition of substance abuse, or with the label of having a SUD, can lead to what has been termed the "double negative" which in turn can perpetuate substance use (Li & Moore, 2001).

SUD has often been cited in the literature as a risk factor for the onset of disability. Higher rates of SUD may be differentiated by whether the substance abuse predates or follows the onset of disability (Kolakowsky-Hayner et al., 1999, 2002; Li & Moore, 1998). Persons with SUD are more likely to experience a disabling injury, particularly a traumatic injury where risk-taking behaviors can have a marked influence on incidence (Corrigan, Rust, & Lamb-Hart, 1995; Heinemann & Hawkins, 1995; Kolakowsky-Hayner et al., 1999; McKinley et al., 1999; Rice et al., 1989; Tate, 1993; Tate, Forchheimer, Krause, Meade, & Bombardier, 2004). Thus, preinjury alcohol and drug problems are important predictors of a SCI (Kolakowsky-Hayner et al., 1999, 2002). An example of the nature of the relationship between disability and onset (i.e., whether the substance abuse predates or follows the onset of disability) will be discussed in the following section.

SPINAL CORD INJURY AND SUD

While alcohol and substance consumption is frequently a problem in terms of traumatic injuries in general, its prevalence is especially high in the realm of SCI due to the demographic characteristics of the SCI population. While males incur over 78% of all SCI (NSCISC, 2004), they also consume 76% of all alcohol (Greenfield & Rogers, 1999) and have a three times higher prevalence of heavy drinking, defined as consuming five or more drinks on the same occasion at least five times during a 30-day period, than do females (SAMHSA/OAS, 2002). This link between SUD and SCI has often been reported in the literature (Heinemann & Hawkins, 1995; McKinley, Kolakowsky, & Kreutzer, 1999; Young, Rintala, Rossi, Hart, & Fuhrer, 1995) and it is commonly accepted that use of substances is a risk factor for SCI (Burke, Linden, Zhang, Maiste, & Shields, 2001; Tate, 1993).

The long-term health care costs for people with SCI are particularly dramatic. In 2004, estimated lifetime costs ranged from $600,000 to $2.7 million (NSCISC, 2004). People with SCI face many other costs including psychosocial challenges such as elevated rates of depression (Kennedy & Rogers, 2000), divorce (DeVivo, Hawkins, Richards, & Go, 1995) and high unemployment rates (Yerxa & Locker, 1990).

Tate and colleagues (2004) analyzed data from 16 Model Spinal Cord Injury Systems (MSCIS) which included the largest sample of participants with SCI across the United States. They identified persons with SCI at risk for SUD by describing their patterns of alcohol and substance use and abuse in relation to their individual characteristics and were able to identify how these patterns related to medical and psychosocial outcomes after SCI. They concluded that persons with SCI have special and unique alcohol- and substance-related issues (Tate et al., 2004).

The number of persons with SCI and coexisting SUD is higher than in the general population (Tate et al., 2004). Statistics for the general population released by NIAAA indicate that 7.41% of persons aged 18 years and older meet standard diagnostic criteria for alcohol abuse and dependence (NIAAA, 2000). In contrast, Tate and colleagues (2004) found that 17% of participants in the MSCIS database engaged in at-risk drinking behaviors based on the NIAAA criteria. Similarly, the rate found for alcohol abuse based on frequency of CAGE-positive responses is 14.2%. The CAGE (an acronym for cut down, annoyed, guilty, an eye opener) is recognized as among the most efficient and effective screening devices for alcohol abuse.

These elevated levels of at-risk drinking and alcohol abuse subsequent to SCI reflect the prevalence of similarly elevated levels of alcohol and drug use prior to injury. Estimates of substance use (alcohol included) at the time of SCI injury range from 17% to 62% (Heinemann, Mamott, & Schnoll, 1990; McKinley, Kolakowsky, & Kreutzer, 1999; O'Donnell, Cooper, Gessner, Shehan, & Ashley, 1981). Heinemann and colleagues (1990) reported that alcohol use prevalence was 90% for 18- to 25-year-olds and 60% for those older than 25 years. In a study of 103 recently injured persons with SCI, Heinemann examined exposure to and recent use of 10 types of substances and compared this to the prevalence in the general population. Marijuana was used by 51% of younger subjects and by 30% of older ones. General conclusion was that the SCI sample reported greater use of all substances except inhalants (Heinemann & Hawkins, 1995). These studies suggest that preinjury alcohol and drug consumption are linked to use post-SCI. This has been confirmed by numerous studies (Elliot, Kurylo, Chen, & Hicken, 2002; Kolakowsky-Hayner et al., 1999, 2002) where as many as two-thirds of SCI persons have been found to return to drinking within 18 months.

The relationship between illicit drug and alcohol use and the incidence of SCI has been documented in numerous studies. Young and colleagues (1995) reported that more than 30% of persons admitted to hospitals with a diagnosis of SCI tested positive for illicit drugs. Moreover, it is accepted that there is a causal and not simply a correlational relationship between the use of alcohol and drugs and motor vehicle accidents leading to SCI. For example, Cushman and colleagues (1991) found that alcohol intoxication leads to a reduction in response time, leading to an increase in accidents. In addition, they found an association between both alcohol and drug use and the failure to wear seat belts.

What is less well appreciated is the extent to which SUD can be a result of SCI and its treatment. In a 1992 study, Heinemann and colleagues found that while 70% of subjects reported having experienced substance abuse, for 52% this occurred following their injuries. Additionally, abuse of prescribed medications was quite prevalent. A 1998 profile of medication usage among persons with SCI found that on average the population takes over eight medications from five therapeutic categories. Researchers concluded that level of medication usage is elevated beyond what is generally considered at risk for "medical misadventure" (Hope & Kailis, 1998).

In 1992 study Heinemann and colleagues found that abuse of prescription medication was significantly elevated among persons who were depressed and had not adjusted to their disabilities. Unfortunately, studies of SUD all too frequently discount the importance of misuse of prescribed medications. For SCI, a population with a predisposed vulnerability, due to both prior lifestyle and postinjury psychological vulnerabilities, this is especially imprudent.

Alcohol abuse has been cited as a barrier to effective rehabilitation. Research has shown that alcohol abuse is correlated with longer lengths of stays, poor rehabilitation outcomes, decreased life satisfaction, depression, anger, anxiety, and increased risk for seizures, pressure ulcers, urinary tract infections, and reinjury (Heinemann & Hawkins, 1995; Krause, Coker, Charlifue, & Whiteneck, 1999; McKinley, Kolakowsky, & Kreutzer, 1999; Tate, 1993). Furthermore, alcohol abuse has been associated with poor ratings of health and impaired self-care activities up to 18 months after the onset of disability (Bombardier & Rimmele, 1998; Tate, 1993). Tate and colleagues (2004) found that those having alcohol abuse problems and those who report being substance users reported worse outcomes after injury: worse pain, more pressure ulcers, and lower satisfaction with life.

Findings from the Tate and colleagues (2004) study confirm the myriad of psychosocial difficulties (e.g., behavioral, physiologic, environmental) associated with SCI and SUD and as a result the importance of having physicians, psychologists, and/or social workers discuss their substance and alcohol dependency issues with patients, during admission and initial evaluation assessments. Careful screening for dependency problems should be conducted in determination of the appropriate protocol for treatment of pain during rehabilitation, given the high potential for SUD with traditional pain medications. Follow-up assessments after discharge from the rehabilitation program are equally important to prevent the recurrence of dependency problems. The outpatient team must be informed about SUD issues, if they are to coordinate patient care that promotes healthy lifestyle behaviors in the community. Beyond these treatment issues, from a physiologic perspective as central nervous system depressants, both alcohol and substances may further negatively impact one's perception and self-report of his/her satisfaction with life.

LESSONS LEARNED FROM SARDI

Since 1990, Wright State University (WSU) has been home to the Substance Abuse Resources and Disability Issues (SARDI). The mission of SARDI is to improve the quality of life for persons with disabilities, especially those affected by substance abuse. This is accomplished through several services, including participatory action research, evaluation, training, and clinical intervention. Much of the research in SARDI has been supported through the National Institute on Disability and Rehabilitation Research (NIDRR) via Rehabilitation Research and Training Center (RRTC) awards. SARDI has conducted RRTC research for the past decade, and much of this research has focused on employment-related issues facing persons with disabilities and coexisting substance use disorders. Recently funded research projects in the RRTC on Substance Abuse, Disability, and Employment include the following:

1. *Development of a substance abuse screening instrument* to be developed primarily for state vocational rehabilitation programs that serve a total of over 500,000 persons with disabilities per year.
2. *Randomized clinical trial of Individualized Placement and Support (IPS),* a proven model for employing persons with severe mental illness, will be tested with persons with other disabilities. A randomized clinical trial (RCT), in concert with the TBI Network at Ohio State University (OSU), will test this model among persons with substance use disorders and traumatic brain injuries or other disabilities.
3. *Policy study of state vocational rehabilitation programs.* There is considerable state-to-state variation in the proportion of persons with substance abuse diagnoses served by vocational rehabilitation programs. This study will investigate policy and practices that contribute to this unusually large variation.
4. *Analysis of unsuccessful vocational rehabilitation closures.* Approximately one half billion dollars per year are expended by vocational rehabilitation programs on cases that are not successfully closed. A multistate study will investigate reasons for these unsuccessful closures, with the primary hypothesis being that

hidden substance abuse is a significant contributor to unsuccessful cases.

The SARDI program and its associated RRTC operate on the principle that providing direct clinical services is an important method for directly testing theories while being grounded in the reality of service delivery at the community level. This is an important method for bridging the gap between research and practice. To this end, SARDI operates the Consumer Advocacy Model (CAM), a community-based outpatient alcohol, drug, and mental health treatment service located in Dayton, Ohio, that was specifically established to assist people with coexisting disabilities.

Initially established on a model for addressing TBI and substance abuse at the TBI Network through Ohio State University (OSU), it has been expanded to serve persons with any disability or combination of disabilities. The program has been cofunded by the Centers for Disease Control (CDC), NIDRR, the Ohio Rehabilitation Services Commission (ORSC), the Ohio Department of Alcohol and Drug Addiction Services (ODADAS), and the Ohio Department of Mental Health. CAM was recognized by the Substance Abuse and Mental Health Services Administration (SAMHSA) as being a model program that provides exemplary methods for financing dual disorder service programs.

Over the past 10 years, research findings and clinical experiences have led SARDI researchers to the following observations:

PERSONS WITH DISABILITIES AND SUD RISK:

- In contrast with other sectors of our society at risk for SUD, persons with disabilities and their advocates have struggled with establishing a visible constituency with policy and law-makers regarding the SUD issue. Without this presence, it is difficult to adequately effect systems change to address prevention and treatment services (e.g., independent living centers, VR programs, and others have been slow to embrace this topic). The reasons for this include conflicts over whether SUD is a critical issue for persons with disabilities, as well as fear of stigma should this topic be publicized (McCarty, 2002).
- Persons with disabilities have a history of limited or inadequate access to health care services. A growing body of preliminary research and anecdotal evidence suggests that a significant proportion of persons with the most severe disabilities are either denied access to SUD treatment altogether, or when enrolled, treatment providers do not understand functional limitations of

disabilities and the associated need for accommodations (RRTC, 2002 Conference Proceedings).

- Psychosocial factors such as acceptance of disability and satisfaction with life are positively correlated with successful reductions in substance abuse; whereas, high sensation seeking and anger are inversely correlated with SUD (Li & Moore, 2001).
- National data indicate that youth in special education, by their senior year in high school, tend to use more illicit drugs and tobacco than nondisabled peers. This is in spite of age of drug use onset being a year or more later than for nondisabled peers. Very few resources exist to adequately address these risks, due in part due to the philosophy of integrating students into larger classrooms where they have less access to prevention messages (Hollar & Moore, 2004).

PERSONS WITH DISABILITIES AND SUD TREATMENT SERVICES:

- Engagement in treatment for persons with disabilities is more tenuous, and therefore it is more incumbent on treatment centers to be consumer friendly and less confrontational, at least during initial stages of treatment. A "treatment engagement" strategy that has been successful for persons with TBI is to provide gift certificates as an incentive to attend scheduled appointments. Unfortunately, this practice often is not permitted by state agencies (Corrigan, Bogner, Lamb-Hart, Heinemann, & Moore, 2005).
- A longer duration but lower intensity of treatment works best for many persons with coexisting conditions, due in part to daily stresses experienced by consumers and long-term needs for support (Moore & Lorber, 2004).
- The SUD treatment course may be more difficult and prognosis more guarded for persons with disabilities, as coexisting conditions increase the need for additional support services; however, some statewide data suggest that persons with coexisting disabilities, as a group, successfully complete treatment at rates comparable to the general population (Moore & Weber, 2000).
- Case management can be a critical component of successful recovery from SUD for persons with disabilities (Heinemann, Corrigan, & Moore, 2004).
- A high percentage of persons who are identified as having a physical or mental disability in SUD treatment exhibit considerable problems with cognition and memory. This may be the most common functional limitation of consumers who require

accommodations (Allen, Moore, & Sample, 1999; Doninger et al., 2003; Moore & Allen, 2004).

- Successful treatment takes time and repeated contacts in many cases. Personal satisfaction with life and "acceptance of two disabilities" appear to be positively correlated with recovery, while ratings of anger and thrill-seeking tolerance are negatively correlated with recovery (Moore & Li, 1998; RRTC, 2002).
- It may be necessary to establish Medicaid and other programmatic waivers at the state level in order to successfully provide treatment to persons with more severe coexisting conditions that involve SUD (Moore & Lorber, 2004).

PERSONS WITH DISABILITIES AND EMPLOYMENT

The RRTC program at SARDI has had considerable focus on the VR system. Findings from the national RSA 911 VR Case Services Data indicate that persons with SUD and a coexisting disability have more difficulty achieving successful employment than persons with just SUD (Moore & Li, 1994b). For example, in 2001, the "successfully rehabilitated" (status code 26) rates for persons with a single disability of SUD was 33.2% and 35.9%, respectively (approximately 6% lower than the VR average for one disability). In addition, persons with a SUD and another non-SUD disability experienced successful employment rates of only 30.5% (approximately 9% lower than others with two non-SUD disabilities). Surprisingly, the highest rate of successful employment involving SUD was for those with both a primary and secondary condition of SUD (e.g., alcoholism plus drug addiction), with 39.8% of this group achieving successful employment (nearly the same rate as the mean for any two non-SUD disabilities) (Moore & Li, 1994b). Although the effect sizes for the cohort are "small" in the above comparison, the differences in these statistics translate into employment versus unsuccessful rehabilitation for many thousands of individuals across the country every year.

A target population of persons with SUD and a coexisting disability in the RRTC research program is consistent with another important area of inquiry—how to address employment services for persons with disabilities whose SUD is "hidden" from the rehabilitation system and employers. Findings indicate that nearly one quarter of consumers with SUD are not identified as such by VR (13.9% versus 23.5%) (RRTC, 2002). An earlier study employing two standardized SUD screening instruments found even higher rates (31%) of SUD at

VR intake (DiNitto & Schwab, 1993). Additional findings include the following:

- Practitioners in VR believe that the problematic use of alcohol and other drugs by people who apply for and receive services has a substantial impact on their ability to be effective in coordinating and delivering services that will result in a positive outcome, employment, and they want tools to help them overcome the barriers to success.

- Great variability exists in how providers of rehabilitation services identify and address SUD. Factors such as special ADA qualification language for alcoholism and drug addiction rehabilitation amendment act provisions on consumer choice VR practices, counselor attitudes, and lack of services or reimbursement for addressing SUD seem to cause this variability. The rehabilitation programs with the most proactive policies appear to have a history of either special arrangements with the SUD treatment system to share resources or personnel, or there is one person within the rehabilitation agency with a special interest in substance abuse who has championed the service needed (Moore & Weber, 2000).

- When compared to chronic and debilitating disabilities such as mental illness, SUD may have even a greater influence on the inability to work than the "primary" diagnosis of mental illness (Glenn, Ford, Moore, & Hollar, 2003).

- Although disabilities with traumatic etiologies appear to place persons at higher risk for SUD, persons with conditions such as multiple sclerosis appear to have higher than average rates of alcohol abuse (Bombardier et al., 2004).

- Approximately one in five consumers of VR services has a drunk driving arrest or has been referred to SUD treatment (Moore & Li, 1994).

- Persons of color and women have unique treatment needs and cultural perspectives that must be addressed to be effective when addressing SUD and coexisting disabilities (RRTC, 2002; Ford & Li, 1996).

FUTURE DIRECTIONS
FOR PRACTICE AND RESEARCH

This section focuses on treatment-related issues for persons with disabilities and suggests future research avenues. We provide an example of an innovative approach to employing persons with disabilities and co-occurring SUD through the novel intervention mentioned above: the Individualized Placement and Support (IPS) model.

A wide variety of alcohol and drug education and treatment programs has been developed and implemented in the United States. Their target audiences vary, including children who do not yet have significant personal drinking histories as well as those who are at risk and those with addiction problems. Similarly these programs differ in terms of their formats and the philosophies that guide them. The oldest, most well known and arguably most successful program is Alcoholics Anonymous (AA), developed in the late 1930s. AA's target audience is people with alcohol addiction. This 12-step program focuses on community, spirituality, and commitment to abstinence. Numerous studies have been done of AA's efficacy, and while randomized studies are difficult to conduct, the evidence has generally been favorable (Fiorentine & Hillhouse, 2000). AA's broad appeal and acceptance of others makes this an excellent treatment option for those with disabilities.

One noteworthy injury prevention program is entitled Think First. While not focused solely on alcohol, Think First aims at avoidance of behaviors that are associated with the onset of SCI and TBI, including driving under the influence, riding with drunk drivers, and not wearing seatbelts and bicycle helmets. Studies of the program suggest that the Think First program is effective in increasing knowledge of risk factors for SCI and TBI among both elementary school and high school aged children (Avolio, Ramsey, & Neuwelt, 1992; Gresham et al., 2001). The program's effects on behaviors and incidence of injury have not been determined.

Models Systems data from Tate and colleague's study (2004) indicated that motor vehicle crashes (MVCs) account for the highest percentage of injuries among nondrinkers and all types of drinkers. Among at-risk drinkers, MVCs accounted for 51.2% of the SCI cases. These results support those from other studies that report MVCs to be the main cause of SCI among at-risk drinkers. Among both at-risk drinkers and substance users, a disproportionately high number acquired their SCI in sports-related events. These findings suggest that in addition to driving safety programs, it is important that education programs be developed that can be used in both schools and work sites, focusing on prevention and safety for younger persons with sports interests.

One of the projects in the RRTC on Substance Abuse, Disability, and Employment is a RCT evaluating the principles of the IPS intervention, a form of supported employment established for persons with severe mental illness and persons with SUD who have coexisting disabilities. IPS is described by the Center for Mental Health Services

(CMHS/SAMHSA) as a scientifically supported practice for improving employment outcomes for persons with mental illness. It is being implemented at two innovative sites: the TBI Network, affiliated with the OSU College of Medicine and Public Health, and at CAM. The TBI Network serves an outpatient population of approximately 150 active consumers, all of who have TBI and SUD. The CAM program serves approximately 280 outpatient consumers with SUD and a coexisting disability (e.g., TBI, physical disability, mental illness, developmental disability, deafness).

The IPS model is predicated on the belief that work skills training prior to job placement is not efficient or effective for persons with more severe disabilities, but rather real work experience with domain- and job-specific support is the best method for connecting and maintaining these persons with jobs. The basic principles of IPS include: (a) Vocational rehabilitation is an integral part of mental health (including SUD) treatment; (b) The goal is competitive employment in work settings integrated into a community's economy, not segregated in sheltered work settings; (c) Consumers are expected to obtain jobs directly, rather than first engaging in lengthy pre-employment training; (d) VR services are continuous and based on work experience in the community; (e) Follow-along services from mental health providers are time un-limited, based on consumer need (i.e., services not restricted to 90 days post-employment as with state-based VR); and (f) The choice of work site and related services are based on consumer preference and choice.

The high prevalence and incidence rates of SUD among persons with disabilities and the costs to society require continued research in this area. Innovative interventions and in particular prevention programs to decrease risks for persons with disabilities are needed. Finally, bridging the gap between research and practice is of particular importance.

QUESTIONS FOR
DISCUSSION AND/OR FURTHER STUDY

Service Domain

1. What are the unique psychosocial issues facing persons with disabilities who have coexisting substance use disorders?
2. Describe the "double negative" and how you would address this as a practitioner.
3. Provide an example of how a bio-psychosocial domain, for example, demographic, personal/psychological, medical/disability related, or

environmental, might influence the functioning and well-being of a person with a disability and co-occurring substance use disorder.

Research Domain

4. Research suggests that persons with quadriplegia, traumatic brain injury, or mental illness have significantly higher alcohol abuse than did other disability groups. What are the factors that might account for higher rates in these three groups?

Policy Domain

5. There is considerable state-to-state variation in the proportion of persons with substance abuse diagnoses served by vocational rehabilitation (VR) programs. From a policy perspective, what can be done to develop a uniform system within VR to diagnose and serve persons with co-occurring disabilities?
6. A growing body of research suggests that persons with the most severe disabilities are either denied access to SUD treatment altogether, or when enrolled, treatment providers do not understand functional limitations or the need for accommodations. What SUD treatment program policies might contribute to this situation?

REFERENCES

Allen, J. B., Moore, D., & Sample, E. B. (1999). *Relationship between substance abuse severity indicators and cognitive performance in a dual-diagnosis population.* Meeting of the American Neuropsychiatric Association, New Orleans, LA.

American with Disabilities Act. (1990). Information and technical assistance on the American with Disabilities Act. Retrieved March 2006, updated Feb. 2006 from http://www.usdoj.gov/crt/ada/adahom1.htm

Avolio, A. E., Ramsey, F. L., & Neuwelt, E. A. (1992). Evaluation of a program to prevent head and spinal cord injuries: A comparison between middle school and high school. *Neurosurgery, 31*(3), 557–561.

Bombardier, C. H., & Rimmele, C. T. (1998). Alcohol use and readiness to change after spinal cord injury. *Archives of Physical Medicine & Rehabilitation, 79*(9), 1110–1115.

Brodwin, M. G., Tellez, F., & Brodwin, S. K. (2002). *Medical, psychosocial, and vocational aspects of disability* (2nd ed.). Athens, GA: Elliott & Fitzpatrick.

Burke, D. A., Linden, R. D., Zhang, Y. P., Maiste, A. C., & Shields, C. B. (2001). Incidence rates and populations at risk for spinal cord injury: A regional study. *Spinal Cord, 39*(5), 274–278.

Corrigan, J. D., Bogner, J., Lamb-Hart, G., Heinemann, A.W., & Moore, D. (2005). Increasing substance abuse treatment compliance for persons with traumatic brain injury. *Psychology of Addictive Behaviors, 19*(2), 131–139.

Corrigan, J. D., Rust, E., & Lamb-Hart, G. L. (1995). The nature and extent of substance abuse problems among persons with traumatic brain injuries. *Journal of Head Trauma Rehabilitation, 10*(3), 29–45.

Cushman, L. A., Good, R. G., & States, J. D. (1991). Characteristics of motor vehicle accidents resulting in spinal cord injury. *Accident Analysis and Prevention, 23*(6), 557–560.

DeVivo, M. J., Go, B. K., & Jackson, A. B. (2002). Overview of the national spinal cord injury statistical center database. *Journal of Spinal Cord Medicine, 25*, 335–338.

DeVivo, M. J., Hawkins, L. N., Richards, J. S. & Go, B. K. (1995). Outcomes of post-spinal cord injury marriages. *Archives of Physical Medicine & Rehabilitation, 76*(2), 130–138.

DiNitto, D. M., & Webb, D. K. (1998). Compounding the problem: Substance abuse and other disabilities. In C. A. McNeece & D. M. DiNitto (Eds.), *Chemical dependence: A systems approach* (2nd ed., pp. 347–390). Boston: Allyn and Bacon.

DiNitto, D. M., & Schwab, A. J. (1993). Screening for undetected substance abuse among vocational rehabilitation clients. *American Rehabilitation, 2*, 12–20.

Doninger, N. A., Heinemann, A. W., Bode, R. K., Sokol, K., Corrigan, J. D., & Moore, D. (2003). Predicting community integration following traumatic brain injury with health and cognitive status measures. *Rehabilitation Psychology, 48*(2), 67–76.

Drake, R., Becker, D. R., Bond, G. R., & Mueser, K. (2003). A process analysis of integrated and non-integrated approaches to supported employment. *Journal of Vocational Rehabilitation, 18*, 51–58.

Elliot, T. R., Kurylo, M., Chen, C., & Hicken, B. (2002). Alcohol abuse history and adjustment following spinal cord injury. *Rehabilitation Psychology; 47*, 278–290.

Fiorentine, R., & Hillhouse, M. P. (2000). Exploring the additive effects of drug misuse treatment and twelve-step involvement: Does twelve-step ideology matter? *Substance Use & Misuse, 35*(3), 367–397.

Ford, J. (2001). *The culture of disability.* (NAADD Report, 4(1), 3.) San Francisco, CA: National Association on Alcohol, Drugs and Disability.

Ford, J., & Li, L. (1996, March). *Factors related to illicit drug use by women with disabilities.* Paper presented at the meeting of the Women's Health Conference, American Psychological Association (APA). Washington, DC.

Glenn, M. K., Ford, J., Moore, D., & Hollar, D. (2003). Employment issues as related by individuals living with HIV or AIDS. *Journal of Rehabilitation, 69*(1), 30–36.

Greenfield, T. K., & Rogers, J. D. (1999). Who drinks most of the alcohol in the US? The policy implications. *Journal of Studies on Alcohol, 60*(1), 78–89.

Greer, B. G., Roberts, R., & Jenkins, W. M. (1990). Substance abuse among clients with other primary disabilities: Curricular implications for rehabilitation education. *Rehabilitation Education, 4*, 33–44.

Gresham, L. S., Zirkle, D. L., Tolchin, S., Jones, C., Maroufi, A., & Miranda, J. (2001). Partnering for injury prevention: Evaluation of a curriculum-based intervention program among elementary school children. *Journal of Pediatric Nursing, 16*(2), 79–87.

Groah, C., Goodall, P., Kreutzer, J., Sherron, P., & Wehman, P. H. (1990). Addressing substance abuse issues in the context of a supported employment program. *Cognitive Rehabilitation, 8*, 8–12.

Heinemann, A. W., Corrigan, J. D., & Moore, D. (2004). Case management for traumatic brain injury survivors with alcohol problems. *Rehabilitation Psychology, 49*(2), 156–166.

Heinemann, A. W., & Hawkins, D. A. (1995). Substance abuse and medical complications following spinal cord injury. *Rehabilitation Psychology, 40*, 125–140.

Heinemann, A. W., Keen, M., Donahue, R., & Schnoll, S. (1988). Alcohol use by persons with recent spinal cord injury. *Archives of Physical Medicine & Rehabilitation, 69*, 619–624.

Heinemann, A. W., Mamott, B. D., & Schnoll, S. (1990). Substance use by persons with recent spinal cord injuries. *Rehabilitation Psychology, 35*, 217–238.

Heinemann, A. W., McGraw, T. E., Brandt, M. J., Roth, E., & Dell'Oliver, C. (1992). Prescription medication misuse among persons with spinal cord injuries. *International Journal of the Addictions, 27*(3), 301–316.

Helwig, A. A., & Holicky, R. (1994). Substance abuse in persons with disabilities: Treatment considerations. *Journal of Counseling and Development, 72*(3), 227–233.

Hindman, M. H., & Widem, P. (1980). The multidisabled: Emerging response. *Alcohol Health & Research World, 5*(2), 5–10.

Hollar, D., & Moore, D. (2004). Relationship of substance use by students with disabilities to long-term educational, employment, and social outcomes. *Substance Use & Misuse, 39*(6), 931–962.

Hope, M. E., & Kailis, S. G. (1998). Medication usage in a spinal cord injured population. *Spinal Cord., 36*(3), 161–165.

Kennedy P., & Rogers, B. A. (2000). Anxiety and depression after spinal cord injury: A longitudinal analysis. *Archives of Physical Medicine & Rehabilitation, 81*(7), 932-937.

Kessler, R. C., Nelson, C. B., McGonagle, K. A., Edlund, M. J., Frank, R. G., & Leaf, P. J. (1996). The epidemiology of co-occurring addictive and mental disorders: Implications for prevention and service utilization. *American Journal of Orthopsychiatry, 66*, 17–31.

Kolakowsky-Hayner, S. A., Gourley, E. V., III, Kreutzer, J. S., Marwitz, J. H., Cifu, D. X., & Mckinley, W. O. (1999). Pre-injury substance abuse among persons with brain injury and persons with spinal cord injury. *Brain Injury, 13*(8), 571–581.

Kolakowsky-Hayner, S. A., Gourley, E. V., III, Kreutzer, J. S., Marwitz, J. H., Meade, M. A. & Cifu, D. X. (2002). Post-injury substance abuse among persons with brain injury and persons with spinal cord injury. *Brain Injury, 16*(7), 583–592.

Krause, J. S., Coker, J., Charlifue, S., & Whiteneck, G. G. (1999). Health behaviors among American Indians with spinal cord injury: Comparison with data from 1996 Behavioral Risk Factor Surveillance System. *Archives of Physical Medicine & Rehabilitation, 80*, 1435–1440.

Kunz, J. L. (1997). Alcohol use and reported visits to health professionals: An exploratory study. *Journal of Studies on Alcohol, 58*, 474–479.

Li, L., & Moore, D. (1998). Acceptance of disability and its correlates. *The Journal of Social Psychology, 138*(1), 13–25.

Li, L., & Moore, D. (2001). Disability and illicit drug use: An application of labeling theory. *Deviant Behavior: An Interdisciplinary Journal, 22*, 1–21.

Linkowski, D. C. (1971). A scale to measure acceptance of disability. *Rehabilitation Counseling Bulletin, 4*, 236-244.

Marinelli, R. P., & Dell Orto, A. (1999). *The psychological and social impact of disability* (4th ed.). New York: Springer Publishing Company.

McCarty, D. (2002). Assessing the sociopolitical environment for treatment, rehabilitation, and employment. In E. Wolkstein (Ed.), *Second National Conference on Substance Abuse and Coexisting Disabilities*. Dayton, OH: Wright State University RRTC on Drugs and Disability.

McKinley, W. O., Kolakowsky, S. A., & Kreutzer, J. S. (1999). Substance abuse violence and outcome after traumatic spinal cord injury. *Archives of Physical Medicine & Rehabilitation, 78*, 306–312.

Moore, D., & Allen, J. (2004). Effectiveness of cognitive skills training for dually diagnosed persons with mental illness. *ODMH Research Briefs 2003*. Columbus, OH: Ohio Department of Mental Health Services.

Moore, D., Greer, B. G., & Li, L. (1994). Alcohol and other substance use/abuse among people with disabilities. *Journal of Social Behavior & Personality, 9*(5), 369–382.

Moore, D., & Li, L. (1994a). Alcohol use and drinking-related consequences among consumers of disability services. *Rehabilitation Counseling Bulletin, 38*(2), 124–133.

Moore, D., & Li, L. (1994b). Substance use among applicants for vocational rehabilitation services. *Journal of Rehabilitation, 60*, 48–53.

Moore, D., & Li, L. (1998). Prevalence and risk factors of illicit drug use by people with disabilities. *The American Journal on Addictions, 7*(2), 93–102.

Moore, D., & Lorber, C. (2004). Clinical characteristics and staff training needs of two substance use disorder treatment programs specialized for persons with disabilities. *Journal of Teaching in the Addictions, 3*(1), 3–20.

Moore, D., & Polsgrove, L. (1991). Disabilities, developmental handicaps, and substance misuse: A review. *The International Journal of the Addictions, 26*(1), 65–90.

Moore, D., & Siegal, H. (1989). Double trouble: Alcohol and other drug use among orthopedically impaired college students. *Alcohol Health & Research World, 13*, 118–123.

Moore, D., & Weber, J. (2000, November). *An analysis of statewide substance use treatment episode data and persons with coexisting disabilities.* Paper presented at the meeting of the American Public Health Association Annual Conference, Boston, MA.

Mueser, K., Drake, R. E., & Miles, K. M. (1997). The course and treatment of substance use disorder in persons with severe mental illness. In L. S. Onken, J. D. Blaine, S. Genser, & A. M. Horton (Eds.), *Treatment of drug-dependent individuals with comorbid mental disorders* [NIDA Research Monograph 172]. Rockville, MD: National Institute on Drug Abuse.

Mueser, K. T., Becker, D. R., & Wolfe, R. (2001). Supported employment, job preference, job tenure and satisfaction. *Journal of Mental Health, 10*(4), 411–417.

Mullahy, J., & Sinelar, J. (1996). Employment, unemployment and problem drinking. *Journal of Health Economics, 4*, 409–434.

National Association on Alcohol, Drugs, and Disability (NAADD). (1999). *Access limited: Substance abuse services for people with disabilities: A national perspective.* San Mateo, CA: Author.

National Institute on Alcohol Abuse and Alcoholism. (2000). *10th Special report to the US Congress on alcohol and health: highlights from current research from the Secretary of Health and Human Services* (NIH Publication no. 00–1583l). Washington, (DC): US Department of Health and Human Services.

National Spinal Cord Injury Statistical Center (NSCISC). (2004). *Spinal cord injury facts and figures at a glance.* Retrieved March 2006, updated June 2005 from http://www.spinalcord.uab.edu/show.asp?durki=21446

O' Donnell, J. J., Cooper, J. E., Gessner, J. E., Shehan, I., & Ashley, J. (1981). Alcohol, drugs, and spinal cord injury. *Alcohol Health Research World, 82*, 27–29.

Regier, D. A., Farmer, M. E., Rae, D. S., Locke, B. Z., Keith, S. J., Judd, L. L., et al. (1990). Comorbidity of mental disorders with alcohol and other drug abuse. *Journal of the American Medical Association, 264*(19), 2511–2518.

Rice, D. P., MacKenzie, E. J., and associates (1989). *Cost of injury in the United States: A report to congress.* San Francisco, CA: Institute for Health & Aging, University of California and Injury Prevention Center, The Johns Hopkins University.

Rice, D. P. (1995). Economic costs of substance abuse. *Proceedings of the Association of American Physicians, 111*, 119–125.

Rehabilitation Research and Training Center. on Drugs and Disability (1998). Educational and health survey. In *Substance use disorder treatment for people with physical and cognitive disabilities: Treatment improvement protocol (TIP)*. Rockville, MD: Center for Substance Abuse Treatment (CSAT/SAMHSA) and the National Clearinghouse on Alcohol and Drug Information.

Rehabilitation Research and Training Center on Drugs & Disability. (2002). In E. Wolkstein, (Ed.), *Proceedings of the Second National Conference on Substance Abuse and Coexisting Disabilities: Facilitating Employment for a Hidden Population*. Dayton, OH: Wright State University.

Smart, J. (2001). *Disability, society, and the individual*. Gaithersburg, MD: Aspen.

Substance Abuse and Mental Health Services Administration (SAMHSA). (1998). *National admissions to substance abuse treatment services: The Treatment Episode Data Set (TEDS)* [1992B1996]. U.S. Department of Health and Human Services. Retrieved April 2005, from http://www.samhsa.gov/

Substance Abuse and Mental Health Services Administration (SAMHSA). (1999). *Substance abuse: People with disabilities at high risk* [TIP 29]. U.S. Department of Health and Human Services. Retrieved November 2005, from http://www.samhsa.gov/

Substance Abuse and Mental Health Services Administration/Office of Applied Studies (SAMHSA/OAS). (2002). *The NHSDA Report: Substance use, dependence or abuse among full-time workers*. Rockville, MD: U.S. Department of Health and Human Services. Retrieved November 2005, from http://www.samhsa.gov/

Tate, D. G. (1993). Alcohol use among spinal cord injured patients. *Archives of Physical Medicine & Rehabilitation, 72*, 192–199.

Tate, D. G., Forchheimer, M., Krause, J. S., Meade, M. A., & Bombardier, C. (2004). Patterns of alcohol use and abuse in persons with spinal cord injury: Risk factors and correlates. *Archives of Physical Medicine & Rehabilitation, 85*, 1837–1847.

Yerxa, E. J., & Locker, S. B. (1995). Quality of time use by adults with spinal cord injuries. *American Journal of Occupational Therapy, 44*(4), 318–326.

Young, M. E., Rintala, D. H., Rossi, C. D., Hart, K. A., & Fuhrer, M. J. (1995). Alcohol and marijuana use in a community-based sample of persons with spinal cord injury. *Archives of Physical Medicine & Rehabilitation, 76*(6), 525–532.

Wright, B. A. (1983). *Physical disability: A psychological approach* (2nd ed.). New York: Harper & Row.

Zucker, R. A., Bingham, C. R., Fitzgerald, H. E., Schulenberg, J. E., Wadsworth, K. N., Burchart, A. T., et al. (1996). Longitudinal research on alcohol problems: The flow of risk, problems, and disorder over time. *Alcoholism: Clinical and Experimental Research, 20*, 93A–95A.

SECTION III

Employment

INTRODUCTION TO
SECTION III: EMPLOYMENT

The barriers to employment for persons with disabilities (PWD) are substantial and complex. One need look no further than the approximately 70% unemployment rate for persons with significant disabilities to comprehend the gravity of the situation. This figure is a stark contrast with the goal of full participation among PWD as espoused by the World Health Organization, the Centers for Disease Control and Prevention (Healthy People 2010), persons with disabilities, rehabilitation psychologists, and others.

The barriers fall into a variety of domains, including laws and regulations, such as income limits for Medicaid eligibility. Physical/environmental barriers are prevalent and often easily recognized, such as lack of transportation infrastructure or inaccessible businesses. Employer-related barriers are often less visible, such as unwillingness to make work accommodations, or outright discrimination. Individual obstacles include body structure or function limitations, although these are rarely the primary barrier to work. Other individual barriers may not be noticed or recognized, such as depression or fatigue.

Conversely, there are a number of positive developments in employment for persons with disabilities, including policy changes, such as the Ticket to Work Act. There are also new models for helping persons with disabilities prepare to enter or reenter the workforce, such as "job clubs." Increasingly, interventions to promote employment target employers, communities, and policy makers and not solely consumers. The promise of these types of interventions is heightened with consumer participation in the identification of the barriers to be addressed and the specific interventions being developed. In the long run, only these types of integrated interventions will result in increased employment for this population.

In addition, empirical research is being implemented and considered in policy development, employer-based interventions, and consumer-based interventions. Much more research is needed, however, to bring forward consistently effective employment-related policies and interventions. In particular, public policy changes are rarely examined comprehensively or over an adequate time to effectively assess their effects on employment rates for persons with disabilities. Furthermore, as Bruyère and colleagues point out, the interplay between disability policy and private sector trends has not been fully considered.

The two comprehensive chapters addressing employment among persons with disabilities offer insight into new integrated models for promoting entry into the workforce, recent trends in the literature, and the gaps in knowledge, research, and policy that require additional attention.

Susanne Bruyère and her colleagues examine U.S. disability employment policy, identify gaps between present and needed knowledge, and suggest specific areas in which the best tools and perspectives of social science research can be brought to bear upon employment and disability policy issues. They note that disability employment policies affect not only people with disabilities and their families, but also those who provide employment or disability-related services. Policies are designed to affect society broadly by improving educational and work opportunities of Americans With Disabilities. They argue that policy analysis should integrate the skills and knowledge of psychologists and rehabilitation researchers with those of economists, lawyers, policy analysts, organizational behaviorists, program evaluation experts, computational modelers, and others. The authors review research that examines the effects of the Americans With Disabilities Act of 1990, Ticket to Work and Work Incentives Improvement Act, Workforce Investment Act of 1998, Individuals with Disabilities Education Act, and the Rehabilitation Act of 1973.

Christopher Wagner and his colleagues examine issues that are important to vocational rehabilitation consumers and providers. They evaluate employment services using a stages-of-change model in order to review the evidence base for early-stage practices, including outreach and marketing, assessment and career counseling, and development of employer partnerships; preparation-stage activities, including job-skills training and job-seeking training, job development, and placement; action-stages services, such as job coaching and supportive services; and maintenance services related to career stability and enhancement. They review the supported employment literature as a method that bridges various stages. They observe the benefits of community integration, employer partnerships, flexible and user-oriented services and practices, a career enhancement orientation, and services for individuals experiencing mid-career health impairments. They conclude that practices that support individualized employment in community workplaces facilitate positive outcomes. Needed is additional research that will refine our knowledge of supported practices and the best packaging of these practices for specific consumer groups and settings.

CHAPTER SEVEN

Employment and Disability Policy: Recommendations for a Social Sciences Research Agenda

Susanne M. Bruyère
William A. Erickson
Sara A. VanLooy
Elaina Sitaras Hirsch
Judith A. Cook
Jane Burke
Laura Farah
Michael Morris

PURPOSE AND OVERVIEW OF THE CHAPTER

The purpose of this chapter is to present research that has examined the impact and efficacy of U.S. employment and disability policy, identify the gaps between present and needed knowledge, and suggest specific areas in which the best tools and perspectives of social science research can be brought to bear upon employment and disability policy issues.[1]

Many different approaches could be used in this analysis. Disability employment policies affect not only people with disabilities and their families and employers, but also those who provide employment or

143

disability-related services. They are designed to affect society broadly by improving educational and work opportunities for the one in seven Americans who have some kind of disability. Their impact can be felt in many areas, and our research must cross disciplinary boundaries to focus on these different aspects. Analyses should integrate the skills and knowledge of psychologists, rehabilitation researchers, and clinicians with those of economists, lawyers, policy analysts, organizational behaviorists, program evaluation experts, computational modelers, and others. For example, Livermore, Stapleton, Nowak, Wittenburg, and Eiseman (2000) performed a comprehensive review from an economic perspective of existing policies and programs affecting the employment of people with disabilities.[2]

This chapter will provide an overview of research that has examined the effect of several major laws regarding employment and disability. To allow a more meaningful discussion, we limited our analysis to five pieces of legislation that we believe have major public policy implications. They are as follows: the Americans With Disabilities Act of 1990 (ADA), Ticket to Work and Work Incentives Improvement Act (TWWIIA), Workforce Investment Act of 1998 (WIA), Individuals with Disabilities Education Act (IDEA), and the Rehabilitation Act of 1973 (as amended).[3] For a broader discussion of the implications of other employment legislation for rehabilitation professional practice, see Bruyère and Brown (2003).

What follows is a summary of research to date on each law, including the type or focus of studies conducted, methods used, and preliminary findings. As would be expected given the wide scope of the selected legislation, we found a broad array of research approaches, including analyses of civil rights protections (nondiscrimination and equal access), analyses of the efficacy of various provisions for employment service delivery systems, economic research examining incentives to employment and the impact of health care access, and the impact of employer accommodations and other factors on the employment process choices of employers and individuals with disabilities. The overview of identified research is followed by a conclusion and recommendations for further research.

OVERVIEW OF RELATED RESEARCH

Americans With Disabilities Act of 1990

Title I of the Americans With Disabilities Act of 1990 (ADA) extended protections against discrimination in employment to people with disabilities.[4] The goal of the ADA employment provisions is to provide equal rights to people with disabilities, thus increasing their labor market opportunities. Title I prohibits job-related discrimination on the basis of disability, and requires that employers provide reasonable accommodations. Reasonable accommodation is a modification or adjustment to a job, the work environment, or the way things usually are done that enables a qualified individual with a disability to enjoy an equal employment opportunity. These regulations apply to private employers with at least 15 employees and are enforced by the Equal Employment Opportunity Commission (EEOC).

Research on the results of the ADA falls primarily into three categories: economic and employment studies examining the impact of the ADA, employer and reasonable accommodation research, and administrative record and ADA legal dispute studies.

Economic and Employment Studies

There have been a variety of economic studies performed to determine the efficacy of the ADA in raising employment rates and income for individuals with disabilities. Collignon (1997) suggests that the best economic indicators regarding employment and income would be total earnings, the percentage of people with disabilities with paid employment, the proportion who earn above the minimum wage, and the percentage of those below the poverty line. An early study by Blanck (1994) examined employment histories from 1990 to 1993 of adults with mental retardation. He found no change in the employment integration of this group over the early ADA period, but earned income levels increased, especially for the younger participants. However, he also noted that 90% of participants who were not employed or were employed in nonintegrated settings in 1990 remained in those settings in 1993—what he termed the "black hole effect."

Other research, however, suggests that the ADA has had an impact on changing employer behavior regarding accommodation, perhaps assisting in retention of workers with disabilities who are already in the workplace. Burkhauser, Butler, and Weathers (2001) examined the affect of employer accommodation and the ease of access and Social Security Disability Insurance (SSDI) benefit rates on the timing of SSDI applications following the onset of a disability. Retrospective data from the Health and Retirement Study (HRS) together with matching state level data on SSDI allowance rates and individual level Social Security administrative record data on the generosity of SSDI benefits was used. The results showed that employer accommodation significantly slows a worker's application for SSDI benefits, while easier access to and more generous SSDI benefits increase the speed of application following the onset of a health condition.

DeLeire (2000a, 2000b) analyzed Survey of Income and Program Participation (SIPP) panel data from 1984 through 1993. After adjusting for age, education, marital status, race/ethnicity, industry, and occupation, his results implied that the employment rates for men with disabilities fell 4.1% relative to men without disabilities following the enactment of the ADA. His analysis found that there was no relationship between the ADA and the relative wages of men with disabilities, as relative wages remained flat during the period from 1986 to 1995. He suggests that ADA mandates that resulted in increased costs to employers may have contributed to the decline in employment rates. A similar argument for a causal relationship between the ADA and unemployment of individuals with disabilities is made by Acemoglu and Angrist (1998). Their analysis of CPS data suggests that the ADA reduced the hiring of people with disabilities but did not affect separations. Schwochau and Blanck (2000) argue that both of these studies fail to take into account the characteristics of individuals classifying themselves as disabled and how this may translate into differences in employment patterns. They suggest that a combination of incentives and disincentives along with changes in the economy explains why the employment rate of people with disabilities appears to be declining.

Are these declines in employment rates actually due to the ADA or are there other possible explanations? Bound and Waidmann (2000) examined employment rates using data from the National Center for Health Statistics' National Health Interview Survey for the years 1969–1997, SSA information, and the number of individuals receiving SSDI. They concluded that the growth of the SSDI program that occurred over the same period as the implementation of the ADA could account for much of the decline in the relative employment of disablesd men and women. Burkhauser, Daly, Houtenville, and Nargis (2002) found a similar result in their analysis of CPS data. It was determined that the share of household income from SSDI or SSI received by the working age work-limited disability population dramatically increased and fully offset declines in their labor earnings as a share of income. Goodman and Waidman (2003) examined findings by Bound and Waidman (2000) and Autor and Duggan (2003) and concluded that SSDI expansions did lead to changes in employment rates. Burkhauser and Stapleton (2003) felt that the weight of evidence they examined favored the expansion of SSDI and SSI as the more likely cause for the undeniable declines in employment, but many questions remain to be answered.

Schumacher and Baldwin (2000) examined data from the 1990 and 1993 SIPP, controlling for job conditions. They found large wage differentials between male workers with and without disabilities, and also that workers with disabilities are more likely to make involuntary job changes, possibly because of employer prejudice or job mismatch, as two potential hypotheses. Baldwin and Johnson found evidence of discrimination against women (1995) and men (2000) with disabilities in their analysis of SIPP data.

Yelin (1997) examined employment trends for men and women with disabilities and concluded that women had experienced increases in employment, while men's rates dropped. His analysis also found that people with disabilities experienced disproportionate growth in part-time work.

Employer Research

Blanck (1991) performed a survey of 47 employers of various sizes after the passage of the ADA, but just prior to the implementation of the Title I employment provisions. He found the majority (68%) of employers surveyed were not aware of the ADA. In an early postimplementation survey of 618 employers in Georgia, Newman and Dinwoodie (1992) found that only 11% expected an increase in the number of individuals with disabilities in their workforce, while almost a quarter said the issue of hiring an employee with a disability never came up or they avoided hiring them. Clearly, further research on employer attitudes towards applicants and employees with disabilities is vital to better understand the response to the ADA (Walters & Baker, 1996).

A survey of human resource (HR) professionals in both private and federal sectors by Bruyère (2000) found that organizations have made significant efforts to make changes in attitudes toward persons with disabilities, but that this was reported as among the most difficult changes to make. In a review of recent literature regarding employer attitudes towards disabilities and the ADA, Hernandez, Keys, and Balcazar (2000) found that employers generally have expressed positive attitudes towards people with disabilities. However, they also found that employers tend to be less positive when more specific attitudes are assessed, and that the employment provisions of the ADA provoke misgivings. Several studies cited positive attitudes towards employees with disabilities who were placed by vocational, employment, and supported-employment programs. A small-scale study by Gerber (1992) examined employer ADA knowledge as it related to learning disabilities. Price and Gerber (2001), in duplicating this study, had more positive findings; however, most employers still had little awareness or knowledge of "hidden" disabilities. Most employers wanted employees with learning disabilities to self-disclose, but had little knowledge of how to accommodate them.

Drum (1998) interviewed key personnel in state governments and found that many saw a lack of representation of people with disabilities, and felt it was an unintended consequence of institutional HR processes.

Drum suggests that it is important to understand the beliefs and attitudes of public administrators towards people with disabilities because of their impact on employment.

Reasonable Accommodations and Employer Research

Earlier surveys of employers found most to be quite positive regarding the ADA, although some questioned if the responses were truly representative of actual behavior. The Global Strategy Group surveyed a random sample of 300 CEOs and HR managers in Fortune 500 companies for the President's Committee on Employment of People with Disabilities (PCEPD) (PCEPD, 1995a). They found that 73% of the top industries were hiring people with disabilities, and 54% of those who make hiring decisions for these companies said that the ADA had a positive impact on their corporations. A Harris poll conducted in 1995 for the National Organization on Disability found that 70% of 404 senior corporate executives support the ADA and almost 90% supported policies to increase the number of people with disabilities in their companies (PCEPD, 1996). Eighty-seven percent of employers who had hired persons with disabilities said they would encourage other companies to do likewise in a 1995 poll conducted by Mason-Dixon for the Florida Chamber of Commerce Foundation's Disability Awareness Project (PCEPD, 1995b).

Costs associated with accommodations commonly come up as a major concern (Harger, 1993; McKee, 1993; Roessler & Sumner, 1997). The Job Accommodation Network (1999) reports that the majority (71%) of accommodations cost less than $500. An earlier study that examined accommodations provided in response to the Rehabilitation Act of 1973 (Berkeley Planning Associates, 1982) reported that 81% of accommodations were less than $500. Blanck (1996) found that 99% of accommodations made by Sears Roebuck and Co. cost less than $1,000. Interestingly, despite the oft-repeated concerns regarding costs, a survey by Bruyère (2000) of over 800 private sector employers performed in 1998 found that 16% or fewer saw the cost of accommodations, training, and additional supervision as a barrier to employment or advancement for people with disabilities. Employer tax incentives, which reduce costs, were viewed as one of the least effective means of reducing barriers.

People with mental health disabilities have frequently been found to have received less accommodation. As Billitteri (1997) states, "many employers . . . have been more inclined to install wheelchair ramps and Braille elevator controls than to adjust for depression or obsessive-compulsive disorder" (p. 795). Scheid (1998) surveyed 117 randomly selected businesses regarding the ADA. Fifteen percent had specific policies for hiring those with mental disabilities and 38% had actually done so, although nearly 60% held what Scheid defined as "patronizing or potentially discriminating attitudes," and supported policies that focused responsibility on the mental health or rehabilitation community. In another employer survey, Bruyère (2000) found a lack of training for mental illness accommodations, although a majority expressed interest in more information regarding that topic. A study by MacDonald-Wilson, Rogers, Massaro, Lyass, and Crean (2002) of individuals in supported employment found that job coaches were vital to employment success, but the coaches needed additional training to provide effective accommodations for individuals with psychiatric disabilities. Jones (1997) examined legal issues related to limiting access to mental health care by insurance plans, particularly those provided by employers under the ADA and the Mental Health Act of 1996.

In a survey of 813 HR representatives of private employers, Bruyère (2000) found that the vast majority had made some accommodations in the employment process, and half reported proactively recruiting employees with disabilities. Most employers found it easy to accommodate, but they tended to be less familiar with accommodations for auditory and visual impairments.

Research by Bruyère and Erickson includes a survey of private employers on their awareness of Web accessibility issues in employment and HR processes. According to Bruyère and Erickson (2001), applications for employment, benefits, and staff training are increasingly becoming Web based, raising potential ADA concerns regarding their accessibility to users with disabilities. An evaluation of E-recruiting sites and job boards found that the majority were inaccessible to applicants with certain disabilities (Erickson, 2002). Many of the major accessibility issues encountered on these sites could have been corrected without significant difficulty for the Web designers.

Administrative Remedies and Legal Disputes

One of the greatest concerns of businesses regarding the ADA is its potential to result in expensive discrimination charges (Harger 1993; Litvan, 1994). However, Bruyère (2000) found that the majority of employers had not experienced discrimination claims. The most common claims were of wrongful discharge and failure to accommodate, experienced by 19% and 14% of private employers, respectively.

McMahon, Shaw, and Jaet (1995) analyzed the EEOC charges filed in the first calendar year of the ADA. Overall, 84% of complaints involved currently employed individuals, with the remaining 13.6% related to job acquisition. The majority of the charges (70%) involved matters of job retention. Reasonable accommodation accounted for only about 19% of charges. Individuals with a physical distinguishing disability (disfigurement, missing limb, etc.) and those with visual or hearing impairments were more likely to be involved in hiring discrimination, harassment, and promotion complaints, but least involved with discharge issues.

A study by Ullman, Johnson, Moss, and Burris (2001) examined the effects of the EEOC three-tiered charge policy, implemented in June 1995, on claimants with psychiatric disabilities. Charges with evidence suggesting a high probability of discrimination are classified as "category A" and fully investigated. The investigators found that category A cases had the highest total benefits rate and also that psychiatric illnesses were significantly less likely to be classified in the upper two tiers than other disabilities. Two major concerns are noted: that the EEOC has never validated the accuracy with which its staff assigned priority to cases, and the fact that psychiatric disabilities are frequently assigned the lowest priority, perhaps due to bias or lack of training on the part of the EEOC investigators.

Moss, Ullman, Starrett, Burris, and Johnsen (1999) examined the outcomes of the 145,794 ADA employment charges filed and closed by March 1998. They found that only 15.7% brought some sort of benefit to the charging parties and less than 2% resulted in new hires or reinstatements. The proportion of charges resulting in beneficial outcomes was also found to have decreased in recent years. Charges closed by local Fair Employment Practice Agencies (FEPA) were more likely to lead to some benefit (23.3%) than those closed by the EEOC (11.5%). However, in determinations resulting in monetary benefits, EEOC-handled charges received a median benefit of $5,646 compared to $2,400 for FEPA.

Moss and Johnsen (1997) examined the administrative complaint process within five EEOC offices. They found that many charges were given extensive investigation, but that there were numerous problems with the process, including understaffing, insufficient investigative time, and inadequate funds. In a more recent study, Moss, Burris, Ullman, Johnsen, and Swanson (2001) discovered major differences in outcomes depending on the investigating field office. They suggest that many problems were related to the lack of resources required to sufficiently pursue investigations, which they refer to as an "unfunded mandate."

Results in the courts suggest that the law is being interpreted quite narrowly. Lee (2001) analyzed 267 ADA lawsuits decided by federal appellate courts through July 1998, and determined that the plaintiffs won in only 4% of the cases, and the vast majority (89%) resulted in a summary judgment for the employer.

Lee (2001) and Diller (2000) note that much litigation has centered on whether the individual qualifies as disabled for ADA purposes, and that courts frequently find the plaintiffs are not covered under the ADA.

Feldblum (2000) and Hahn (2000) both discuss the definition of disability in extensive detail as it relates to the ADA and federal court decisions. Petrila and Brink (2001) point out that courts have increased the burden on individuals to prove disability, which can be particularly difficult for those with mental illness.

The National Council on Disability (2002) summarized Supreme Court decisions regarding the ADA in a recent paper. They state that "the Supreme Court has issued a number of decisions that have dramatically changed the way the ADA is interpreted, in most cases contrary to what Congress had intended" (p.1). The decisions of the court have been generally favorable to litigants with disabilities regarding the interpretation of the language of the ADA and what it covers, requires, and the scope of defenses produced. However, the results of cases concerning who can invoke the ADA's protection have been mixed—some decisions have taken an inclusive view, while others have been quite restrictive of the definition of disability under the ADA.

The ADA provides employment disability nondiscrimination protections, and represents one legislated approach to promote equitable access to the workplace for persons with disabilities. While employer attitudes towards people with disabilities appear to be a continuing problem, the cost of accommodation and the changes to employer policies and practices necessitated by the regulatory requirements of this law appear to be of much less concern to employers than originally thought. One of the foremost issues discussed regarding the impact of the ADA has been whether this civil rights legislation for people with disabilities has resulted in higher or lower rates of employment. While most agree that employment rates among people with disabilities fell in the 1990s, there is little agreement as to the reason.

TICKET TO WORK AND WORK INCENTIVES IMPROVEMENT ACT OF 1999

The Ticket to Work and Work Incentives Improvement Act (TWWIIA), signed into law on December 17, 1999, was passed to provide beneficiaries and recipients of Supplemental Security Income (SSI), Social Security Disability Insurance (SSDI), or both, the incentives and supports needed to prepare for, attach to, or advance in work.[5] The goals of TWWIIA are to reduce and remove certain barriers to employment for individuals who receive SSI and SSDI, and to encourage beneficiaries and recipients to access services and supports to assist them in pursuing employment. At the heart of the Act was a desire by Congress to increase options available to beneficiaries of the Social Security Administration's (SSA) disability programs, by expanding upon the existing network of service providers available and creating a more comprehensive set of supports for people with disabilities considering work.

The Ticket Program permits an individual to choose from an array of service providers (called Employment Networks or ENs), placing control over provider selection in the hands of the consumer. The EN can be a private organization or public agency that agrees to work with SSA to provide vocational rehabilitation, employment, and/or other support services to assist a SSA beneficiary/recipient to prepare for, attach to, and remain at work.

Title II of TWWIIA governs the provision of health care services to workers with disabilities, and attempts to reduce the disincentives to employment for people with disabilities posed by the threat of loss of health care benefits by encouraging states to improve access to Medicare and Medicaid. According to Cheek (2001), as of late 2001, approximately 28 states had adopted some type of Medicaid Buy-In for Employed Persons with Disabilities (MA-EPD). Cheek discusses and compares three different buy-in options, including one under the Balanced Budget Act (BBA) and two options under the Ticket Act designed to allow states to develop a Medicaid eligibility category targeted for employed persons with disabilities making more than the standard allowable limit.

Schecter (1997) examined Disability Insurance (DI) beneficiaries who returned to work. He found that most did so because of financial needs and did not attribute their return to work to an improvement in their health. Those who returned to work were more likely to be young and better educated. However, the work they returned to tended to be for fewer hours, lower pay, and required less exertion than their pre-DI employment.

Because the legislation was enacted in 1999, little research on its effects has been conducted to date. Efforts are now under way to evaluate various components of TWWIA. The most ambitious of these is SSA's effort to design, and eventually conduct, a comprehensive evaluation of the Ticket to Work component of the law. The draft design for this evaluation calls for a thorough review of implementation, an extensive analysis of participants, rigorous estimation of its effects on employment, earnings, program exits, and program costs, and investigation into other potential effects.[6] To the extent feasible, the evaluation will assess how other policies and programs (e.g., the Medicaid Buy-in) affect Ticket to Work (TTW) activities implementation. CMS has awarded Medicaid Infrastructure Grants to 38 states and has awarded Demonstration grants to 4 states.[7] Each of these grants has its own monitoring and evaluation plans and funding. Some effort is also allocated, via the grants, to state-to-state technical assistance. General Accountability Office (GAO) has recently produced a report on other countries' efforts to improve employment outcomes for people with disabilities and these efforts' relevance to TTW and other U.S. efforts.[8]

The implementation of the Ticket legislation also is tied to the Workforce Investment Act (WIA), in that Ticket recipients can use this benefit within the One Stop Career service structure created by WIA.

WORKFORCE INVESTMENT ACT OF 1998 (WIA)

The purpose of the Workforce Investment Act of 1998 (WIA)[9] is to consolidate workforce preparation and employment services into a unified system of support that is responsive to the needs of job seekers, employers, and communities. Under Title I of the Act, a framework is provided for the delivery of workforce investment activities at the state and local level that provides services in an effective and meaningful way to all customers, including those with disabilities.

WIA created a workforce development system that encourages and facilitates One-Stop service delivery; this employment and training system was intended to serve every job seeker through a central location that provides access to multiple programs. WIA and the Department of Labor's Employment and Training Administration stress the need for access when addressing the needs of people with disabilities and WIA mandates a partnership in the One-Stop system with Vocational Rehabilitation. What follows is a compilation of some of the research to date on issues affecting the involvement of persons with disabilities in WIA programs and activities.

The General Accounting Office (GAO) conducted a series of studies regarding early implementation challenges in 2001 (U.S. General Accounting Office, October 2001), and more recently has evaluated the need for improvements in performance measures (U.S. General Accounting Office, 2002a), and youth service strategies (U.S. General Accounting Office, 2002b). The GAO study of WIA performance measures was conducted between December 2000 and August 2001. In general, WIA's performance measurement system captures some useful information, but the lack of clear definitions of what and who is being tracked for many measures limits their usefulness in drawing conclusions about program success. Without clear definitions and processes, the measures will not provide Congress with a true picture of how well the programs are performing.

The study of youth service strategies was conducted between February 2001 and February 2002. GAO's findings recognized that WIA aims to fundamentally change the way services for at-risk youth are provided—but implementation challenges remain. Although neither GAO study focused specifically on youth or adults with disabilities, they both raise relevant questions about the need for further policy guidance and evaluation of key system components in its early stages of development.

The Rehabilitation Research and Training Center (RRTC) on Workforce Investment and Employment Policy for Persons with Disabilities[10] has conducted a series of studies that are more specifically directed at understanding issues affecting full access and effective and meaningful participation of job seekers with disabilities. Morris and Farah (February 2001) conducted a review of the WIA plans submitted by each of the 50 states and the District of Columbia. The purpose of the review was to establish a research baseline for evaluating state implementation efforts to provide participation of individuals with disabilities. Two policy documents were used as a framework: (1) *The Emerging Disability Policy Framework: A Guidepost for Analyzing Public Policy* (Silverstein, 2000a), and (2) *A Description of the Workforce Investment Act Legal Framework from a Disability Policy Perspective* (Silverstein, 2000b). The framework provides a structure that can be used to design, implement, and evaluate public policies and programs to ensure meaningful inclusion of people with disabilities in mainstream society.

In order to receive federal financial assistance under the Workforce Investment Act, a state must submit a state plan to the U.S. Department of Labor. The RRTC developed a template based on the Emerging Disability Policy Framework for analyzing each state plan to identify specific approaches, activities, policies, procedures, and strategies related to effective and meaningful participation by persons with disabilities in the system proposed. The general findings were that the plans vary significantly in their descriptions of policy goals, program design, interagency collaboration, and performance accountability. Individual plans were inconsistent in their attention to detail across the 14 areas analyzed. More than 80% of the state plans include persons with disabilities and/or representatives of public and private agencies, such as vocational rehabilitation programs that serve persons with disabilities, in the state plan development process. However, the majority of plans did not describe in detail the nature and scope of their involvement.

Storen, Dixon, and Funaro (2002) conducted a study to ascertain the accessibility status of One-Stop Centers and the ways that workforce development systems are serving people with disabilities. Working with The Heldrich Center, they surveyed One-Stop managers and operators throughout the country—a population familiar with day-to-day operations at One-Stops and policy discussions at the Workforce Investment Board (WIB) level. The survey asked the following: how partnerships between workforce development agencies and disability-specific agencies are working; whether people with disabilities are largely being referred to disability-specific organizations or included in general WIA services; if One-Stops are physically accessible; whether all information technology (IT) services available in One-Stops is accessible to people with disabilities; and if staff and administrators of One-Stop systems feel prepared to meet the needs of job seekers with disabilities.

The survey results showed that many One-Stops are relying heavily on their partners to create an effective system for job seekers with disabilities. Advocacy organizations for people with disabilities are a major provider of technical assistance, and 70% of respondents agree that Vocational Rehabilitation (VR) or other disability-specific organizations will handle most of the people with disabilities who enter the workforce development system. Of the respondents, 51% were very satisfied with their relationship with VR. All of these outcomes create a positive picture of One-Stop's interactions with those organizations that serve the disability community.

At the same time, fewer respondents indicated that outreach to people with disabilities is an important strategy for creating an effective One-Stop system, and 30% of respondents disagreed with the statement "my One-Stop has sought to serve people with disabilities by conducting specific outreach activities to attract customers with disabilities." Outreach to employers regarding hiring people with disabilities was also less important in the respondents' minds. A majority reported that they usually refer job seekers to disability-specific organizations when it is determined that the customer has a disability, though at least half also offer job seeker accessible and appropriate services in the general One-Stop system.

Furano and Dixon (2002) examined how the One-Stop system serves people with disabilities. Representatives of disability-specific organizations who are partners in their state or local One-Stop system were surveyed by phone. Major areas for improvement highlighted by this survey of disability-specific agencies were: performance management, accessibility, and outreach to job seekers and employers.

Accessibility is also a significant concern, particularly because the large majority of One-Stop managers and operators believed their centers were physically accessible and a significant number also indicated that they provide enough accessible virtual tools. Representatives from disability agencies believed this was an area that still needed improvement, and very few reported that their One-Stop system is completely accessible.

Elliott, Tashjian, Neenan, Levine, and Chewning (2002) assessed how early WIA implementation is affecting the Vocational Rehabilitation (VR) program at both the state and local levels.[11] In addition, Research Triangle Institute (RTI) has reviewed pertinent statutory, regulatory, and policy materials. Researchers interviewed key federal officials to obtain their perspectives on implementation of WIA and to refine the study's research questions. RTI also conducted site visits to a sample of states and local One-Stop centers in each state over the course of the study in order to conduct interviews with officials of state and local WIBs, state directors of VR, and other One-Stop and VR personnel, partners, and consumers.

Results from this RTI study indicate that most VR program representatives believed that closer coordination and collaboration among related workforce programs and services would probably result in a net benefit to present and potential VR consumers. Respondents indicated that the development of One-Stop systems at local levels had provided VR programs with enhanced entrée to programs and employers. The program has also benefited from increased exposure to additional service providers and resources. Although many thought it was too early to judge the effectiveness of WIA participation in enhancing employment and earnings outcomes for VR consumers, VR program personnel generally held high expectations in this regard. Many clearly indicated that enhancing these outcomes would be the ultimate test of WIA's effectiveness.

As discussed, one of the focuses of WIA is providing effective services to transitioning youth. The Individuals with Disabilities Education Act (IDEA) also addresses this important emphasis to support movement toward employment for youth with disabilities.

INDIVIDUALS WITH DISABILITIES EDUCATION ACT (IDEA)

Under the Individuals with Disabilities Education Act (IDEA), states are required to provide a free appropriate public education for students with disabilities at the elementary and secondary level (U.S. Department of Education, 2002).[12] In the 1999–2000 school year, 562,744 students ages 14–21 exited from special education programs in the United States (U.S. Department of Education, 2002, Table AD1). The number of special education students graduating with diplomas is 56.2% (U.S. Department of Education, 2002)—far below the 75% of their peers in regular education who receive diplomas (National Center for Education Statistics, 2000).

IDEA mandates that students with disabilities have an Individualized Education Program (IEP) that includes a statement of transition needs, and that schools provide transition services for students with disabilities age 16 and older. Hasazi, Furney, and DeStefano (1999), in a study of sites implementing these transition planning requirements, found that the federal mandate for transition planning and services has played a critical role in promoting promising transition practices. However, they found that interviewees (all of whom were transition service providers) believed that much more needed to be done and that "representative" (i.e., typical) sites faced challenges from lack of resources, funding, and pressures from educational reformers. Frank and Sitlington (2000) compared outcomes for students in the high school class of 1985 in Iowa with students in the class of 1993, one year after graduation. They found that the 1993 graduates had substantially better postschool outcomes in several areas. However, their unemployment rates and postsecondary education enrollment rates were still significantly lower than those of their nondisabled peers.

Three recent surveys of the literature on the transition from school to work for youth with disabilities are available: Kohler and Chapman (1999) conducted a comprehensive review of several qualitative and smaller-scale quantitative studies on specific practices and/or concepts that might influence a youth's transition. Harvey (2001) examined studies that attempted to assess the efficacy of vocational education for students with disabilities by examining employment as an outcome. Wittenburg and Maag (2002) summarized available empirical evidence on the transitional experience of youths with disabilities, limiting their review to studies that used large national or state databases, and focusing on economic and social outcomes, including employment, postsecondary education enrollment, and independent living.

Kohler and Chapman (1999) included 20 studies that met their criteria: studies pertaining to the transition from school to adult life, that focused on students with special needs, that were of topics related to transition practices, and that were research-oriented. They hoped to find examples of empirical research relevant to the topic of transition from school to adult life, focusing on studies published between 1990 and 1997, with particular emphasis on practices in five categories outlined by the National Transition Alliance (Kohler, 1996).

Twelve of the 20 studies examined addressed practices related to Student-Focused Planning and Development. Few of these established any strong relationship between interventions and outcomes. Seven of the 20 studies dealt with the practice of life skills instruction or social skills training. These studies generally suggested there is some evidence of the effectiveness of this type of training. One (Benz, Yovanoff, & Doren, 1997) found that high social skills were predictive of postschool employment. Six studies also looked at student self-awareness and self-advocacy training (Aune, 1991; Durlak, Rose, & Bursuck, 1994; Kohler, 1994; National Center for Disability Services, 1994; Posthill & Roffman, 1991; Wehmeyer & Lawrence, 1995). Aune (1991) found that a large majority of students who completed such a program expressed increased knowledge of services available to them, accommodations they would require, and how to request them. However, many surveyed students were reluctant to approach others to ask for accommodation. Studies that examined student participation in independent living skills training found that these skills did assist graduates in living independently (Posthill & Roffman, 1991), but high levels of these skills were not predictive of later employment (Benz et al., 1997).

While several studies examined the IEP process, only one (Benz et al., 1997) examined the relationship between specific interventions and outcomes. These researchers examined whether access to career planning and guidance, career awareness training, assigned work-based experience, and student/parent agreement about student's work and schooling goals would predict competitive employment and/or productive engagement. The results suggested that two or more work experiences during school were related to competitive employment and that career awareness was not predictive of competitive employment, although it was found to be predictive of productive engagement.

The 1990 IDEA amendments mandate student participation in the IEP and transition planning process. Kohler and Chapman found five studies that either referred to the planning process as "student-centered" or said that student involvement in decision making formed an integral component of the process (Aune, 1991; Gugerty, 1994; Kohler, 1994; Morgan & Hecht, 1990; Wehmeyer & Lawrence, 1995). Career counseling services were also explicitly provided to students in four studies (Aune, 1991; Benz et al., 1997; Kohler, 1994; Morgan & Hecht, 1990). Results from these studies again reflect more of an implied contribution from the package of intervention practices than a direct test of the effect of these practices.

On the topic of the practice of assessment, the majority of studies of assessments were conducted with students to examine vocational variables such as student interests, skills, values, and achievement (Aune, 1991; Kohler, 1994; Morgan & Hecht, 1990; Peters, Templeman, & Brostrom 1987), and/or learning needs (Wehmeyer & Lawrence, 1995). Unfortunately, while these practices are explicitly mentioned or referred to in the documents, a direct test of their effectiveness on transition outcomes was not made.

Overall, Kohler and Chapman found that most of the studies examined were notable for the lack of details provided about specific interventions and practices. Most of the analyzed studies did not take an empirical approach to establishing connections between a practice and specific outcomes. Instead they affirmed that a technique was or was not used, listed outcomes, and implied the outcomes were due to the interventions applied.

Harvey (2001) examined 15 studies of vocational education outcomes and found that 11 of the 15 reported that at least 60% of students with disabilities participated in vocational education while in high school. Wagner (1991) found that 65% of students with disabilities from the National Longitudinal Transition Survey (NLTS) had taken a vocational education course in their most recent year of high school.

The majority of studies in the Harvey review reported postschool employment rates for students with disabilities of 50% or higher (Harvey, 2001). Studies that compared employment rates for students with disabilities who had participated in vocational education with the rates for those who had not usually found higher levels of postschool employment for those who had participated. Hasazi, Johnson, Hasazi, Gordon, and Hull (1989) and Wagner (1991) reported levels of postschool employment 13% to 48% higher than those who did not take vocational education.

Conclusions about the efficacy of vocational education for students with disabilities were mixed, however. Harvey (2001) found that, of the studies examined, nearly half concluded that vocational education was a poor predictor of overall postschool employment and satisfaction. However, the Schlalock, Holl, Elliott, and Ross (1992) study indicated that hours in vocational programming was a positive predictor of more weeks employed, more hours worked per week, wages per hour, and annual salary. And Wagner (1991), who used NLTS data, concluded that secondary vocational education is an intervention that has the potential to improve academic performance while still in school and employment performance after leaving school.

Wittenburg and Maag (2002) found that the majority of research at the national level on the characteristics and outcomes of special education students relies on data from the NLTS.

Wagner, Blackorby, Cameto, Hebbeler, and Newman (1993b) included a variety of descriptive statistics on the basic demographic, work, and economic characteristics of special education students. The majority of special education students participated in competitive employment at some point (56%) and approximately one fourth enroll in postsecondary education. D'Amico (1991) examined competitive employment rates for students with disabilities. This study found that participation in vocational education during the last year of secondary school was associated with higher employment rates, and if the vocational education included work experience, students were more likely to be in competitive employment. Several other NLTS studies examined the complex factors that may influence postsecondary outcomes, particularly of subgroups with specific demographic and/or impairment characteristics (Blackorby, Hankock, & Siegel, 1993; Blackorby & Wagner, 1996; Heal & Rusch, 1995; Wagner, 1992; Wagner, Blackorby, Cameto, & Newman, 1993a).

A small number of other data collection efforts have gathered information on special education students at the state level. While these surveys are not as comprehensive as the NLTS, some provide more recent information on postschool outcomes.

A three-state study in Oregon, Nevada, and Arizona included a sample of special education students who were interviewed during their last year of high school and at a follow-up one year later. These data included a variety of specific measures, such as test scores, that were not readily available in other surveys. Several researchers used these data to examine postsecondary enrollment rates and employment success (Benz et al., 1997; Doren & Benz, 1998; Halpern, Yovanoff, Doren, & Benz, 1995). For example, Halpern and colleagues (1995) found several school-related factors, such as transition planning and satisfaction with instruction, outweighed the effect of demographic factors in predicting postsecondary education enrollment. Benz et al. (1997) found significant differences across men and women in postschool employment after controlling for several characteristics, including test scores and high social and job search skills.

A recent New York state survey in five cities (Buffalo, New York, Rochester, Syracuse, and Yonkers) included interviews with special education students one year after they completed high school in 1997. The New York State Education Department (1999) used this survey to determine the critical programmatic indicators, including transition planning, which may have contributed to student success. They found that former special education students who reported benefits from transition planning exhibited better academic and employment outcomes.

Wittenburg and Maag (2002) found that the existing papers from the NLTS and state surveys illustrate that a number of factors influence postschool outcomes, including individual characteristics, family characteristics, education/rehabilitation characteristics, and work characteristics. However, it is not possible to disentangle the precise effect of specific individual factors on outcomes. In addition, it is difficult to determine whether key outcomes or factors vary significantly because of differences in sample selections and data definitions used in each study.

As did Kohler and Chapman (1999), Wittenburg and Maag (2002) found little research that attempted to assess the impact of specific approaches and interventions. They also found that with a few exceptions, most available studies do not provide information on recent outcomes. This limitation is particularly important given that several recent policy changes may substantially affect transition decisions of youth with disabilities.

Further research on the efficacy of service delivery to youth with disabilities is discussed below, as a part of the analysis of the Rehabilitation Act's provisions that relate to state vocational rehabilitation services.

REHABILITATION ACT OF 1973 (AS AMENDED)

The Congressional intent for the Rehabilitation Act of 1973 (Public Law 93–112) was to develop and implement, through research, training, services, and the guarantee of equal opportunity, comprehensive and coordinated programs of vocational rehabilitation and independent living for individuals with disabilities in order to maximize their employability, independence, and integration into the workplace and the community.

The standards for determining employment discrimination under the Rehabilitation Act are the same as those used in Title I of the Americans With Disabilities Act. The following are the four sections that govern employment nondiscrimination and affirmative action included in Title V of the Rehabilitation Act.

- Section 501 requires affirmative action and nondiscrimination in employment by federal agencies of the executive branch.[13]
- Section 503 requires affirmative action and prohibits employment discrimination by federal government contractors and subcontractors with contracts of more than $10,000.[14]
- Section 504 of the Rehabilitation Act prohibits discrimination on the basis of disability in programs and activities, public and private, that receive federal financial assistance or under any program or activity conducted by any Executive agency or by the United States Postal Service.[15]
- Section 508 requires federal electronic and information technology to be accessible to people with disabilities, including employees and members of the public.
- Title 3 provides funding for the construction and staffing of rehabilitation centers and facilities that are designed to provide a variety of services, including vocational rehabilitation, to individuals with disabilities.

What follows is a brief overview of some of the research performed in the Rehabilitation Act areas described above.

Federal Employment and the Rehabilitation Act

Studies have used both administrative records and surveys to examine the effects of the Rehabilitation Act and issues related to employment of people with disabilities. A study by Lewis and Allee (1992) analyzed a sample of federal personnel records for the effect of disability status on grade level, entry level, and promotion probabilities from 1977 through 1989. They found that employees with disabilities entered the federal workforce at lower grade levels than comparable nondisabled employees but that this discrepancy had diminished in the later years, especially for those with nonsevere disabilities. The grade gap between comparable disabled and nondisabled federal employees was found to have widened during the 1980s. After controlling for starting grade, they concluded that a disability was a greater obstacle to promotion than being a woman or a racial/ethnic minority and the disadvantage was greater for those with severe disabilities.

A study by Bruyère and Horne (1999) surveyed 403 federal agency representatives (mostly Human Resources and EEO) regarding the employment of people with disabilities. A parallel survey (Bruyère, Erickson, & Horne, 2002) of 1,001 federal supervisors was performed as follow-up. Over 90% of the respondents reported making some accommodations for employees with disabilities. The most common barriers to employment and advancement of people with disabilities noted by both groups included attitudes and stereotypes about people with disabilities, lack of related experience and lack of skill and training on the part of the employee with a disability, and supervisors' lack of knowledge about accommodations. The most common disability claims were failure to provide reasonable accommodations and failure to promote. About one quarter of the supervisors reported having been trained in Section 508 requirements.

Vocational Rehabilitation and the Rehabilitation Act

Much of the research performed in Vocational Rehabilitation (VR) that is reviewed here is based on analysis of administrative and survey data. Studies have focused on a variety of issues including: consumer characteristics and satisfaction with VR services, employment outcomes, service trends, and outcomes of sheltered, supported, and competitive employment.

One of the most comprehensive employment studies included a six-year longitudinal study of the Vocational Rehabilitation (VR) service program. The U.S. Department of Education Rehabilitation Services Administration (RSA) followed a random national sample of approximately 8,500 VR recipients over a period of three years through the use of annual surveys and case file information.[16] Part of the purpose of this survey was to collect data that could be used to help understand the relationship between outcomes and differences in the types of people served by the agencies, including demographic characteristics, disability type, functional limitations, SSI/SSDI recipients, work experience, and attitudes. Research based on this data has examined: the characteristics and perspectives of vocational rehabilitation customers (Hayward & Tashjian,

1996), characteristics and outcomes of former vocational rehabilitation customers with employment outcomes (Hayward, 1998), and clients' satisfaction with VR services and employment outcomes (Hayward & Schmidt-Davis, 2000).

This most recent report focused on transitional youth, who account for 13.5% percent of the total VR customer population. They most often applied to VR for services that would help them to enter the labor force. The majority of youth VR consumers (63%) achieved an employment outcome as a result of VR services. Approximately three quarters of the consumers said they were very or mostly satisfied with the services they received, with those who achieved employment showing greater satisfaction than those who had not.

VR consumer satisfaction was also found to be quite high in a 1995 survey by the Missouri State Rehabilitation Advisory Council as part of the Program Evaluation Committee (Kosciulek, Vessell, Rosenthal, Accardo, & Merz, 1997). They found that 80% felt they had been served in a timely manner, 69% said that their counselor helped them to understand their disability and its potential effect on future work, 82% felt that they were involved in making choices about their goals and services, 76% strongly agreed that VR helped (or will help) get them a job. It must be noted that the response rate of 17% for this survey, although dramatically better than the previous survey of 4%, is quite poor and may have resulted in a biased sample.

Other studies have focused on specific disabilities and VR. One recent study examined employment outcome trends for people with severe developmental disabilities using state VR services, focusing on the type of employment (Gilmore, Schuster, & Butterworth, 2000). They analyzed the administrative database (RSA-911) from 1985 to 1995, focusing on successful "closure" (employment) and the use of competitive and supported employment, compared to sheltered workshops. They found no significant changes in the total number of successful closures; however, fewer clients went into sheltered workshops. The number of hours worked remained the same, but earnings dropped after adjusting for inflation over the period. Outcomes regarding earnings were best for those who were in competitive employment compared to supported or sheltered workshops.

Mank, Cioffi, and Yovanoff (1998) examined employment outcomes related to the severity of mental retardation and "behavioral challenges" (e.g., aggressiveness towards others, harm to oneself, etc.). Data was collected for 462 individuals on a variety of job features, including how typical the job was compared to that of nondisabled employees. Generally the trend was of lesser outcomes for those with more severe disabilities and behavioral challenges. However, they also noted that there were exceptions to this rule. Fewer hours of direct support were provided to individuals with severe mental retardation who had higher outcomes. It is hypothesized that perhaps this might be related to the finding that job situations with coworker training was also related to better outcomes for persons with more severe disabilities and/or perhaps the "job fit" was better. They suggest additional research is needed to follow individuals' employment features and outcomes over time and to explore in more detail the nature of coworker training and involvement and its relation to outcomes.

Kaye (1998) examined the 1995 RSA administrative records and determined that 46% of all persons exiting the VR system had been employed for at least 60 days. The majority were competitively employed (85%) compared to less than one fifth before rehabilitation. Only 18% reported being able to support themselves through earnings, but the majority did report earnings as their primary source of support.

A longitudinal study of VR administrative records (R300/911) found a disparity between individuals with severe physical disabilities when compared to those with psychiatric disabilities (Andrews et al., 1992). There was a nearly 20% increase between 1977 and 1984 in the number of those with severe physical disabilities obtaining competitive employment, while there was a 3.4% decrease for those with severe psychiatric disabilities.

People who report a work disability are nearly twice as likely to report being self-employed (14.7%) than those without a disability (8%), according to research performed by Arnold, Seekins, and Ravesloot (1995). They found that rural VR counselors were more likely to use self-employment than urban-based counselors, perhaps in response to the more limited opportunities available in rural areas. In a follow-up, Arnold (2001) surveyed 330 self-employed people with disabilities, exploring their experiences to see what might be done to improve VR services' support for this type of employment outcome. Forty-three percent gave flexible hours and/or working conditions as one of the reasons they chose self-employment to accommodate their disability. Sixteen percent reported utilizing state Vocational Rehabilitation agency money to help fund the initial investment for their business.

Wehman and Revell (1998) performed a national survey of 54 state/territorial supported employment systems and examined the growth of supported employment over a 10-year period. During 1993 to 1995, supported employment (SE) showed rapid growth—16%—and was expanding among people with mental illness. Wages were predominantly above minimum wage and typically better than earnings of those in nonsupported employment and especially above that of sheltered workshops. VR expenditures indicated that persons with disabilities were increasingly choosing supported employment, and state funding agencies were securing supported employment services through a variety of funding methods and emphasizing service to those with significant disabilities.

Rogers (1997) performed a cost-benefit analysis of SE programs for individuals with psychiatric disabilities and considered them to be more cost-effective compared to other programs such as sheltered workshops. It was also determined that SE was more expensive than the alternative vocational programs, reducing the overall benefit to below the actual cost of the program. However, Landis (1999) studied net effects and service costs of community mental health center clients and found that after adjusting for economic fluctuation and controlling for individual functioning, the cost of SE was no greater than that of sheltered workshops and that the customers showed greater improvement in role performance in the SE programs.

In evaluating VR success it is also important to consider other factors outside of the program itself. Misra and Tseng (1986) conclude that local labor market variations can have an effect on VR success given the strong correlation they found between unemployment rates and VR closure rates.

CONCLUSIONS AND RECOMMENDATIONS FOR FURTHER RESEARCH

Above, we summarized research that examined the impact and efficacy of U.S. employment and disability policy. Here, we will identify and discuss existing gaps in current knowledge, and suggest specific areas in which future research is needed.

Across the five pieces of legislation, the greatest amount of research has been conducted on the Americans With Disabilities Act of 1990. Considerable work has been done on analysis of claims and legal outcomes, employer attitudes, and problems encountered in implementing the ADA. Cook and Burke suggest that further "qualitative, ethnographic studies of consumers' and employers' experiences in using protections of the ADA are needed to understand the full range of effects of this new law on relationships between workers and employers" (2002, p. 26).

The controversies over the extent and nature of the ADA's impact on employment of people with disabilities highlight the importance of the use of economic modeling and national data sets to capture longitudinal employment trends and state differences for specific populations of people with disabilities. However, they also highlight the importance of a responsible application of these methodologies, with an understanding of the strengths and limitations of each of the respective data sets used, and when they are best applied to answer specific employment and disability questions. Given a changing economy, the facts revealed by more attentive tracking of policies' effects on persons with disabilities, and the interplay between employment and disability, public policy changes are imperative.

Another area for further analysis will be the increasing use of information technology in the employment process, and its impact on applicants and current employees with disabilities, as well as the implications for an aging workforce. Although efforts have begun in this area, much more is needed to fully understand what changes are occurring and how people with disabilities may be negatively affected and possibly advantaged. Given the federal government's position as a leader in IT access and greater experience in this area, a well-conceived research agenda that incorporates study of both the federal and private sectors is needed. This will allow us to understand how initiatives such as Section 508 of the Rehabilitation Act, targeted to federal sector workplaces and their use of IT, can be extended to encouraging accommodation in the private sector business world.

Overall, despite the recent implementation of TWWIIA, a tremendous investment is being made in evaluating its various provisions. What appears to be lacking is a systematic effort to look at the effects of all of the law's provisions, and, more broadly, the joint effects of the implementation of TWWIIA and initiatives authorized under WIA, IDEA, and other legislation. In particular, it is important to know how these efforts interact with each other. Do some new programs that appear to be successful when evaluated in isolation have offsetting effects on other programs, resulting in little or no progress toward the goals of better employment outcome and increased economic independence (Walker, 2002)?

The studies of WIA previously presented capture a system in the early stages of implementation. Future research needs to follow the impact on job seekers with disabilities in the workforce investment system over a longer period of time. With only limited state performance data to date, it is still too early to assess long-term results (U.S. Department of Labor, 2000). Another question we should be examining is, "How do the outcomes for people with disabilities from underserved communities compare to other people with disabilities at One-Stop Job Centers?" (Walker, 2002).

A whole new area of inquiry that deserves attention is the relationship between Employment Networks and the One-Stop system, and the effect of Tickets to Work on individual training accounts. There are great opportunities to expand service and support choices for adults with disabilities. The interrelationship and impact of coordinated service delivery between WIA and TWWIIA is a major area for future policy research that also deserves attention. SSA and the U.S. Department of Labor are jointly planning a new initiative to assist individuals with disabilities who want to go to work through the creation of a new support position. Disability Program Navigators at One Stop Career Centers will link people with disabilities with employers, Benefits Planning, Assistance, and Outreach (BPA&O) programs, and other needed employment supports. Navigators will also provide information on SSA's work incentives and return to work initiatives, including the Ticket to Work Program.[17] Another opportunity for intergovernmental program support suggested by Golden, O'Mara, Ferrell, and Sheldon (2002) includes possible collaboration between Public Housing Authorities currently administering a Family Self-Sufficiency Program to become an Employment Network under TWWIIA.

With the reauthorization of IDEA, it is timely to discuss needed research, and there may be an opportunity to influence program evaluation. There is an increasing awareness across public policy forums of the importance of appropriate preparation of young people with disabilities for the workplace. A direct test of specific interventions and transition outcomes has not been made. Nonetheless, the correlations found in these studies do provide some information on the transition process, and possible factors that could enhance it. Transitional youth make up 13.5% of total VR customers, so this is another area in which the interplay between laws becomes very important (Hayward and Schmidt-Davis, 2000). The application of large national data set analysis in this policy arena appears to be useful. Wittenburg and Maag (2002) found that existing research conducted using the NLTS and state surveys illustrate that several factors are correlated to postschool outcomes. They suggest that this information can be used to inform several types of policy decisions regarding transition

Analysis of the research conducted to date on the Rehabilitation Act allows us to examine employment and disability-related policy from a number of perspectives. Although analyses have been conducted examining the efficacy of VR services, further research is needed. The availability of the data from the Longitudinal Survey of Vocational Rehabilitation Services Program (LSVRSP), as well as the possibility of linking this data with other national longitudinal administrative data sets, provides an excellent opportunity for further analysis.

There are a variety of areas for potential VR-related research. Research is needed to understand the individual, agency, and service variables that affect performance, as well as potential interactions between these variables. It is vital to identify the most cost-effective methods for serving individuals with significant disabilities, as well as ways of providing services to obtain the best possible employment outcomes for the customers. This might also include examining the allocation of resources within state VR services to determine the optimal service configuration to enhance employment outcomes for their respective customers. Research regarding third-party funding agreements and their effectiveness on quality and quantity of employment outcomes would also be of great value to the VR community and their customers. Research is also needed to determine effective models, services, and resources related to the vocational rehabilitation of people with disabilities from diverse cultures (Walker, 2002).

As the largest employer in the United States, the federal government as an employer represents an under-exploited source of information on the impact of employment disability nondiscrimination and civil rights legislation on employer practices. Significantly more might be done to further explore the impact of such very specific employer-directed workplace provisions as those directives initiated in the Executive Orders to enhance the hiring of persons with disabilities (100,000 over the next five years), the requirement for specific written reasonable accommodation policies, and the requirement for departments to explore flex-place schemes to accommodate part-time offsite employment for persons with disabilities or chronic illness who cannot do full-time employment in the work setting (Office of Personnel Management, n.d.).

An overarching principle in this chapter is the importance of multiple approaches to address employment and disability research questions. This typically involves combining quantitative and qualitative methods so that the findings of each enhance the other (Cook and Burke, 2002). Such research could benefit also from having a New Paradigm[18] disability advocacy approach applied to these efforts. NIDRR's New Paradigm, which has been made part of the objectives for NIDRR-funded research, is a framework for disability research that treats disability as the product of an interaction between characteristics of the individual and characteristics of the natural, built, cultural, and social environments. This paradigm recognizes the critical role played by a person's environment in determining the ability to work and live independently.

Consistent with this philosophy is the use of Participatory Action Research (PAR), which emphasizes research as a joint product of discussion between professional researchers and practitioners and consumers (Whyte, 1991). PAR research in the disability field involves members of the target group to be studied in topic choice, study design, and execution of the research (Bruyère, 1993). The Consumer-Directed Theory of Empowerment (CDTE) is a similar approach, with the philosophy that people with disabilities should be treated as informed consumers who have control over the policies and practices directly affecting their lives (Kosciulek, 1999a). PAR suggests that people with disabilities should be made a part of research into disability issues; the resulting research findings can then influence policy development in ways that are consistent with a consumer-directed philosophy (Kosciulek, 1999b).

We have discussed the value of applying economic analyses of large national data sets to our increased understanding of the effect of employment and disability policy. Such scrutiny enables us to examine the impact of policies at the national, state, and individual levels. However, as pointed out by Cook and Burke (2002), "Research on economics and education among individuals with disabilities will require recruitment and training of research and policy economists in disability and recovery processes. This will require advanced graduate and postgraduate support for multiple years of advanced study and research" (p. 23). This same recommendation can apply to the other disciplinary areas that we would like to integrate into our inquiry as well, and the need for similarly targeted training to employ these other lenses to best effect when applying them to the disability agenda.

We also urge continued collaboration among disability advocates and professional associations that represent disability and rehabilitation professions. To be consistent with a participatory action research (PAR) approach, it is vital that any disability-focused research includes the perspectives of persons with disabilities. Therefore, any such collaboration must have at its nexus the participation of disability advocacy associations, particularly those with public policy and legislative advocacy interests. In addition, a comprehensive look at employment and disability policy, and its resulting implications for service delivery and practice, would be most effective if standards of practice and care associations are included in the collaboration in design and implementation of research.

Much research has been done on selected pieces of the laws chosen for study here, but much also remains to be done. Even those laws that have been in place for a number of years have not had their impact and implications for employment and disability policy fully investigated. The Conference sponsored by the National Institute on Disability and Rehabilitation Research and the American Psychological Association in 2002, which spawned this chapter, afforded an excellent opportunity to begin this process. But it is only the beginning, and it will be imperative that we continue on in this effort to realize the gains that need to be made in having employment and disability policies that are designed and evaluated using the best tools and methods from a wide variety of contributing disciplines.

QUESTIONS FOR DISCUSSION AND/ OR FURTHER STUDY

Service Domain

1. How has the federal mandate for transition planning and services played a critical role in promoting promising transition practices?

2. What are the goals of the Ticket to Work and Workforce Investment Act and what might be some implications of TWWIIA regarding the provision of services?

Research Domain

3. Describe the three broad types of research that predominantly characterize the research on the Americans With Disabilities Act since its passage in 1990. Give examples of studies conducted under each area.
4. Describe the information gathered about the Vocational Rehabilitation (VR) service program from the six-year longitudinal study conducted of this program.

Policy Domain

5. What policies and other factors might have affected the employment rate of people with disabilities in the 1990s? How and why might they have affected it?
6. What were the most common barriers to employment and advancement of people with disabilities noted by both human resource and EEO professionals and supervisors in the research conducted on disability employment nondiscrimination in the Federal Sector workforce?

NOTES

1. The authors would like to acknowledge the contributions of the following individuals who assisted with the literature review and contributed information for this manuscript: Anne Sieverding, Research Assistant for the Cornell University Program on Employment and Disability; David Stapleton, Director, Cornell Center for Policy Research; and David Wittenburg, Senior Research Associate, Urban Institute.
2. See http://digitalcommons.ilr.cornell.edu/edicollect/79/ (retrieved March 17, 2006) for a copy of this paper.
3. See http://www.ilr.cornell.edu/ped/il/independence/ for "Independence," an online primer on public policy relating to employment of people with disabilities.
4. See the U.S. EEOC web site at http://www.eeoc.gov/policy/ada.html for more information.
5. See the SSA web site at http://www.ssa.gov/work/Ticket/ticket.html or more information on the Work Incentives Improvement Act.
6. Further information about the Ticket to Work evaluation is at http://www.mathematica-mpr.com/htmlreports/ttwtext.htm (retrieved March 17, 2006).
7. For further information see http://www.cms.hhs.gov/TWWIA/03_MIG.asp (retrieved March 17, 2006).
8. GAO-01–153, "SSA Disability: Other Programs May Provide Lessons for Improving Return-to-Work Efforts," January 12, 2001.

9. Workforce Investment Act of 1998, WIA, Public Law 105–220. See http://www.doleta. gov/regs/statutes/wialaw.txt for further information.
10. See the University of Iowa Law, Health Policy, and Disability Center Web site at http:// disability.law.uiowa.edu/ for further information
11. Go to the Research Triangle Institute (RTI) Web site at: http://www.rti.org to see this report.
12. According to the IDEA Amendments of 1997, "child with a disability" is defined as a child who needs special education and related services because of mental retardation, hearing impairments (including deafness), speech or language impairments, visual impairments (including blindness), serious emotional disturbance, orthopedic impairments, autism, traumatic brain injury, other health impairments, or specific learning impairments. Children aged three through nine who experience developmental delays in physical development, cognitive development, communication development, social or emotional development, or adaptive development may also be included at the discretion of the State and the local educational agency.
13. 29 U.S.C §791; http://www4.law.cornell.edu/uscode/29/791.html
14. 29 U.S.C. §794; http://www4.law.cornell.edu/uscode/29/793.html
15. 29 U.S.C. §794; http://www4.law.cornell.edu/uscode/29/794.html
16. Further information and data from this survey is available for download on line from www.lsvrsp.org
17. For further information, see the Social Security Administration Web site at http://www. ssa.gov/pressoffice/disabilityinfo-pr.htm, for the Social Security Administration (SSA) press release entitled "Social Security announces new initiatives to promote employment opportunities for people with disabilities," October 16, 2002.
18. See http://www.ncddr.org/rpp/lrp_ov.html to read the U.S. Department of Education National Institute on Disability and Rehabilitation Research Long Range Plan.

REFERENCES

Acemoglu, D., & Angrist, J. (1998). *Consequences of employment protection: The case of the Americans With Disabilities Act.* (Working Paper No. 6670). National Bureau of Economic Research, Cambridge, MA.

Andrews, H., Barker, J., Pittman, J., Mars, L., Struening, E., & LaRocca, N. (1992). National trends in vocational rehabilitation: A comparison of individuals with physical disabilities and individuals with psychiatric disabilities. *Journal of Rehabilitation, 58,* 7–18.

Arnold, N. (2001) First national study of people with disabilities who are self-employed. Retrieved March 17, 2006, from http://rtc.ruralinstitute.umt.edu/SelEm/SelEmRePrgRpt.htm.

Arnold, N., Seekins, T., & Ravesloot, C. (1995). Self-employment as a vocational rehabilitation outcome in rural and urban areas. *Rehabilitation Counseling Journal, 39,* 94–106.

Aune, E. (1991). A transition model for postsecondary-bound students with learning disabilities. *Learning Disabilities Research and Practice, 6,* 177–187.

Autor, D., & Duggan, M. (2003). The rise in disability recipients and the decline in unemployment. *Quarterly Journal of Economics, 118,* 157–205.

Baldwin, M., & Johnson, W. (1995). Labor market discrimination against women with disabilities. *Industrial Relations, 34,* 555–577.

Baldwin, M., & Johnson, W. (2000). Labor market discrimination against men with disabilities. *Southern Economic Journal, 66*(3), 548–566.

Benz, M. R., Yovanoff, P., & Doren, B. (1997). School-to-work components that predict post school success for students with and without disabilities. *Exceptional Children,* 63(2), 151–165.

Berkeley Planning Associates. (1982). A *study of accommodations provided to handicapped employees by federal contractors: Final report* (report prepared for the U.S. Department of Labor, contract no. J-E1–0009). Washington, DC: Author.

Billitteri, T. (1997). Mental health policy: The issues. CQ *Researcher, Congressional Quarterly Inc.,* 7(34), 795–797.

Blackorby, J., Hankock, G. R., & Siegel, S. (April 1993). *Human capital and structural explanations of post-school success for youth with disabilities: A latent variable exploration of the National Longitudinal Transition Study.* Paper presented at the annual meeting of the American Educational Research Association, Atlanta, GA.

Blackorby, J., & Wagner, M. (1996). Longitudinal post-school outcomes of youth with disabilities: Findings from the National Longitudinal Transition Study. *Exceptional Children,* 62(5), 399–413.

Blanck, P. (1991). The emerging work force: Empirical study of the Americans With Disabilities Act. *Journal of Corporation Law,* 16(4), 693–803.

Blanck, P. (1994). Employment integration, economic opportunity, and the Americans With Disabilities Act: Empirical study from 1990–1993. *Iowa Law Review,* 79(4), 853–923.

Blanck, P. (1996). Transcending title I of the Americans With Disabilities Act: A case report on Sears, Roebuck and Co. *Mental and Physical Law Reporter,* 20(2), 278–286.

Bound, J., & Waidmann, T. (2000). Accounting for recent declines in employment rates among the working-aged disabled (Working Paper No. 7975). Cambridge, MA: National Bureau of Economic Research. Retrieved March 17, 2006, from http://www.nber.org/papers/w7975

Bruyère, S. (1993). Participatory Action Research: Overview and implication for family members of persons with disabilities. *Journal of Vocational Rehabilitation,* 3(2), 62–68.

Bruyère, S. (2000). *Disability employment policies and practices in private and federal sector organizations.* Ithaca, NY: Cornell University, School of Industrial and Labor Relations Extension Division, Program on Employment and Disability.

Bruyère, S., & Brown, J. (2003). Legislation impacting employment for persons with disabilities. In E. Szymanski and R. Parker (Eds.), *Work and disability: Issues and strategies in career development and job placement* (pp. 27–52). Austin, Texas: Pro-Ed.

Bruyère, S., & Erickson, W. (2001). *E-Human resources: A review of the literature and implications for people with disabilities.* Ithaca, NY: Cornell University, School of Industrial and Labor Relations Extension Division, Program on Employment and Disability.

Bruyère, S., & Horne, R. (1999). *Disability policies and practices in U.S. federal agencies.* (Report by the Presidential Task Force on the Employment of Adults with Disabilities.) Ithaca, NY: Cornell University, School of Industrial and Labor Relations Extension Division, Program on Employment and Disabilities.

Bruyère, S., Erickson, W., & Horne, R. (2002). *Survey of the federal government on supervisor practices in employment of people with disabilities.* (Report by the Presidential Task Force on Employment of Adults with Disabilities). Ithaca, NY: Cornell University, School of Industrial and Labor Relations Extension Division, Program on Employment and Disability.

Burkhauser, R. V., Butler, J. S., & Weathers, R. (2001). How policy variables influence the timing of Social Security Disability Insurance applications. *Social Security Bulletin,* 64(1), 52–83.

Burkhauser, R. V., Daly, M., Houtenville, A., & Nargis, N. (2002). Employment of working age people with disabilities in 1980s and 1990s: What current data can and cannot tell us. *Demography,* 39(3), 541–555.

Burkhauser, R. V., & Stapleton, D. (2003). A review of the evidence and its implications for policy change. In D. Stapleton & R. V. Burkhauser (Eds.), *The decline in employment of people with disabilities: A policy puzzle* (pp. 369–405). Kalamazoo, MI: W. E. Upjohn Institute for Employment Research.

Cheek, M. (2001). *Medicaid buy-in programs for employed persons with disabilities: Going forward.* Washington, DC: The Center for Workers with Disabilities.

Collignon, F. (1997, January). Is the ADA successful? Indicators for tracking gains. *Annals of the American Academy of Political and Social Science, 549,* 129–147.

Cook, J., & Burke, J. (2002). *Public policy and employment of people with disabilities: Exploring new paradigms.* Unpublished manuscript. University of Illinois at Chicago, Department of Psychiatry, National Research and Training Center on Psychiatric Disability.

D'Amico, R. (1991). The working world awaits: Employment experiences during and shortly after secondary school. In M. Wagner, Newman, R. D'Amico, E. D. Jay, P. Butler = Nalin, C. Mardec, & R. Cox (Eds.), *Youth with disabilities: How are they doing? The first comprehensive report from the National Longitudinal Study of Special Education Students.* Menlo Park, CA: SRI International.

DeLeire, T. (2000a). The wage and employment effects of the Americans With Disabilities Act. *Journal of Human Resources, 35*(4), 693–715.

DeLeire, T. (2000b). The unintended consequences of the American with Disabilities Act. *Regulation, 23*(1), 21–24.

Diller, M. (2000). Judicial backlash, the ADA, and the civil rights model. *Berkeley Journal of Employment and Labor Law, 21*(1), 19–53.

Doren, B., & Benz, M. R. (1998). Employment inequity revisited: Predictors of better employment outcomes of young women with disabilities in transition. *Journal of Special Education, 31*(4), 425–442.

Drum, C. (1998). The social construction of personnel policy: Implications for people with disabilities. *Journal of Disability Policy Studies, 9*(1).

Durlak, C. M., Rose, E., & Bursuck, W. D. (1994). Preparing high school students with learning disabilities for the transition to post-secondary education: Teaching the skills of self-determination. *Journal of Learning Disabilities, 27*(1), 51–59.

Elliott, B., Tashjian, M., Neenan, P., Levine, D., & Chewning, L. (2002, March). *Implementation of the Workforce Investment Act: Adult literacy and disability perspectives* (First Interim Report for the Vocational Rehabilitation Program for the Rehabilitation Services Administration, U.S. Department of Education.) Research Triangle Park, NC: Research Triangle Institute.

Erickson, W. (2002). *A review of selected e-recruiting websites: Disability accessibility considerations.* Ithaca, NY: Cornell University, School of Industrial and Labor Relations Extension Division, Program on Employment and Disability.

Feldblum, C. (2000). Definition of a disability under federal anti-discrimination law: What happened? Why? And what can we do about it? *Berkeley Journal of Employment and Labor Law, 21*(91), 91–165.

Frank, A., & Sitlington, P. (2000, June). Young adults with mental disabilities—does transition planning make a difference? *Education and Training in Mental Retardation and Developmental Disabilities, 35*(2), 119–134.

Funaro, A., & Dixon, K. A. (2002, June). *How the one-stop system serves people with disabilities: A nationwide survey of disability agencies* (Report for the Rehabilitation Research and Training Center on Workforce Investment and Employment Policy for Persons with Disabilities.) New Brunswick, NJ: Rutgers, the State University of New Jersey, John J. Heldrich Center for Workforce Development.

Gerber, P. J. (1992). At first glance: Employment for people with learning disabilities at the beginning of the ADA era. *Learning Disability Quarterly, 15*(4), 330–332.

Gilmore, D., Schuster, J., & Butterworth, J. (2000). An analysis of trends for people with MR, cerebral palsy, and epilepsy receiving services from state VR agencies: Ten years of progress. *Rehabilitation Counseling Bulletin, 44*(1), 30–38.

Golden, T. P., O'Mara, S., Ferrell, C., & Sheldon, J. (2002). *Supporting career development and employment for individuals with disabilities: The role of benefits planning, assistance and outreach and protection and advocacy for beneficiaries of social security.* Ithaca, NY: Cornell University, School of Industrial and Labor Relations Extension Division, Program on Employment and Disability.

Goodman, N., & Waidman, T. (2003). SSDI and the employment rate of people with disabilities. In D. Stapleton & R. Burkhauser (Eds.), *The decline in employment of people with disabilities: A policy puzzle* (pp. 339–405). Kalamazoo, MI: W. E. Upjohn Institute for Employment Research.

Gugerty, J. (1994). Characteristics of services provided by two-year colleges that serve students with learning or cognitive disabilities in highly effective ways. *Issues in Special Education and Rehabilitation, 9*(1), 79–87.

Hahn, H. (2000). Accommodations and the ADA: Unreasonable bias or biased reasoning? *Berkeley Journal of Employment and Labor Law, 21*(1), 166–192.

Halpern, A. S., Yovanoff, P., Doren, B., & Benz, M. R. (1995). Predicting participation in postsecondary education for school leavers with disabilities. *Exceptional Children, 62*(2), 151–164.

Harger, D. (1993). Drawing the line between reasonable accommodation and undue hardship under the Americans With Disabilities Act: Reducing the effects of ambiguity on small businesses. *Kansas Law Review, 41,* 783–807.

Harvey, M. (2001). The efficacy of vocational education for students with disabilities concerning post-school employment outcomes: A review of the literature. *Journal of Industrial Teacher Education, 38*(3), 25–44.

Hasazi, S., Furney, K., & DeStefano, L. (1999). Implementing the IDEA transition mandates. *Exceptional Children, 65*(4), 555–566.

Hasazi, S., Johnson, R., Hasazi, J., Gordon, L., & Hull, M. (1989). Employment of youth with and without handicaps following high school: Outcomes and correlates. *Journal of Special Education, 23*(3), 243–255.

Hayward, B. (1998). *Longitudinal study of the vocational rehabilitation service program, third interim report: Characteristics and outcomes of former VR consumers with an employment outcome.* Research Triangle Park, NC: Research Triangle Institute. Retrieved April 12, 2002, from http://www.rti.org/pubs/Interim3.Pdf

Hayward, B., & Schmidt-Davis, H. (2000). *A longitudinal study of the vocational rehabilitation service program, fourth interim report: Characteristics and outcomes of transitional youth in VR.* Research Triangle Park, NC: Research Triangle Institute. Retrieved April 12, 2002, from http://www.rti.org/pubs/interim4.pdf

Hayward, B., & Tashjian, M. (1996). *A longitudinal study of the Vocational Rehabilitation service program, second interim report: Characteristics and perspectives of VR consumers.* Research Triangle Park, NC: Research Triangle Institute. Retrieved April 12, 2002, from http://www.rti.org/pubs/interim2.pdf

Heal, L. W., & Rusch, F. R. (1995). Predicting employment for students who leave special education high school programs. *Exceptional Children, 6*(5), 472–487.

Hernandez, B., Keys, C., & Balcazar, F. (2000). Employer attitudes toward workers with disabilities and their ADA employment rights: A literature review. *Journal of Rehabilitation, 66*(4), 4–16.

Job Accommodation Network. (1999). *Accommodation benefit/cost data, tabulated through July 30, 1999.* Retrieved March 10, 2003, from http://www.jan.wvu.edu/media/Stats/BenCosts0799.html

Jones, C. (1997, April). Legislative subterfuge? Failing to insure persons with mental illness under the Mental Health Parity Act and the Americans with Disability Act. *Vanderbilt Law Review, 50*(3), 753–793.

Kaye, S. (March 1998). Vocational rehabilitation in the United States. *Disability Statistics Abstract,* Number 20. Retrieved March 17, 2006, from http://dsc.ucsf.edu/publication.php?pub_id=5.

Kohler, P. D. (1994). On-the-job training: A curricular approach to employment. *Career Development for Exceptional Individuals, 17*(1), 29–40.

Kohler, P. (1996). *Taxonomy for transition programming.* Champaign: Transition Research Institute, University of Illinois.

Kohler, P., & Chapman, S. (1999). *Literature review on school-to-work transition.* Champaign, IL: University of Illinois at Urbana–Champaign, Transition Research Institute. Retrieved March 17, 2006, from http://www.ed.uiuc.edu/sped/tri/stwpurpose.htm.

Kosciulek, J. (1999a). The consumer-directed theory of empowerment. *Rehabilitation Counseling Bulletin, 42*(3), 196–213.

Kosciulek, J. (1999b). *Implications of consumer direction for disability policy: Development and rehabilitation service delivery.* Paper presented at the Mary Switzer Memorial Seminar, East Lansing, MI. Retrieved July 31, 2002, from the Switzer Memorial Seminar Series Web site, http://www.mswizter.org/sem99/papers/kosciulek.html

Kosciulek, J., Vessell, R., Rosenthal, R., Accardo, D., & Merz, C. (1997). Consumer satisfaction with vocational rehabilitation services. *Journal of Rehabilitation, 63*(2), 5–9

Landis, J. (1999). Estimating net effects and costs of service options for persons with serious mental illness. *Psychiatric Services, 50*(6), 735–738.

Lee, B. (2001). The implications of ADA litigation for employers: A review of federal appellate court decisions. *Human Resource Management, 40*(1), 35–50.

Lewis, G., & Allee, C. (1992). The impact of disabilities on the federal career success. *Public Administration Review, 52*(4), 389–397.

Litvan, L. M. (1994, January). The disabilities law: Avoid the pitfalls. *Nation's Business, 82,* 25.

Livermore, G. A., Stapleton, D. C., Nowak, M. W., Wittenburg, D. C., & Eiseman, E. D. (2000). *The economics of policies and programs affecting the employment of people with disabilities.* Ithaca, NY: Cornell University, School of Industrial and Labor Relations Extension Division, Program on Employment and Disability.

MacDonald-Wilson, K., Rogers, S., Massaro, J., Lyass, A., & Crean, T. (2002). An investigation of reasonable accommodations for people with psychiatric disabilities: Quantitative findings from a multi-site study. *Community Mental Health Journal, 38*(1), 35–49.

Mank D., Cioffi, A., & Yovanoff, P. (1998). Employment outcomes for people with severe disabilities: Opportunities for improvement. *Mental Retardation, 36*(3), 205–216.

McKee, B. (1993). The disabilities labyrinth. *Nation's Business, 81*(4), 18–23.

McMahon, B., Shaw, L., & Jaet, D. (1995). An empirical analysis: Employment and disability from an ADA litigation perspective. *NARPPS Journal, 10*(1), 3–14.

Misra, S., & Tseng, M. (1986). Influence of the unemployment rate on vocational rehabilitation outcomes. *Rehabilitation Counseling Bulletin, 29*(3), 158–165.

Morgan, D., & Hecht, J. (1990). *Report on the methodology for the West End special education transition program evaluation.* Riverside, CA: California Educational Research Cooperative. (ERIC Document Reproduction Service No. ED 327 021.) Retrieved March 17, 2006, from http://cerc.ucr.edu/publications/PDF_Transfer/Special_Education/se003_report_on_the_methodology/se003_report_on_the_methodology.pdf.

Morris, M., & Farah, L. (2001, February). *Review of state plans for the Workforce Investment Act from a disability policy framework.* Iowa City, IA: The University of Iowa, Rehabilitation Research and Training Center on Workforce Investment and Employment Policy for Persons with Disability, with assistance from Robert Silverstein of the Center for the Study and Advancement of Disability Policy for the Presidential Task Force on Employment of Adults with Disabilities.

Moss, K., Burris, S., Ullman, B., Johnsen, M., & Swanson, J. (2001). Unfunded mandate: An empirical study of the implementation of the Americans With Disabilities Act by the Equal Employment Opportunity Commission. *Kansas Law Review, 50*(1), 1–110.

Moss, K., & Johnsen, M. (1997). Employment discrimination and the ADA: A study of the administrative complaint process. *Psychiatric Rehabilitation Journal, 21,*111–121.

Moss, K., Ullman, M., Starrett, B., Burris, S., & Johnsen, M. (1999). Outcomes of employment discrimination charges filed under the Americans With Disabilities Act. *Psychiatric Services, 50*(8), 1028–1035.

National Center for Disability Services. (1994). *A demonstration project to teach self-determination skills to youth with disabilities* (Final Report). Albertson, NY: National Center for Disability Services.

National Center for Education Statistics. (2000). *Dropout rates in the United States: 1998.* U.S. Department of Education, Office of Educational Research and Improvement (NCES 2000–022). Retrieved March 17, 2006, from http://nces.ed.gov/pubsearch/pubsinfo.asp?pubid=2000022.

National Council on Disability. (2002). Americans With Disabilities *Supreme Court decisions interpreting the Americans With Disabilities Act.* Washington, DC: Author. Retrieved July 2, 2002, from http://www.ncd.gov/newsroom/publications/supremecourt_ada.html.

New York State Education Department. (1999). *The post school status of former special education students in the big five cities* (Vocational and Educational Services for Individuals with Disabilities [VESID] Report.) Albany, NY: Author. Retrieved March 17, 2006, from http://www.vesid.nysed.gov/specialed/transition/rp0299/word/0299rri.htm.

Newman, J., & Dinwoodie, R. (1992). Impact of the Americans With Disabilities Act on private sector employers. *Journal of Rehabilitation Administration, 20*(1), 3–13.

Office of Personnel Management. (n.d.). *Federal employment of people with disabilities: Laws and Executive Orders.* Washington, DC: Author. Retrieved March 17, 2006, from http://www.opm.gov/disability/hrpro_5-01.asp.

Peters, J. M., Templeman, T. P., & Brostrom, G. (1987). The school and community partnership: Planning transition for students with severe handicaps. *Exceptional Children, 53*(6), 531–536.

Petrila, J., & Brink, T. (2001). Mental illness and changing definitions of disability under the Americans With Disabilities Act. *Psychiatric Services, 52*(5), 626–630.

Posthill, S. M., & Roffman, A. J. (1991). The impact of a transitional training program for young adults with learning disabilities. *Journal of Learning Disabilities, 24*(10), 619–629.

President's Committee on Employment of People with Disabilities. (1995a). *ADA survey by Global Strategy Group, Inc.* Washington, DC: Author.

President's Committee on the Employment of People with Disabilities. (1995b). *Mason-Dixon Poll, January 1995, State of Florida Division of Vocational Rehabilitation, National Organization for Disabilities.* Washington, DC: Author.

President's Committee on the Employment of People with Disabilities. (1996). *What does business really think about the ADA?* Washington, DC: Author. Retrieved March 17, 2006, from http://www.dol.gov/odep/archives/ek96/business.htm.

Price, L., & Gerber, P. (2001). At second glance: Employees with disabilities in the Americans With Disabilities Act era. *Journal of Learning Disabilities, 34*(3), 202.

Roessler, R., & Sumner, G. (1997). Employer opinions about accommodating employees with chronic illness. *Journal of Applied Rehabilitation Counseling, 28,* 29–34.

Rogers, S. (1997). Cost-benefit studies in vocational services. *Psychiatric Rehabilitation Journal, 20*(3), 25–33.

Schecter, E. (1997). Work while receiving disability insurance benefits: Additional findings from the New Beneficiary Follow-up Survey. *Social Security Bulletin, 60,* 3–17.

Scheid, T. (1998). The Americans With Disabilities Act, mental disability, and employment practices. *Journal of Behavioral Health Services & Research, 25*(3), 312–324.

Schlalock, R., Holl, C., Elliott, B., & Ross, I. (1992). A longitudinal follow-up of graduates from a rural special education program. *Learning Disabilities Quarterly, 15*(1), 29–38.

Schumacher, E., & Baldwin, M. (2000). *The Americans With Disabilities Act and the labor market experience of workers with disabilities: Evidence from the SIPP.* Evanston, IL: Joint Center for Poverty Research. Unpublished manuscript. Retrieved March 17, 2006, from http://www.jcpr.org/wp/WPprofile.cfm?ID=187.

Schwochau, S., & Blanck, D. (2000). The economics of the Americans With Disabilities Act, part III: Does the ADA disable the disabled? *Berkley Journal of Employment and Labor Law, 2*(27), 271–313.

Silverstein, R. (2000a). Emerging disability framework: A guidepost for analyzing public. *Policy Iowa Law Review, 85*(5), 1691.

Silverstein, R. (2000b, January 27). *A description of the Workforce Investment Act from a disability policy perspective.* Washington, DC: George Washington University Medical Center, Center for the Study and Advancement of Disability Policy in the School of Public Health and Health Services.

Storen, D., Dixon, K. A., & Funaro, A. (2002, February). *One-Stop accessibility: A nationwide survey of One-Stop Centers on services for people with disabilities.* New Brunswick, NJ: Rutgers, the State University of New Jersey, John J. Heldrich Center for Workforce Development (for the Rehabilitation Research and Training Center on Workforce Investment and Employment Policy for Persons with Disabilities).

Ullman, M., Johnson, M., Moss, K., & Burris, S. (2001). The EEOC charge priority policy and claimants with psychiatric disabilities. *Psychiatric Services, 52*(5), 644–649.

U.S. Department of Education. (2002). *Twenty-fourth annual report to Congress on the implementation of the Individuals with Disabilities Education Act.* Washington DC: Author. Retrieved June 6, 2005, from http://www.ed.gov/about/reports/annual/osep/2002/appendix-a-pt2.pdf

U.S. Department of Labor. (2000). *WIA: State Plan Annual Reports PY 2000.* Washington, DC: Employment and Training Administration of the U.S. Department of Labor.

U.S. General Accounting Office. (2002a, February). *Workforce Investment Act: Improvements needed in performance measures to provide a more accurate picture of WIA's effectiveness* (GAO-02-275). Washington, DC: U.S. Government Printing Office.

U.S. General Accounting Office. (2002b, April). *Workforce Investment Act: Youth provisions promote new service strategies, but additional guidance would enhance program development* (GAO-02-413). Washington, DC: U.S. Government Printing Office.

U.S. General Accounting Office. (2001, October). *Workforce Investment Act: Better guidance needed to address concerns over new requirements* (GAO-02-72). Washington, DC: U.S. Government Printing Office.

Wagner, M. (1991). *The benefit of secondary vocational education for young people with disabilities: Findings from the national longitudinal transition study of special education students* (Report No. EC 300 485). Menlo Park, CA: SRI International, Contract 300–87–0054. (ERIC Document No. ED 334 739)

Wagner, M. (1992). *Being female—A secondary disability? Gender differences in the transition experiences of young people with disabilities.* Menlo Park, CA: SRI International.

Wagner, M., Blackorby, J., Cameto, R., & Newman, L. (1993a). *What makes a difference? Influences on post school outcomes of youth with disabilities.* Menlo Park, CA: SRI International.

Wagner, M., Blackorby, J., Cameto, R., Hebbeler, K., & Newman, L. (1993b). *The transition experiences of young people with disabilities: A summary of findings from the National Longitudinal Transition Study of Special Education Students.* Menlo Park, CA: SRI International.

Walker, S. (2002, May). *Diversity matters: Infusing issues of people with disabilities from underserved communities into a trans-disciplinary research agenda in the behavioral and social sciences.* Paper prepared for the Bridging the Gap Conference, Washington, DC: Howard University Research and Training Center for Access to Rehabilitation and Empowerment Opportunities.

Walters, S., & Baker C. (1996). Title I of the Americans With Disabilities Act: Employer and recruiter attitudes toward individuals with disabilities. *Journal of Rehabilitation Administration, 20*(1), 15–23.

Wehman, P., & Revell, G. (1998). Supported employment: A decade of rapid growth and impact. *American Rehabilitation, 24*(1), 31–43.

Wehmeyer, M., & Lawrence, M. (1995). Whose future is it anyway? Promoting student involvement in transition planning. *Career Development for Exceptional Individuals, 18*(2), 69–83.

Whyte, W. (Ed.). (1991). *Participatory action research.* Newbury Park, CA: Sage Publications.

Wittenburg, D., & Maag, E. (2002). School to where? A literature review on economic outcomes of youth with disabilities. *Journal of Vocational Rehabilitation, 17*(4), 265–280.

Yelin, E. (1997). The employment of people with and without disabilities in an age of insecurity. *Annals of the American Academy of Political and Social Science, 549,* 117–128.

CHAPTER EIGHT

Evidence-Based Employment Practices in Vocational Rehabilitation

Christopher C. Wagner
Amy J. Armstrong
Robert T. Fraser
David Vandergoot
Dale F. Thomas

The essential goal of vocational rehabilitation (VR) services is to assist individuals with disabilities to successfully obtain and maintain competitive employment in a field of interest, in order to support increased autonomy and full participation in society (Bolton, Bellini, & Brookings, 2000). Over the past 15 years, the VR process has been subject to some relatively dramatic changes. Changes have included legislation-driven policy that addresses best practices, consumer choice, and service-based outcomes (Rehabilitation Act Amendments), and restructures the employment service system (Workforce Investment Act) to a One-Stop service model. Social Security Administration policies have established the Ticket to Work and Work Incentives Improvement programs that address benefits and employment. The Ticket to Work program vicariously affects employment outcomes by attempting to reduce disincentives to employment, thereby eliminating systems barriers that may affect individuals' decisions to seek employment. As of 2002, the federal Rehabilitation Services Administration no longer considers sheltered employment to represent a successful employment closure. This places an emphasis on community-based competitive employment outcomes, especially for individuals with significant disabilities.

The VR system has seen a prioritization of services for individuals with significant disabilities in the majority of states (Thomas & Whitney-Thomas, 1996). Due to the funding challenges to the VR system and fluctuations in agency ability to purchase services, some former community rehabilitation providers have moved away from VR contracting in pursuit of other entrepreneurial endeavors. In this context, some return-to-work strategies have also changed markedly. For example, Menz (1997) reports a tenfold increase in the use of the supported employment interventions for individuals with severe disabilities between the years 1986 and 1993.

The labor market also has gone through significant changes. The profound decrease in manufacturing has had a marked influence on individuals with disabilities, prompting their movement to service work, particularly for women (Trupin, Sebasta, Yelin, & LaPlante, 1997). These positions typically do not have opportunity for career growth, salary increases, or benefits. The dramatic increase in temporary and part-time work has resulted in a corresponding lack of career-oriented employment (Trupin et al., 1997). Another trend has been the overt outsourcing of personnel services by national companies. With unemployment periodically dropping to 3% to 4% in recent years (although currently higher), there has been increasing competition for quality employees.

When the economy is weak, people with disabilities often experience sustained unemployment due to a labor market scenario in which many marginalized and nonmarginalized job seekers compete with one another for extant jobs. Highly educated and skilled workers are in greater demand, yet many individuals with disabilities are not competitive for these jobs because of a lack of postsecondary education (NCES, 1999) and the additional barriers to employment that individuals with disabilities face. These additional barriers include lack of available appropriate jobs, lack of transportation, inadequate training, and risk of losing health benefits (Loprest & Maag, 2001). Over the past decades, the number of recipients of Disability Insurance (SSDI) and Supplemental Security Income (SSI) disability benefits has grown dramatically. Approximately 4.9 million workers were receiving SSDI in December, 1999, and 3.7 million working age individuals were receiving SSI, accounting for an expenditure exceeding $60 billion (Kregel & Head, 2002).

Even when competitive for jobs, some individuals with disabilities may prefer part-time work based upon the severity of their impairments and in order to maintain both Social Security Disability Income (SSDI) subsidy and medical coverage. In spite of the work incentives instituted by the Social Security Administration (SSA) such as trial work periods, continuing eligibility for Medicare, IRWE, PASS, and the Ticket to Work and Work Incentives Improvement Act of 1999, beneficiaries still experience a fear of losing benefits (Loprest & Maag, 2001).

Unfortunately, even in a strong economy with low unemployment rates, unemployment for individuals with significant disabilities remains high. It is currently estimated that the employment rate of individuals with significant disabilities is 35% (thus, unemployment is approximately 65%); this serves as a sharp contrast to the approximately 81% of individuals without disability who are working (National Organization on Disability, 2004). The Americans with Disabilities Act, although perhaps preventing job termination for individuals with disabilities (Murdick, 1997), may have had some negative impact on the hiring of individuals with disabilities, specifically men (Acemoglu & Angrist, 2001). However, the number of contextual variables involved makes this difficult to determine (e.g., the increase in movement to Social Security subsidy, a decrease in elementary manufacturing jobs for men).

The extent to which these contextual variables affect employment outcomes is unknown. The increase in temporary work, telecommuting, and self-employment in our society may open new doors while simultaneously decreasing the availability of career jobs with benefits. Similarly, the type of work sought by rehabilitation participants may continue to shift toward part-time and self-employment options, requiring rehabilitation professionals either to change their goals for consumers or to experience a mismatch between their goals and the priorities of consumers (Callahan, Shumpert, & Mast, 2002; Drebing et al., 2004).

EMPLOYMENT OUTCOMES MEASUREMENT ISSUES

Securing and maintaining employment is the most tangible outcome for VR programs (Thomas, Menz, & Rosenthal, 2001). Employment outcomes can provide a meaningful way to compare the effectiveness of similar programs (Gibbs, 1991; Johnston & Granger, 1994; Thomas & Menz, 1997) and are often used to justify the time, human resources, and dollars invested in rehabilitation efforts (Berkowitz, 1985; Johnston, Hall, Carnavale, & Boak, 1995).

The employment outcome research does not use a standard means of reporting employment outcomes (McAweeney, Forchheimer, & Tate, 1997; Thomas & Menz, 1997; Vogel, Bishop, & Wong, 1998). In fact, analyses of literature reveal a wide variability in the types of data reported. For example, Bolton (2001) reviewed 22 assessment instruments commonly used to measure rehabilitation outcomes focusing upon employment, independent living, and community participation. This variability in measurement makes meaningful comparison of programs or services difficult (Cifu et al., 1997; Thomas et al., 2001).

The lack of a standardized employment outcome measure has been identified as a substantial gap in the VR literature for almost two decades (Vandergoot, 1987). In fact, the employment outcome literature often fails to define even the most basic aspects of the obtained job (Kay, 1993). For example, researchers may not specify whether employment is permanent or temporary, full-time or part-time, or if the employment is subsidized by other entitlement programs or government initiatives (Johnston, 1991). These are important variables, pertaining to both the quality and comparability of outcomes. Researchers also use different criteria to measure job success, thus making comparisons among programs difficult. Efforts are needed to begin to understand employment outcome reporting (Thomas & Menz, 1997) and to bridge this gap.

Variables proposed for reporting outcome measurements include:

- Number of hours worked and wages earned (Stodden & Browder, 1986)
- Income and satisfaction with income (Gilbride, Thomas, & Stensrud, 1998)
- Standard timeframes, particularly important for individuals who have cyclical difficulty maintaining work such as those with brain injury (Johnston et al., 1995) or psychiatric disability (Bond & McDonel, 1991)
- Job satisfaction (Gilbride, Thomas, & Stensrud, 1998; Koch & Merz, 1995)
- Employment benefits received and worker satisfaction with benefits (Bell, Lysaker, & Milstein, 1996; Gilbride, Thomas, & Stensrud, 1998)
- Potential to experience advancement (Gilbride, Thomas, & Stensrud, 1998; Sands, Kozleski, & Goodwin, 1992)
- Consumer involvement in choosing an employment goal and specific services (Rumrill & Garnette, 1997)
- The need for and nature and extent of job accommodations (Zuckerman, 1993)
- The consumer's level of improvement in standard of living or quality of life (Bolton, 2001; Fabian, 1991; Felce & Perry, 1995)

One example of cross-site comparison of outcomes using a standard metric is the effort to evaluate more than one hundred Projects With Industry (PWI) programs funded by the Rehabilitation Services Administration. These indicators tend to be focused on quantity and quality of job placement program compliance. Program indicators for the PWI program include: numbers placed with or without severe disabilities, numbers served who were unemployed more than six months at intake, numbers served with severe disabilities who were unemployed six months at intake, and change in weekly earnings from intake. These indicators have been used across PWI programs to assess comparative effectiveness and efficiency. More emphasis is needed to examine the applicability of these and other indicators in assessments of public and private rehabilitation providers.

A FRAMEWORK FOR REHABILITATION PLACEMENT EMPLOYMENT OUTCOMES RESEARCH

Use of an organizational framework to consolidate findings can clarify trends in the available research (Vandergoot, 1987). For purposes of the present review, findings will be discussed in relation to the rehabilitation participant, the counselor, the employer, and the services provided. These categories of consideration are not exhaustive, but do address major issues of relevance and lead to specific recommendations for agency administrators, rehabilitation providers, and researchers.

The Vocational Rehabilitation Client/Consumer

There are a number of issues relating to employment outcomes that specifically relate to the consumer, including demographics, specific types of disabilities, consumer involvement in the rehabilitation process confidence, or expectancies regarding potential outcomes. However, reviewing the relationship of specific types of disabilities to outcomes is beyond the scope of this summary, so we limit our discussion here to historical factors and client expectancies.

DEMOGRAPHICS AND HISTORICAL FACTORS

The prediction of outcomes using demographic and historical variables has long been a subject of study in VR (Bolton, Bellini, & Brookings, 2000). Gender may predict outcome, with men having greater employment success (Rabren, Hall, & Brown, 2003). Older individuals are also less likely to achieve employment success (Ponsford, Olver, Curran, & Ng, 1995). Race and ethnicity also have been related to outcome, with minority and underprivileged backgrounds sometimes predicting less provision of services and less successful outcomes (Kreutzer et al., 2003; Moore, 2001a, 2001b; Moore, Alstron, Donnell, & Hollis, 2003; Moore, Feist-Price, & Alston, 2002), although findings in this regard are mixed (Cifu et al., 1997; Rabren, Hall, & Brown, 2003). Lack of high school education may also hinder employment outcomes (Kreutzer et al., 2003). Past work experience (Dean, 1991; Keyser-Marcus et al., 2002; Majunder, Walls, Fullmer, & Misra, 1997) also appears to relate strongly to outcome.

In a broad study that controlled for a number of variables, Bolton, Bellini, and Brookings (2000) incorporated a composite "Scale of Social Disadvantage" comprised of these variables (including age, education, marital status, financial assistance, family income at referral, employment status, and three disability status items) to determine contribution to employment outcomes of demographic factors relative to the contributions of functional limitations and services provided. These demographic and historical factors generally predicted competitive employment outcomes and salary at closure across an array of disability groups including orthopedic, chronic medical, psychiatric, mental retardation, and learning disabilities, above and beyond the contributions of provision of services and functional limitations. These authors argue that ease of collection of historical variables combined with their value in predicting outcomes makes the modest effort involved worthwhile, even if these variables are generally not modifiable.

Self-Efficacy

Consumer choice and empowerment are major emphases in the VR system. Eden and Aviram (1993) demonstrated a link between increasing general self-efficacy (perceived ability to achieve goals) and increasing job search behavior—although the focus was not specifically on individuals with disabilities. Regenold, Sherman, and Fenzel (1999) found that self-efficacy predicted attainment of employment goals among individuals with psychiatric disabilities in a supported employment program. Similarly, Caplan, Vinokur, Price, and van Ryn (1989) demonstrate a link between increases in specific self-efficacy (confidence in achieving job-related goals) and earnings among re-employed participants (again, not specifically individuals with disabilities). Self-efficacy, and even improved employment outcomes, may be fostered by professionals holding positive opinions of the talents, skills, and spirit of consumers (Gowdy, Carlson, & Rapp, 2003). Further evaluation of strategies regarding consumer involvement in the VR process could prove useful, as could studies of factors that facilitate consumer confidence, hope, and self-efficacy.

REHABILITATION PRACTITIONERS AND THE CLIENT-COUNSELOR RELATIONSHIP

Few formal evaluations have been done regarding the impact of counselor traits, although several studies are instructive. Koch (2001) found that VR consumers prefer meaningful involvement in services with a facilitative counselor possessing expert knowledge, specific information about all available VR processes, active participation in plan development, and some commitment of effort to personal development issues. McCarthy and Leierer (2001) found that rehabilitation consumers prefer counselors who display clear commitment to the program participant by communicating the importance of the counseling endeavor.

In earlier research by Zadny and James (1977a, 1977b), there was a relationship between counselors who felt knowledgeable about labor market information and placement outcome. There appears to be a demand, particularly within the PWI movement, for counselors with a thorough understanding of the labor market, current business practices, and the relationship between impairments and job functions (Fraser, 1999). There is also an interest within the PWI movement in recruiting counselors with the capacity to conduct vocational assessments linked to current job market demands and with business communication skills and marketing ability (Fraser, 1999). State agencies are using a variety of placement staffing strategies, yet little research exists as to their respective effectiveness in terms of employment outcomes (Gilbride & Stensrud, 2003).

Several factors influence how current placement activities should be considered and conducted, including rehabilitation counselor competencies such as knowledge of the labor market, employer needs and employer-centered services, legislation, and holistic consumer supports, as well as consumer expectations for employment outcomes and choice (Gilbride & Stensrud, 2003). Ford and Swett (1999) note that placement competencies have changed in recent years. It has become important to be able to educate consumers about available choice, to understand the One Stop system, and grasp Social Security benefit situations and additional funding options. These studies provide a basis for the direction of future research in the measurement and impact of counselor competencies, such as provision of relevant information, facilitative style, and investment in client outcomes.

Regarding the client-counselor relationship, Schelat (2001) found that summary scores on a measure of working alliance (including the elements of goals, tasks, and bonds) strongly predicted the likelihood of successful VR closures. Lustig and colleagues (Lustig, Strauser, Rice, & Rucker, 2002; Lustig, Strauser, Weems, Donnell, & Smith, 2003) found that positive working alliance predicted employment outcomes, expectancies regarding future employment, and job satisfaction. One research group (Chan, Shaw, McMahon, Koch, & Strauser, 1997; McMahon, Shaw, Chan, & Danczyk-Hawley, 2004; Shaw, McMahon, Chan, & Hannold, 2004) has already developed assessment tools and a training protocol designed to improve the match between rehabilitation providers and consumers regarding the expectancies about the rehabilitation endeavor and to improve the working alliance.

Further study regarding the role of the counselor-consumer working alliance in VR practices would be valuable. This could be followed by the investigation of the relative contribution to the alliance of specific elements of counselor-consumer agreement on relevant tasks, goals, and bonds. Also beneficial would be investigation or brief, effective therapeutic approaches focusing upon increasing counselor empathy and warmth, enhancing consumer engagement, addressing resistance to change, and increasing self-efficacy. Motivational interviewing (Miller & Rollnick, 2002; Wagner & McMahon, 2004) is one such approach with considerable evidence (much of it from controlled clinical trials) demonstrating effectiveness with such wide-ranging issues as substance abuse, medication adherence, exercise behavior, smoking cessation, and problem gambling.

EMPLOYMENT SERVICES

Gilbride, Stensrud, and Johnson (1994) report that nearly all job development and placement work is provided by one of four sources: general rehabilitation counselors, placement specialists, contracted providers, and supported employment programs. Gilbride and Stensrud (2003) indicate that most agencies use a combination of these service providers, that the categories are not mutually exclusive, and that although providers often operate in these different roles, they generally use similar approaches. Gilbride (2000) reports that generalist rehabilitation counselors provide over half of placement services, and that among other providers the use of specialists is increasing (relative to contract and supported employment providers), from a level of 20% in 2000 to an anticipated level of approximately 30% in 2005. Earlier research (Stevens, Boland, & Ransom, 1982) indicated that using placement specialists resulted in higher levels of employment outcome. The extent to which such a finding applies today is unknown, although concerns have been raised about the cost efficiency of high use of specialists (Vandergoot, 1987) and the possibility that, as use of specialists grows, the placement knowledge and skills of generalist providers will decrease (Gilbride, 2000). In any case, further research is needed on the relative advantages of specific services being provided by professionals in specific roles.

A cursory review of the employment services literature will reveal a vast array of employment services and models. Because similar services often are offered under different models and labels, and because purportedly different services often overlap in their basic tasks, differentiation of services for the purpose of review is challenging. To facilitate the process of review, we organize services into a sequential framework for this chapter. As the rehabilitation process centers on facilitating change, we draw upon the well-known stages of change model (Prochaska, DiClemente, & Norcross, 1992) to organize the effort into the phases of precontemplation, contemplation, preparation, action, and maintenance. Although the model was initially developed to describe stages of individual change (i.e., not contemplating change, considering making changes, deciding to make changes and preparing to implement plans, implementing plans, and sustaining new behaviors over time), it has been used for several years as a model to organize and sequence services for substance-related problems (DiClemente & Valasquez, 2002; Ingersoll, Wagner, & Gharib, 2000). To the best of our knowledge, no one has used the stages of change model to organize VR interventions, although it is fairly consistent with a number of stage-based individualistic career counseling models. However, because it is somewhat more general than career counseling models, it allows for better integration of employer-oriented services.

Precontemplation phase rehabilitation services focus on developing awareness and interest, and are primarily outreach in nature, marketing rehabilitation services to potential consumers and potential employers. Contemplative services are those that involve the tasks of contemplating the needs, desires, and abilities of both consumer and employer, along with the available opportunities for both in a potential future relationship. These services include assessment of client abilities and interests, exploration of job and career options, and, on the business side, development of rehabilitation-business relationships, assessment of employer needs, and development of potential job opportunities. Preparatory services include consumer education and skill training efforts, job-seeking skills training and support on the consumer side. On the employer side, preparatory activities include formal job analysis, consultation regarding potential accommodations and work modifications, and exploration of natural supports available to future employees placed in the setting. Action phase activities include job placement and on-the-job training, mentoring and coaching, as well as facilitation of the development of relationships between the new employee and others in the worksite, including both supervisors and coworkers. Maintenance activities include an array of support and assistive services, job retention services, and career enhancement services.

OUTREACH AND MARKETING

Marketing and outreach to individuals with disabilities continues to be a priority for rehabilitation providers. Individuals with disabilities may not be aware of the existence of providers and the services they offer. In a sobering assessment, Bruyère (2000) reports that only approximately 5% of individuals with disabilities utilized disability-specific employment programs to locate employment.

Employers apparently are also unaware of vocational rehabilitation services, or have an inadequate understanding of the services provided (Janni, Reenewitz, May, & Dallas, 1992). Kirchner, Johnson, and Arkans (1997) indicated that few employers report being contacted by VR. Additionally, employers may not know how to access referrals or may be distrustful due to less than desirable experiences with agency performance after placement (Stensrud, 1999). There appears to be no "single brand identity" for the public rehabilitation system as a personnel resource to our country's employers. If employment outcome is the goal, an agency's hiring resource identity merits substantive attention. Research addressing education and outreach initiatives and their impact on employment access would be beneficial to the VR system and to individuals with disabilities.

Zadny (1980) indicated that the employers who are contacted the most are those that hire the most, yet Young, Rosati, and Vandergoot (1986) found that only 30% of employers surveyed had been contacted even once by a rehabilitation agency. The nature of marketing contacts may be important as well. Direct contact may be better understood and received by employers than relatively ineffective mail marketing or more global media public-relations approaches (Vandergoot, 1987).

TABLE 8.1 Stages of Change and Vocational Rehabilitation Services

Stage	Consumer	Employer
Precontemplation	Consumer outreach	Marketing to businesses
Contemplation	Assessment Career counseling	Development of employer relationships
Preparation	Job development and placement	Job development and placement
	Job and job-seeking training	Development of workplace supports
Action	Job coaching Supportive services	Early employment assistance/consultation
Maintenance	Job retention and career enhancement services	Long-term problem resolution consultation

ASSESSMENT AND CAREER COUNSELING

Assessment practices in VR include interviews, standardized tests, transferable skills analysis, work samples, and situational assessments. Assessment that focuses on consumer skills, interests, preferences, and support needs may lead to better outcomes than assessment that focuses on deficits or limitations (Sarkees-Wircenski & Wircenski, 1994). Ideally, the actual assessment processes used should be directly derived from the specific goals of assessment for each individual. Various theories have been developed to assist in matching individuals with jobs, but some have recently called into question the usefulness of theories in light of the complexities involved in accurately predicting employment success for people with disabilities (Parker & Schaller, 2003), referring to extant theories as "overly simplistic and fundamentally flawed" (p. 167).

Similar concerns over traditional standardized paper-and-pencil testing led to the development of practices relying more on work samples and situational assessments (LeBlanc, Hayden, & Paulman, 2000). These practices assess direct performance of vocational tasks. The tasks may be real or simulated, in controlled settings or in the workplace, and may be performed discretely or over a period of days. Rao and Kilgore (1992) used situational assessment to predict employment outcome of individuals with brain injuries with an accuracy between 70% and 85% (Rao & Kilgore, 1992). LeBlanc, Hayden, and Paulson (2000) found no individual neuropsychological test that could accurately predict the vocational performance of individuals with closed head injury in a work setting, and concluded that situational assessment is critical in predicting real-world employment outcomes. Relatedly, O'Neill (2002) found that higher performing VR offices serving individuals with brain injuries used more community-based vocational assessments and psychosocial services, while low-producing offices more frequently used facility-based neuropsychological and psychological evaluations.

Career counseling involves the entire process of assessment, development of vocational goals and career plans, implementation of plans, and, in recent models, follow-up activities such as assistance with post-employment adjustment, adaptation, and advancement (Hershenson & Liesener, 2003; Salomone, 1996). As noted previously, a number of career counseling models are stage-based and similar to the more general stages of change model. Hershenson and Liesener (2003) note that vocational professionals are supported in expecting lower career decision-making self-efficacy and a pessimistic attributional style among individuals with disabilities, but should be careful not to assume these will be true of any given individual. They also note that practitioners should accommodate for the different attitudes and career implications that may differentiate individuals with precareer onset disabilities, midcareer onset disabilities, and those with progressive and episodic disabilities.

DEVELOPMENT OF EMPLOYER RELATIONSHIPS

Demand-side approaches to vocational rehabilitation focus on developing lasting relationships with employers that serve to appropriately match employers and employees, rather than focusing on consumer needs while overlooking the needs and preferences of employers. Gilbride and Stensrud (2003) counsel rehabilitation professionals to take care to develop relationships with the right employers, preferably those serving the primary labor market (i.e., jobs with decent wages, benefits, and some degree of worker autonomy) (Hagner, 2000) and those with characteristics that are more amenable to persons with disabilities (Gilbride, Stensrud, Vandergoot, & Golden, 2003). The PWI program attempts to formalize such relationships through Business Advisory Councils that advise rehabilitation professionals on employment opportunities and skills needs. Over the past decade, successful placement of individuals into competitive employment through PWI has exceeded 60% (although 2003 data show a decline to a 53% placement rate). The rates of placement for consumers who were previously unemployed have continued to increase, peaking in 2003 at over 73% (U.S. Department of Education, 2004). Buys and Rennie (2001) identified that elements of effective partnership include a commitment to community responsibility by employers; competency in service delivery by the agencies (responsive, reliable, and consistent); development of trust between agencies and employers; a customer focus by agencies; an exchange of benefits between parties; and a prolonged period of working together.

Developing sound working relationships with employers can be facilitated by viewing employers not simply as outlets for worker placements, but as partners in the process who may have their own idiosyncratic norms, attitudes, interests, needs, and concerns. Viewing things in this way may help to avoid having challenges turn into standoffs. For example, some studies (e.g., Kirchner, Johnson, & Arkans, 1997) indicate that individuals with disabilities perceive discriminatory employer attitudes to be problematic. Likewise, Unger (2002) found that employers had concerns regarding the work potential of employees with disabilities that may be a result of myths or preconceptions and not a result of direct experiences with workers with disabilities. While findings like these may tempt rehabilitation professionals to directly confront negative attitudes, stereotypes, and preconceptions, such advocacy may not serve in consumers' best interests. Instead, it may be beneficial to take a viewpoint that employers' attitudes may simply stem from having little time to devote to personnel issues, and having concern over new initiatives that may further compromise schedules and possibly introduce new complexities into the business environment. This is not to claim that there are no actual discriminatory attitudes in the workplace, but simply that it may be in consumers' bests interests to first extend the benefit of the doubt to employers and assume that such resistance results more from situational factors than internal biases.

In support of assuming this more tolerant viewpoint toward the situation are findings that employers are increasingly expressing more positive attitudes about hiring workers with disabilities (Levy, Jessop, Rimmerman, & Levy, 1993). Although these attitudes may have a social equality component, they may also result from pressure towards or interest in enhancing diversity of their workforce and community image (Nietupski, Harme-Nietupski, Vanerhart, & Fishback, 1996). Alternatively, some employers' interest may result primarily from the possibility of increasing profits by lowering personnel costs. Although this may strike some in the human services fields as callous, this is a central element of modern business practice that is unrelated to the disability status of the workers involved. Rehabilitation professionals who can accept this may paradoxically have more opportunity to influence norms and practices than professionals who do not accept this viewpoint and put their efforts toward confronting it rather than remaining focused on seeking the best feasible outcomes for their customers.

One challenge is that although employers may have increasing willingness to hire individuals with disabilities, such willingness may not regularly translate into action (Hernanadez, Keys, & Balcazar, 2000). There may be a number of factors involved in preventing the transition from contemplation to action regarding this issue, and some research has documented some likely hindrances, as well as potential opportunities. Stensrud (1999) determined that employers may not know how to access the public and private agencies providing employment services to people with disabilities and therefore may not know how to recruit new workers from this pool. Bruyère (2000) found that barriers to employment for individuals with disabilities included lack of supervisor knowledge of accommodation and attitudes and stereotypes. Unger (2002) found that employers value dependable employees, even if performance rate is diminished, and that employers with previous experience with workers with disabilities are more positive about disability issues and amenable to hiring workers with disabilities. Studies also indicate that employers are interested in agencies that can meet their needs (Greenwood, Fletcher-Schriner, & Johnson, 1991), desire clients with both work and interpersonal skills who have been prescreened for their specific job openings, and desire follow-up services (Young et al., 1986). Rehabilitation professionals may be able to directly reduce these barriers to employment through outreach and marketing, developing more employer-friendly referral mechanisms, demonstrating high quality of training and follow-up regarding workers, and providing training and consultation to employers about concerns and possibilities.

In fact, vocational rehabilitation professionals have valuable specialist knowledge to offer employers in relation to a wide array of issues, including accessibility issues, ADA requirements, use of task analysis to explicitly define jobs for hiring purposes, ergonomic design, training of employees to make the best use of on-site supports, worker compensation consulting, disability awareness training, and other issues. Gilbride (2000) documents that over 80% of state rehabilitation agencies provide some sort of employer consultation services. In addition to general consultation, rehabilitation professionals can help employers specifically with conducting job searches and interviews among individuals with disabilities, problem-solving challenges that arise after placement, and long-term follow-up.

JOB DEVELOPMENT AND PLACEMENT

Since World War I, job development and placement have arguably been the prototypical vocational rehabilitation tasks. Many other common VR tasks developed as a means to facilitate placement (e.g., job-seeking skills training, job analysis) (Gilbride & Stensrud, 2003). Over the years, rehabilitation professionals have had an increasing number of tasks requiring their attention and the role of placement in the VR process may have lessened somewhat, yet recent research and writing may be moving placement back toward a more central role. In perhaps the most sophisticated research yet examining the factors contributing to success, Bolton, Bellini, and Brookins (2000) found that among more than 4,600 public rehabilitation consumers, provision of job placement services was the greatest contributor to successful outcome (compared to consumer demographic/historical factors, consumer functional limitations, and other rehabilitation services). This finding builds upon other findings (Moore, Feist-Price, & Alston, 2002; Rumrill, Roessler, & Cook, 1995) to underscore the importance of job placement in the rehabilitation arena.

There are a number of different placement services delivery models, including individual selective job matching, a generic or marketing approach, traditional placement, and networking (Temelini & Fesko, 1996). Expanded approaches can include client-focused preparatory activity, supported employment, or a demand-side placement effort—encouraging the need within the business community (Gilbride & Stensrud, 1992). A networking approach to placement services appears to be both effective and cost-effective (Hagner, 2003; Temelini & Fesko, 1996). This involves networking efforts in building and maintaining employer accounts and involving the consumer in goal setting, networking contacts within the community, and building a social and vocational network. In networking activity, it may be important to develop friends or associates who are work-related contacts, as an important element for employers is that information is received from a trusted intermediary (Hagner, 2003; Owens-Johnson & Hanely-Maxwell, 1999). Networking activities might also be emphasized because many individuals with disabilities secure work on their own. Stoddard, Jans, Ripple, and Kraus (1998) report that 52% of employed adults with disabilities find their jobs via personal contacts and 13% via help-wanted ads, compared to only 5% who found employment using rehabilitation employment services. In addition to networking, Hagner (2003) describes other supported elements of the job development and placement process to include promoting maximum involvement of the job seeker (which in itself is viewed positively by employers), paying attention to stigma (including considering changing renaming of employment agencies if they are likely to reinforce stigma), working with employers to design, carve, and create jobs (including offering job analyses to employers), and using incentives and training/coaching services in ways that "sweeten" the deal versus ways that raise employer concerns about the potential neediness of consumers.

Recent developments such as the federal Ticket to Work and Workforce Investment acts significantly affect job placement. In addition to reducing disincentives related to earnings in the SSDI program, the Ticket to Work Act decentralizes rehabilitation services, shifting power from bureaucracies toward consumers by providing consumers control over which services and providers they use in their rehabilitation efforts. The Workforce Investment Act prescribes consolidation of services into one-stop rehabilitation agencies to reduce duplication of effort, increase consumer ease of using services, and encourage holistic multidisciplinary and multidomain approaches to rehabilitation. One-stop agencies may also be more business-friendly, reducing employer confusion regarding which services are provided where, and increasing the likelihood that employers will seek out and rely upon rehabilitation providers as a source of potential employees (Gilbride & Stensrud, 2003). A challenge is to prevent one-stop agencies from losing a person-centered approach to rehabilitation and focus on career development and becoming employee mills for low-paying high-turnover jobs (Gilbride & Stensrud, 2003).

JOB TRAINING AND JOB SEEKING

Job training services and job-seeking skills training are intended to help consumers move from contemplation of job possibilities to a state of preparedness to obtain work. A variety of training strategies may be used to prepare consumers for specific jobs and for workplace interactions, either in controlled settings or the actual workplace. There is some evidence suggesting that limiting prevocational training and providing training directly in the workplace may lead to better employment outcomes, and this approach has been adopted in supported employment programs (Gowdy, Carlson, & Rapp, 2003).

Job-seeking skills include developing resumes and cover letters, developing job search strategies, finding available job opportunities, selecting and applying to appropriate positions, interviewing with potential employers, and negotiating job offers. Azrin and Philip (1979) developed a structured job club model, providing job-seeking skills instruction while also reinforcing job-seeking behaviors through social support. Research has suggested that job clubs may increase career search self-efficacy (Sterrett, 1998), interviewing skills (Corrigan, Reedy, Thadani, &Ganet, 1995), and placement outcomes (Azrin & Philip, 1979). These models continue to show effectiveness (Brooks, Nackerud, & Risler, 2001) and yet may remain underutilized by rehabilitation providers. Further exploration of which aspects of these approaches are the most successful and with what populations would help to refine these efforts (Ouellette & Dwyer, 1983).

JOB COACHING

The focus of coaching can range from simple skill-based problems to broad challenges in the development of individuals with disabilities into productive, satisfied, and stable workers (Hanley-Maxwell, Owens-Johnson, & Fabian, 2003). Coaching includes direct skill training, development of well-functioning supervisory relationships, assistance in increasing productivity and quality of work, and refinement of job-related social skills and workplace behavior. Coaching can have significant effects. Gray, McDermott, and Butkus (2000) found that coaching of individuals with intellectual disabilities (at a rate of one coach per hundred workers) increased employment by a factor of 10 in an urban setting. If replicated, this finding suggests the approach can be highly effective and highly cost-effective with this subpopulation.

Some have concluded that the individual job coach model is effective, but also expensive (Menz, 1997). One goal of job coaches is to train workers while retaining a focus on development of greater autonomy through instruction and environmental modifications that support greater independence and work functioning. Unfortunately, a naturalistic study of coaching practices indicated that coaches did not decrease involvement with workers over time, but instead maintained steady differences in the amount of on-site presence that appeared unrelated to need, and related instead to worker racial status (Cimera, Rusch, & Heal, 1998).

Parsons, Reid, Green, and Browning (2001) developed an alternating on-site/off-site approach to job coaching of individuals with multiple severe disabilities, in which workers participated in an off-site day program on nonwork days, tailored to specific needs as assessed in the workplace. After development of additional work skills and beneficial work environment modifications in the off-site workshop, these skills and adaptations were integrated back into the workplace with no apparent resulting decrease in work productivity, and with reduced need for continued coaching. Such an approach may have cost-effectiveness benefits as an alternative to the more expensive approach of providing job coaching services primarily on-site, and has potential for reducing stigma for the worker as well (by maximizing worker autonomy while on-site and avoiding the presence of a professional assistant in the workplace when possible) (Hanley-Maxwell, Owens-Johnson, & Fabian, 2003). Farris and Stancliffe (2001) demonstrated some success toward similar goals with a coworker coaching model, which maintained similar outcomes to the professional coaching model, increased the amount of assistance and support workers received on-site, and provided workers with high levels of social involvement in the workplace.

SUPPORTIVE SERVICES

In order to ensure a successful employment experience, several support services and strategies may be considered depending on the needs of the individual. These may include incorporating personal assistance services, accessibility services, and natural, community, and workplace supports. Long-term supports, featured in supported employment programs, may help maximize employment success, integration, and job retention. Extended supports often are critical to the long-term employment success of individuals with severe disabilities, yet they remain among the least analyzed and researched components of employment services (Brook, Inge, Armstrong, & Wehman, 1997).

The Benefits Planning, Assistance, and Outreach (BPA&O) initiative was established by the Ticket to Work and Work Incentives Improvement Act (WIIA) of 1999 to remove employment disincentives associated with a fear of loss of benefits and health care. Benefits planning services include information and referral; problem-solving and advocacy; benefits counseling; long-term benefits assistance; and follow-up services. The Rehabilitation Services Administration is currently investigating the implications of benefits planning and assistance for the roles of rehabilitation professionals and the potential impact on employment of individuals with disabilities.

Personal Assistance Services (PAS) can contribute to integration and empowerment of workers with disabilities (Hagglund, Clark, Mokelke, & Stout, 2004). PAS help individuals with disabilities to accomplish activities of daily living (ADLs) and other tasks. Workplace assistance services include task-related assistance such as lifting or moving items, interpreters for individuals who are deaf, and as assistance with ADLs while at work (Center for Personal Assistance Services, 2004). Unfortunately, while task-related assistance is promoted under the ADA, the ADA does not address PAS in the worksite and individuals may be left to arrange and pay for this on their own (Job Accommodation Network, 2004). Given the high percentage of working-age individuals with self-care difficulties who are not working, work-related PAS services could affect the employability of this population (Bader, 2003).

ACCESSIBILITY, ACCOMMODATIONS, AND ASSISTIVE TECHNOLOGY

Accessibility addresses both structures and services: physical, environmental, and architectural access as well as access to written materials and content such as brochures, websites, and so forth. Approximately 82% of private sector employers and 93% of public sector employers report that they have made facilities accessible (Bruyère, 2000). However, accessibility remains an issue of concern within the one-stop service delivery system (Bader, 2003).

Loprest and Maag (2001) found that 29% of individuals with disabilities reported that transportation was a barrier to finding work. This figure may increase in rural areas where public transportation is not available. Transportation and the development of innovative services have received attention by the federal government, although attempts to increase transportation funding for people with disabilities have not met with much recent success.

In terms of accommodations, Loprest and Maag (2001) determined that one third of nonworking persons with disabilities reported the need for specific accommodations. Bruyère (2000) reports that the most common types of accommodations include: facility accessibility, flexible human resource policies, restructured jobs and work hours, transportation accommodations, written job instructions, and modified work environments. Bruyère found that although considerable progress has been made, barriers remain to the recruitment, hiring, retention, and career advancement of adults with disabilities that warrant consideration.

Assistive technology initially received attention in the 1970s and 1980s (Malik, High, Yuspeh, & Mueller, 1978; Tooman, 1982) in relation to successful placement, but its value for improving employment outcomes is not yet fully established in the research literature and it may remain underutilized in the community (Bader, 2003). However, assistive technology has been cited for increasing employment opportunities for individuals with disabilities (Langton & Ramseur, 2001). Cook (2001) suggests that assistive technology will continue to become a more central part of rehabilitation due to increases in user-friendliness, and improvements in computer software, internet distribution, and intranet networking. Scherer (2002) recommends that rehabilitation professionals focus on facilitating use of technologies among consumers, rather than focusing on the mere availability of technological resources.

Career Stability and Enhancement Services

Millington, Miller, Asner-Self, and Linkowski (2003) call on vocational rehabilitation professionals to "abandon the notion that employment is an event—the event of being hired or of returning to work." They argue that it is in the best interests of consumers to have continuing success as the primary goal of rehabilitation, and that such a focus best serves business needs as well, as it is in stability of work that individuals truly gain greater autonomy and employers are reinforced for viewing this as profitable rather than charitable. They also emphasize that neglecting this focus may contribute to limiting rehabilitation outcomes, citing a U.S. General Accounting Office study (1993) showing that across public VR programs, employment gains generally lasted only about two years. Similarly, Rumrill and Roessler (1999) call for a career development perspective in which the focus is on evaluating employment outcomes utilizing qualitative criteria, providing on the job consultation regarding productivity barriers and reasonable accommodations while concurrently redefining successful closure.

Although there has been much discussion in the literature regarding career stability and enhancement efforts (Crimando, Belcher, & Riggar, 1986), there is relatively little research in these areas to date. In one exception to this trend, Allaire, Niu, and LaValley (2005) used a randomized control design to determine the effectiveness of a job retention program for individuals with chronic rheumatic diseases, finding a significant effect on job retention up to 42 months following the intervention.

Several studies indicate that the career development and postemployment needs of people with disabilities are not being adequately addressed by VR providers. Roessler (2002) states that there is a need for job retention services in rehabilitation based upon the statistics regarding unemployment and job loss rates for people with disabilities. Similarly, Allaire, Niu, and LaValley (2005) reflect that individuals with chronic diseases, who make up a key target for job retention services, are significantly underserved in public VR programs relative to population base and percentage of persons with work limitations. To improve retention outcomes, rehabilitation researchers must identify the key factors impacting employment tenure and the effectiveness of interventions designed to address those factors (Roessler, 2002). Rumrill and colleagues (2000) suggest that VR providers employ career maintenance specialists in an effort to address this service gap.

SUPPORTED EMPLOYMENT

Whereas the previously described services generally focus on one phase of the VR process, supported employment programs are intended to provide ongoing services from assessment through job retention and career stability efforts. Supported employment (SE) is a general model of services designed for working with individuals with significant disabilities, who may substantially benefit from multiple services and extended support. Supported employment is less a package of particular services than a flexible approach to offering individualized assistance, with a bias toward initiating work as soon as possible and providing assistance toward physical and social integration in the workplace, as opposed to a more traditional model of prevocational training services and focus (Hanley-Maxwell, Owens-Johnson, & Fabian, 2003). In light of the stages of change model, it can be viewed as a multistage approach, bridging from precontemplation to maintenance.

SE has been effective in increasing competitive employment, particularly for individuals with significant disabilities (Gamble & Moore, 2003; Twamley, Jeste, & Lehman, 2003; Wehman, Revell, & Kregel, 1998). Gamble and Moore (2003) examined the effect of supported employment in an additive research design (i.e., SE was added to other services) in a sample of over a thousand public vocational rehabilitation clients with traumatic brain injury. Although there was no randomization of services, they statistically controlled for a variety of participant demographic and historical factors and found that supported employment predicted better VR outcomes in regards to case closure status and weekly earnings. Bond (2004) found support for SE services for individuals with mental illness in his review of available controlled trials, summarizing that SE may double or triple rates of employment, which then mediates increases in self-esteem and symptom control. Twamley, Jeste, and Lehman (2003) reviewed the small (nine studies) pool of randomized controlled trials of supported employment services for individuals with schizophrenia and other psychotic disorders, also finding that SE (or the related individual placement and support approach) nearly tripled the number of participants who found competitive work (51% to 18% of controls), for a weighted mean effects size of 0.79. Becker, Smith, Tanzman, Drake, and Tremblay (2001) found that two components of supported employment significantly related to the best employment outcomes for individuals with psychiatric disabilities: community-based services and the use of employment specialists. Bond and colleagues (2001) found that competitive work (versus sheltered or no employment) not only increased satisfaction with services and improved finances, it also promoted improvements in self-esteem and psychiatric symptoms.

Some studies have found that supported employment is a good investment for taxpayers (Cimera, 1998; Schneider, 2003), even providing a net savings to taxpayers because of savings in social security payments and alternative placements. However, Cimera contends that further exploration of how to make these programs even more cost-effective is desirable, especially in light of challenging economic times and dwindling resources of external funders.

SUMMARY

Considerable research has been done over the past decade related to employment practices in vocational rehabilitation that both documents the effectiveness of field-based developments and points the way toward increasingly effective practice for vocational rehabilitation professionals. Nevertheless, much remains unknown, and research outcomes often raise new questions.

A number of rehabilitation trends are consistent with empirical findings. The move from segregation toward integration is one. Research supports rehabilitation practice being done in the community and in the workplace, rather than in rehabilitation agencies and workshops. Rehabilitation professionals increase the likelihood of success by assisting participants to assume as much ownership as possible of the job-seeking process and supporting them in their transition to new employment rather than primarily focusing on prevocational skill preparation and provider-driven placement. Creative efforts are being made to develop approaches that are cost-efficient hybrids of the supported employment approach—capitalizing on the apparent value of providing extended workplace support, while also supporting more autonomy among placed workers, increasing integration into the workplace by using peer coaches, supervisors, and trainers rather than external rehabilitation personnel when possible, and helping employers develop ongoing methods of support and assistance that are similar to those provided to all workers. Viewing workplace supports as falling along a continuum from employer-provided to agency-provided allows for flexible matching between the specific needs of workers with disabilities and the best approach toward providing supports that help without creating dependencies, that support without being paternalistic, and that assist without stigmatizing (Ohtake & Chadsey, 2001).

Greater community integration means not only focusing more on competitive community employment for consumers, but also on community involvement by rehabilitation professionals. A number of employer-focused rehabilitation practices appear useful—including (a) seeking input from employers regarding their needs and preferences, (b) developing of partnerships and consortia, (c) consulting regarding accommodations, hiring practices, and legal issues, and (d) integrating disability-awareness issues into regular on-site training focused on workplace or diversity issues. Demand-side efforts can be mutually beneficial to employers and rehabilitation participants, and rehabilitation professionals may be more effective by capitalizing on this viewpoint versus implicitly reinforcing a viewpoint that businesses should employ workers with disability out of a sense of social responsibility or charity. Consistent with this greater focus on the marketplace, the rehabilitation effort is likely to be more successful to the extent that rehabilitation agencies continue to adopt user-friendly practices—easily accessible services, centralized referral assistance for employers and consumers alike, extended workplace support beyond placement and initial transition, long-term consulting relationships with employers, and career enhancement assistance for workers.

These changes appear to be part of a general transition from a hierarchical model in which rehabilitation professionals controlled or led efforts—assessing potential workers, providing prevocational training, then placing them in segregated workshops that contract to provide goods and services to businesses—toward a less hierarchical model in which the role of rehabilitation professionals is somewhat lessened regarding control over the process while consumers, employers, and coworkers gain greater involvement in the process. Rehabilitation professionals increasingly serve rather than guide consumers—helping them to determine their strengths and challenges, gain confidence in their abilities, match their interests with opportunities in the labor market, own the skill-building and job-seeking process, and use natural and professional supports to increase job satisfaction and develop an advancing career in the primary labor market. Rehabilitation professionals increasingly serve rather than simply access employers—helping them to develop environments, policies, and practices that support increasing integration of workers with disabilities and increase retention of those workers and enhancement of their skills. Rehabilitation professionals also increasingly incorporate natural and formal supports in the workplace, including use of workplace human resources programs and workplace training and supervision efforts, so that standard workplace practices increasingly support workers with disabilities rather than leave support of these workers to rehabilitation personnel.

As the population continues to age, the opportunities and challenges for vocational rehabilitation professionals will increasingly change. Age-related medical conditions will increasingly be represented in the workplace and will change the nature of the needs that the profession addresses. Where, to some degree, research and professional efforts have focused on the developmental needs of individuals who have traditionally been left out of the workplace, the aging of the population will require a greater focus on needed accommodations and adaptations for people who develop impairments mid-career. According to Koch and Rumrill (2003), these issues "have been largely ignored by researchers, practitioners, and policymakers alike over the past three decades" (p. 3).

Obviously, there are many other issues in need of further investigation. It is generally established that individualized employment in community workplaces facilitates development of satisfying careers that are characterized by increased wages and benefits, increased autonomy and empowerment, and increased workplace acceptance and support of individuals with disabilities (Hagner & Cooney, 2003). More research is needed on the best practices for facilitating these outcomes. Appropriate, detailed, and preferably standardized outcome variables need to be developed and used by researchers. Intervention and assistance techniques need to be further refined and investigated for their relative contributions to outcome, providing some direction regarding practical workplace issues (e.g., should placement efforts be given higher priority in allotment of professional effort relative to skills training services?). Practices for increasing consumer participation and investment in, and ownership of, the career development and job-seeking effort also need to be further investigated and refined. Research is needed to identify more effective career stability and enhancement strategies, and more effective supports and accommodations for consumers in the workplace. Effective practices need to be made increasingly efficient and flexible. Rehabilitation providers need guidance on effective and efficient business models, and on matching and combining intervention strategies for greatest effect. More research is needed on the expanding network of individuals, agencies, and business involved in the rehabilitation endeavor, and on effective ways of maximizing impact, increasing coordination of effort, and developing institutionalized practices that reduce barriers and foster empowerment and integration of individuals with disabilities in the workplace environment, with decreased reliance on the efforts of rehabilitation professionals. Finally, further research is needed on the crucial skills required by new rehabilitation professionals and the educational and training practices that best support development of these skills.

QUESTIONS FOR DISCUSSION AND/OR FURTHER STUDY

Service Domain

1. How do the authors use the stages of change model to conceptualize the delivery of vocational rehabilitation services?
2. What employer-focused rehabilitation practices appear to be useful in securing employment opportunities for people with disabilities?
3. What user-friendly practices provided by rehabilitation agencies may increase the placement, and subsequent employment success, of people with disabilities?

Research Domain

4. Describe examples of current research issues and/or gaps that need to be addressed to further explore the employment outcomes of people with disabilities.
5. What challenges may be extant in conducting research exploring best practices and employment outcomes of individuals with disabilities?

Policy Domain

6. In what ways has past research informed the development of legislative policy such as the Rehabilitation Act Amendments, the Work Incentives Act and Ticket to Work initiative, and the Workforce Investment Act?
7. What is the significance of developing a standardized means of reporting employment outcomes?

REFERENCES

Acemoglu, D., & Angrist, J. D. (2001). Consequences of employment protection? The case of the Americans with Disabilities Act. *Journal of Political Economy, 109*(5), 915–957.

Allaire, S. H., Niu, J., & LaValley, M. P. (2005). Employment and satisfaction outcomes from a job retention intervention delivered to persons with chronic diseases. *Rehabilitation Counseling Bulletin, 48,*100–109.

Azrin, N. H., & Philip, R. A. (1979). The job club method for the job handicapped: A comparative outcome study. *Rehabilitation Counseling Bulletin, 23*(2), 144–155.

Bader, B. A. (2003). Identification of best practices in One Stop Career Centers that facilitate use by people with disabilities seeking employment (Doctoral dissertation, Virginia Commonwealth University, 2003). *Dissertation Abstracts , 64,* 1864.

Becker, D. R., Smith, J., Tanzman, B., Drake, R. E., & Tremblay, T. (2001). Fidelity of supported employment programs and employment outcomes. *Psychiatric Services, 52,* 834–836.

Bell, M. D., Lysaker, P. H., & Milstein, R. M. (1996). Clinical benefits of paid work activity in schizophrenia. *Schizophrenia Bulletin, 22*(1), 51–67.

Berkowitz, M. (1985). Benefit cost analysis. In S. Moon, P. Goodhall, & P. Wehman (Eds.), *Proceedings from the First RRTC Symposium on Employment for Citizens Who Are Mentally Retarded: Critical issues related to supported competitive employment.* Richmond: Virginia Commonwealth University, Rehabilitation Research and Training Center.

Bolton, B. F. (2001). Measuring rehabilitation outcomes. *Rehabilitation Counseling Bulletin, 44,* 67–75.

Bolton, B. F., Bellini, J. L., & Brookings, J. B. (2000). Predicting client employment outcomes from personal history, functional limitations, and rehabilitation services. *Rehabilitation Counseling Bulletin, 44,*10–21.

Bond, G. R. (2004). Supported employment: Evidence for an evidence-based practice. *Psychiatric Rehabilitation Journal, 27,* 345–359.

Bond, G. R., Resnick, S. G., Drake, R. E., Xie, H. Y., McHugo, G. J., & Bebout, R. R. (2001). Does competitive employment improve nonvocational outcomes for people with severe mental illness? *Journal of Consulting and Clinical Psychology, 69,* 489–501.

Bond, G., & McDonel, E. C. (1991). Vocational rehabilitation outcomes for persons with psychiatric disabilities: An update. *Journal of Vocational Rehabilitation, 1*(3), 9–20.

Brooke, V., Inge, K. J., Armstrong, A. J., & Wehman, P. (Eds.). (1997). *Supported employment handbook: A customer-driven approach for persons with significant disabilities.* Richmond, VA: Virginia Commonwealth University.

Brooks, F., Nackerud, L., & Risler, E. (2001). Evaluation of the job finding club for TANF recipients: Psychosocial impacts. *Research on Social Work Practice, 11,* 14.

Bruyère, S. (2000). *Disability employment policies and practices in private and federal sector organizations.* Ithaca, NY: Cornell University. Benefit Planning, Assistance, and Outreach Initiative. Retrieved November 23, 2004, from http://www.ilr.cornell.edu/ped/ssa_curriculum/2003_BPAO/2003_TEXT_EDITTED/IntroductionChapter.htm

Buys, N. J., & Rennie, J. (2001). Developing relationships between vocational rehabilitation agencies and employers. *Rehabilitation Counseling Bulletin, 44*(2), 95–103.

Callahan, M., Shumpert, N., & Mast, M. (2002). Self-employment, choice and self-determination. *Journal of Vocational Rehabilitation, 17,* 75–85.

Caplan, R. D., Vinokur, A. D., Price, R. H., & van Ryn, M. (1989). Job seeking, reemployment, and mental health: A randomized field experiment in coping with job loss. *Journal of Applied Psychology, 74,* 759–769.

Center for Personal Assistance Services. (2004). *Personal assistance services.* Retrieved December 15, 2004, from http://www.pascenter.org/home/index.php

Chan, F., Shaw, L. R., McMahon, B. T., Koch, L., & Strauser, D. (1997). A model for enhancing rehabilitation counselor-consumer working relationships. *Rehabilitation Counseling Bulletin, 41,* 122–137.

Cifu, D. X., Keyser-Marcus, L., Lopez, E., Wehman, P., Kreutzer, J. S., Englander, J., et al. (1997, February). Acute predictors of successful return to work 1 year after traumatic brain injury: A multi-center analysis. *Archives of Physical Medical Rehabilitation, 78,* 125–131.

Cimera, R. E. (1998). Are individuals with severe mental retardation and multiple disabilities cost-efficient to serve via supported employment programs? *Mental Retardation, 36,* 280–292.

Cimera, R. E., Rusch, F. R., & Heal, L. W. (1998). Supported employee independence from the presence of job coaches at work sites. *Journal of Vocational Rehabilitation, 10,* 51–63.

Cook, A. M. (2001). Future directions in assistive technology. In M. J. Scherer (Ed)., *Assistive technology: Matching device and consumer for successful rehabilitation* (pp. 269–279). Washington, DC: American Psychological Association, 2002.

Corrigan, P. W., Reedy, P., Thadani, D., & Ganet, M. (1995). Correlates of participation and completion in a job club for clients with psychiatric disability. *Rehabilitation Counseling Bulletin, 39,* 42–53.

Crimando, W., Belcher, K., & Riggar, T. F. (1986). Job retention problems of clients served in rehabilitation facilities. *Journal of Job Placement, 2,* 10–12.

Dean, D. H. (1991, Spring). Comparing employment-related outcomes of the vocational rehabilitation program using longitudinal earnings. *American Rehabilitation, 5–9.*

DiClemente, C. C., & Velasquez, M. W. (2002). Motivational interviewing and the stages of change. In W. R. Miller & S. Rollnick, *Motivational interviewing: Preparing people for change* (2nd ed., pp. 217–250). New York: Guilford.

Drebing, C. E., Van Ormer, E. A., Schutt, R. K., Krebs, C., Losardo, M. B., Penk, W., et al. (2004). Client goals for participating in VHA vocational rehabilitation: Distribution and relationship to outcome. *Rehabilitation Counseling Bulletin, 47,* 162–172.

Eden, D. V., & Aviram, A. (1993). Self-efficacy training to speed reemployment helping people to help themselves. *Journal of Applied Psychology, 78,* 352–360.

Fabian, E. S. (1991). Using quality-of-life indicators in rehabilitation program evaluation. *Rehabilitation Counseling Bulletin, 36,* 344–356.

Farris, B., & Stancliffe, R. J. (2001). The co-worker training model: Outcomes of an open employment pilot project. *Journal of Intellectual & Developmental Disability, 26,* 143–159.

Felce, D., & Perry, J. (1995). Quality of life: Its definition and measurement. *Research in Developmental Disabilities, 16,* 51–74.

Ford, L. H., & Swett, E. A. (1999). Job placement and rehabilitation counselors in the state-federal system. *Rehabilitation Counseling Bulletin, 42,* 354–365.

Fraser, R. T. (1999). Rehabilitation counselor placement-related attributes in the present economy: A Project With Industry perspective. *Rehabilitation Counseling Bulletin, 42,* 343–353.

Gamble, D., & Moore, C. L. (2003). Supported employment: Disparities in vocational rehabilitation outcomes, expenditures and service time for persons with traumatic brain injury. *Journal of Vocational Rehabilitation, 19,* 47–57.

Gibbs, W. E. (1991, Spring). Vocational rehabilitation outcome measures: The probability of employment and the duration of periods of employment. *American Rehabilitation, 40,* 10–13.

Gilbride, D. (2000). Going to work: Placement trends in public rehabilitation. *Journal of Vocational Rehabilitation, 14,* 89–94.

Gilbride, D., & Stensrud, R. (1992). Demand side job development: A model for the 1990s. *Journal of Rehabilitation, 58*(4), 34–39.

Gilbride, D., & Stensrud, R. (2003). Job placement and employer consulting: Services and strategies. In E. M. Szymanski, & R. M. Parker (Eds.), *Work and disability: Issues and strategies in career development and job placement* (2nd ed.). Austin, Texas: Pro-Ed.

Gilbride, D., Stensrud, R., & Johnson, M. (1994). Current models of job placement and employer development: Research, competencies and educational considerations. *Rehabilitation Education, 7,* 215–219.

Gilbride, D., Stensrud, R., Vandergoot, D., & Golden, K. (2003). Identification of the characteristics of work environments and employers open to hiring and accommodating people with disabilities. *Rehabilitation Counseling Bulletin, 46,* 130–137.

Gilbride, D. D., Thomas, J. R., & Stensrud, R. (1998). Beyond Status Code 26: Development of an instrument to measure the quality of placements in the state-federal program. *Journal of Applied Rehabilitation Counseling, 29,* 3–7.

Gowdy, E., Carlson, L., & Rapp, C. (2003). Practices differentiating high performing from low performing supported employment programs. *Psychiatric Rehabilitation Journal, 26,* 232–239.

Gray, B. R., McDermott, S., & Butkus, S. (2000). Effect of job coaches on employment likelihood for individuals with mental retardation. *Journal of Vocational Rehabilitation, 14,* 5–11.

Greenwood, R., Fletcher-Schriner, K., & Johnson, V. (1991). Employer concerns regarding workers with disabilities and the business-rehabilitation partnership: The PWI practitioners' perspective. *Journal of Rehabilitation, 51* (3), 37–45.

Hagglund, K. J., Clark, M. J., Mokelke, E. K., & Stout, B. J. (2004). The current state of personal assistance services: Implications for policy and future research. *NeuroRehabilitation, 19,* 115–120.

Hagner, D. (2000). Primary and secondary labor markets: Implications for vocational rehabilitation. *Rehabilitation Counseling Bulletin, 44,* 22–29.

Hagner, D. (2003). Job development and job search assistance. In E. M. Szymanski & R. M. Parker (Eds.), *Work and disability: Issues and strategies in career development and job placement* (2nd ed., pp. 343–372). Austin, Texas: Pro-Ed.

Hagner, D., & Cooney, B. (2003). Building employer capacity to support employees with severe disabilities in the workplace. *Work: A Journal of Prevention, Assessment and Rehabilitation, 21,* 77–82.

Hanley-Maxwell, C., Owens-Johnson, L., & Fabian, E. (2003). Supported employment. In E. M. Szymanski & R. M. Parker (Eds.), *Work and disability: Issues and strategies in career development and job placement* (2nd ed., pp. 373–406). Austin, Texas: Pro-Ed.

Hernanadez, B., Keys, L., & Balcazar, F. (2000). Employer attitudes toward workers with disabilities and their ADA employment rights: A literature review. *Journal of Rehabilitation, 66*(4), 4–16.

Hershenson, D. B., & Liesener, J. L. (2003). Career counseling with diverse populations: Models, interventions, and applications. In E. M. Szymanski & R. M. Parker (Eds.), *Work and disability: Issues and strategies in career development and job placement* (2nd ed., pp. 373–406). Austin, Texas: Pro-Ed.

Ingersoll, K. S., Wagner, C. C., & Gharib, S. (2000). *Motivational groups for community substance abuse programs.* Richmond, VA: Mid-Atlantic Addiction Technology Transfer Center, Center for Substance Abuse Treatment (Mid-ATTC/CSAT), 2000.

Janni, P., Reenewitz, C., May, G., & Dallas, J. (1992). *Participant follow-up study.* Olympia: Washington State Division of Vocational Rehabilitation.

Job Accommodation Network, Center for Personal Assistance Services. (2004). *Personal Assistance Services (PAS) in the workplace.* Retrieved January 19, 2005, from http://www.jan.wvu.edu/media/PAS.html.

Johnston, M. V. (1991). The outcome of community re-entry programs for brain injury survivors. Part 2: Independent living and productive activities. *Brain Injury, 5,* 155–168.

Johnston, M. V., & Granger, C. V. (1994). Outcome research in medical rehabilitation: A primer and introduction to a series. *American Journal of Physical Medicine and Rehabilitation, 73,* 296–303.

Johnston, M. V., Hall, K., Carnavale, G., & Boak, C. (1995). Functional assessment and outcome evaluation in TBI rehabilitation. In I. J. Horn & N. D. Zasler (Eds.), *Medical rehabilitation of traumatic brain injury.* Philadelphia: Hanley & Belfus.

Kay, T. (1993). Selection and outcome criteria for community-based employment: Perspectives, methodological problems and options. In D. F. Thomas, F. E. Menz, & D. C. McAlees (Eds.), *Community-based employment following traumatic brain injury* (pp. 29–56). Menomonie: University of Wisconsin–Stout, Rehabilitation Research and Training Center.

Keyser-Marcus, L. A., Bricout, J. C., Wehman, P., Campbell, L. R., Cifu, D. X., Englander, J.,et al. (2002). Acute predictors of return to employment after traumatic brain injury: A longitudinal follow-up. *Archives of Physical Medicine and Rehabilitation, 83,* 635–641.

Kirchner, C., Johnson, G., & Arkans, D. (1997). Research to improve vocational rehabilitation: Employment barriers and strategies for clients who are blind or visually impaired. *Journal of Visual Impairment and Blindness, 91,* 377–392.

Koch, L. C. (2001). The preferences and anticipations of people referred for vocational rehabilitation. *Rehabilitation Counseling Bulletin, 44,* 76–86.

Koch, L. C., & Merz, M. A. (1995). Assessing client satisfaction in vocational rehabilitation program evaluation: A review of instrumentation. *Journal of Rehabilitation, 61*(4), 24–30.

Koch, L. C., & Rumrill, P. D., Jr. (2003). New directions in vocational rehabilitation: Challenges and opportunities for researchers, practitioners, and consumers. *Work: A Journal of Prevention, Assessment and Rehabilitation, 21,* 1–3.

Kregel, J., & Head, C. (2002). *Promoting employment for SSA beneficiaries: 2001 annual report of the Benefits, Planning, Assistance and Outreach Program.* Richmond, VA: Virginia Commonwealth University, Benefits Assistance Resource Center.

Kreutzer, J. S., Marwitz, J. H., Walker, W., Sander, A., Sherer, M., Bogner, J., et al. (2003). Moderating factors in return to work and job stability after traumatic brain injury. *Journal of Head Trauma Rehabilitation, 18,* 128–138.

Langton, A. J., & Ramseur, H. (2001). Enhancing employment outcomes through job accommodation and assistive technology resources and services. *Journal of Vocational Rehabilitation, 16,* 27–37.

LeBlanc, J. M., Hayden, M. E., & Paulman, R. G. (2000). A comparison of neuropsychological and situational assessment for predicting employability after closed head injury. *Journal of Head Trauma Rehabilitation, 15,* 1022–1040.

Levy, J. M., Jessop, D. J., Rimmerman, A., & Levy, P. H. (1993). Attitudes of executives in Fortune 500 corporations toward the employability of persons with severe disabilities: Industrial and service corporations. *Journal of Applied Rehabilitation Counseling, 24,* 19–31.

Loprest, P., & Maag, E. (2001). Barriers and supports for work among adults with disabilities: Results from the NHIS-D. Washington, DC: The Urban Institute, Personal Assistance Center. Retrieved November 23, 2004, from http://www.urban.org/UploadedPDF/adultswithdisabilities.pdf

Lustig, D. C., Strauser, D. R., Rice, N. D., & Rucker, T. F. (2002). The relationship between working alliance and rehabilitation outcomes. *Rehabilitation Counseling Bulletin, 46,* 25–33.

Lustig, D. C., Strauser, D. R., Weems, G. H., Donnell, C. M., & Smith, L. D. (2003). Traumatic brain injury and rehabilitation outcomes: Does the Working Alliance make a difference? *Journal of Applied Rehabilitation Counseling, 34,* 30–37.

Majunder, R. K., Walls, R. T., Fullmer, S. L., & Misra, S. (1997). What works. In F. E. Menz, J. Eggers, P. Wehman, & V. Brooke (Eds.), *Lessons for improving employment of people with disabilities from vocational rehabilitation research* (pp. 263–282). Menomonie: University of Wisconsin–Stout, Rehabilitation Research and Training Center.

Malik, K., High, E., Yuspeh, S., & Mueller, J. (1978). Job development and enhanced productivity for severely disabled persons. (Final report, RSA Grant No. 16-P-56803/3-13.) Washington, DC: George Washington University, Medical Research and Training Center.

McAweeney, M. J., Forchheimer, M., & Tate, D. G. (1997, Summer). Improving outcome research in rehabilitation psychology: Some methodological recommendations. *Rehabilitation Psychology, 42*(2), 125–135.

McCarthy, H., & Leierer, S. J. (2001). Consumer concepts of ideal characteristics and minimum qualifications for rehabilitation counselors. *Rehabilitation Counseling Bulletin, 45,* 12–23.

McMahon, B. T., Shaw, L. R., Chan, F., & Danczyk-Hawley, C. (2004). "Common factors" in rehabilitation counseling: Expectancies and the working alliance. *Journal of Vocational Rehabilitation, 20,* 101–105.

Menz, F. E. (1997). Lessons and recommendations. In F. E. Menz, J. Eggers, P. Wehman, & V. Brooke (Eds.), *Lessons for improving employment of people with disabilities from vocational rehabilitation research* (pp. 101–115). Menomonie: University of Wisconsin–Stout, Rehabilitation Research and Training Center.

Miller, W. R., & Rollnick, S. (2002). *Motivational interviewing: Preparing people for change* (2nd ed.). New York: Guilford.

Millington, M. J., Miller, D. J., Asner-Self, K. K., & Linkowski, D. (2003). The business perspective on employers, disability, and vocational rehabilitation. In E. M. Szymanski & R. M. Parker (Eds.), *Work and disability: Issues and strategies in career development and job placement* (2nd ed. pp. 317–342). Austin, Texas: Pro-Ed.

Moore, C. L. (2001a). Racial and ethnic members of under-represented groups with hearing loss and VR services: Explaining the disparity in closure success rates. *Journal of Applied Rehabilitation Counseling, 32,* 15–20.

Moore, C. L. (2001b). Disparities in closure success rates for African Americans with mental retardation: An ex-post-facto research design. *Journal of Applied Rehabilitation Counseling, 32*(2), 30–35.

Moore, C. L., Alston, R. J., Donnell, C. M., & Hollis, B. (2003). Correlates of rehabilitation success among African American and Caucasian SSDI recipients with mild mental retardation. *Journal of Applied Rehabilitation Counseling, 34,* 25–32.

Moore, C. L., Feist-Price, S., & Alston, R. J. (2002). VR services for persons with severe-profound mental retardation: Does race matter? *Rehabilitation Counseling Bulletin, 45*(2), 162–167.

Murdick, N. R. (1997, January). Employment discrimination laws for disability: Utilization and outcome. *Annals of the American Academy of Political and Social Science, 549,* 53–70.

National Organization on Disability. (June 25, 2004). *Landmark disability survey finds pervasive disadvantages.* Retrieved November 24, 2004, from http://www.nod.org/index.cfm?fuseaction=page.viewPage&pageID=1430&nodeID=1&FeatureID=1422&redirected=1&CFID=5172764&CFTOKEN=51487559.

National Center for Education Statistics. (June 1999). *Students with disabilities in postsecondary education: A profile of preparation, participation, and outcomes.* Retrieved November 23, 2004, from www.nces.ed.gov.pubs.

Nietupski, J., Harme-Nietupski, S., VanderHart, N. S., & Fishback, K. (1996). Employer perceptions of the benefits and concerns of supported employment. *Education and Training in Mental Retardation and Developmental Disabilities, 31*(4), 310–323.

Ohtake, Y., & Chadskey, J. (2001). Continuing to describe the natural support process. *Journal of the Association for Persons with Severe Handicaps, 26,* 87–95.

O'Neill, J. (2002, April 24). *Program without walls: A preliminary evaluation of an innovation approach to state agency vocational rehabilitation.* Paper presented at a State of the Science Conference, Washington, DC.

Ouellette, S. E., & Dwyer, C. (1983). An analysis of employment search, development, and placement strategies currently employed with hearing impaired persons in the United States. *Journal of Rehabilitation of the Deaf, 17*(3), 13–20.

Owens-Johnson, L., & Hanley-Maxwell, C. (1999). Employer views on job development strategies for marketing supported employment. *Journal of Vocational Rehabilitation, 12,* 113–123.

Parker, R. M., & Schaller, J. L. (2003). Vocational assessment and disability. In E. M. Szymanski & R. M. Parker (Eds.), *Work and disability: Issues and strategies in career development and job placement* (2nd ed., pp. 155–200). Austin, Texas: Pro-Ed.

Parsons, M. B., Reid, D. H., Green, C. W., & Browning, L. B. (2001). Reducing job coach assistance for supported workers with severe multiple disabilities: An alternative off-site/on-site model. *Research in Developmental Disabilities, 22,* 151–164.

Ponsford, J. L., Olver, J. H., Curran, C., & Ng, K. (1995). Prediction of employment status 2 years after traumatic brain injury. *Brain Injury, 9,* 11–20.

Prochaska, J. O., DiClemente, C. C., & Norcross, J. C. (1992). In search of how people change: Applications to addictive behaviors. *American Psychologist, 47,* 1102–1114.

Rabren, K., Hall, G., & Brown, C. (2003). Employment of transition-age rehabilitation consumers: Demographic and programmatic factors. *Journal of Vocational Rehabilitation, 18,* 145–152.

Rao, N., & Kilgore, K. (1992). Predicting return to work in traumatic brain injury using assessment scales. *Archives of Physical Medicine Rehabilitation, 73,* 911–916.

Regenold, M., Sherman, M. F., & Fenzel, M. (1999). Getting back to work: Self-efficacy as a predictor of employment outcome. *Psychiatric Rehabilitation Journal, 22,* 361–367.

Roessler, Richard T. (2002). Improving job tenure outcomes for people with disabilities: The 3M model. *Rehabilitation Counseling Bulletin, 45,* 207–212.

Rumrill, P. D., Jr., & Garnette, M. R. (1997). Career adjustment via reasonable accommodations: The effects of an employee-empowerment intervention for people with disabilities. *Work: A Journal of Prevention, Assessment & Rehabilitation, 9,* 57–64.

Rumrill, P., & Roessler, R. (1999). New directions in vocational rehabilitation: A career development perspective on closure. *Journal of Rehabilitation, 65*(1), 26–30.

Rumrill, P. D., Roessler, R. T., & Cook, B. G. (1995). Improving career re-entry outcomes for people with multiple sclerosis: A comparison of two approaches. *Journal of Vocational Rehabilitation, 10,* 241–252.

Rumrill, P. D., Jr., Tabor, T. L., Hennessey, M. L., & Minton, D. L. (2000). Issues in employment and career development for people with multiple sclerosis: Meeting the needs of an emerging vocational rehabilitation clientele. *Journal of Vocational Rehabilitation, 14,* 109–117.

Salomone, J. (1996). Career counseling and job placement: Theory and practice. In E. M. Szymanski & R. M. Parker (Eds.), *Work and disability: Issues and strategies in career development and job placement* (2nd ed., pp.365–414). Austin, TX: Pro-Ed.

Sands, D. J., Kozleski, E. B., & Goodwin, L. D. (1992). Quality of life for workers with developmental disabilities: Fact or fiction? *Career Development for Exceptional Individuals, 15*(2), 157–177.

Sarkees-Wircenski, M., & Wircenski, J. (1994). Transition planning: Developing a career portfolio for students with disabilities. *Career Development for Exceptional Individuals, 17*(2), 203–214.

Schelat, R. K. (2001). The predictive capacity of the working alliance in vocational rehabilitation outcomes. *Dissertation Abstracts International, 61,* 3553.

Scherer, M. J. (Ed.). (2002). *Assistive technology: Matching device and consumer for successful rehabilitation.* Washington, DC: American Psychological Association.

Schneider, J. (2003) Is supported employment cost effective? A review. *International Journal of Psychosocial Rehabilitation, 7,* 145–156.

Shaw, L. R., McMahon, B. T., Chan, G., & Hannold, E. (2004). Enhancement of the working alliance: A training program to align counselor and consumer expectations. *Journal of Vocational Rehabilitation, 20,* 107–125.

Stensrud, R. (1999). Reasons for success and failure of supported employment placements. Retrieved January 19, 2005, from Drake University, National Rehabilitation Institute Web site: http://soe.drake.edu/nri/evaluation/employers.html.

Sterrett, E. A. (1998). Use of a job club to increase self-efficacy: A case study of return to work. *Journal of Employment Counseling, 35,* 69–78.

Stevens, P. M., Boland, J. M., & Ransom, S. (1982). Job-development-placement specialists: New perspectives. *Rehabilitation Counseling Bulletin, 25,* 278–281.

Stoddard, S., Jans, L., Ripple, J., & Kraus, L. (1998, June). *Chart work on work and disability in the United States.* (An In-House Information Systems, Inc. report.) Retrieved January 17, 2000, from http:www.inhouse.com/disabilitydata/

Stodden, R. A., & Browder, P. M. (1986). Community based competitive employment preparation of developmentally disabled persons: A program description and evaluations. *Journal of Education and Training of the Mentally Retarded, 21*(1), 43–53.

Temelini, D., & Fesko, S. (1996). *Shared responsibility: Job search practices for the consumer and staff perspective.* Boston: Children's Hospital. (Funded by the National Institute on Disability and Rehabilitation Research, ERIC Document Reproduction Service No. ED410706.)

Thomas, D. F., & Menz, F. E. (1997). Validation of the vocational assessment protocol. *Journal of Head Trauma Rehabilitation, 12*(5), 72–87.

Thomas, D. F., Menz, F. E., & Rosenthal, D. A. (2001). Employment outcome expectancies: Consensus, providers, and funding agents of community rehabilitation programs. *Journal of Rehabilitation, 67*(3), 26–34.

Thomas, D. M., & Whitney-Thomas, J. (1996). Perspectives from consumers and counselors on elements that influence successful vocational rehabilitation system delivery. *Research to Practice, 2*(4), 1–2.

Tooman, M. L. (1982). Placement of severely disabled persons: Multidiscipline team compared to rehabilitation counselors. *Dissertation Abstracts International, 43,* 2895 (UMI No. ADG84–23, 043.)

Trupin, L., Sebasta, D. S., Yelin, E., & LaPlante, M. P. (1997). *Trends in labor force participation among persons with disabilities, 1983–1984.* (Report No. 10.) San Francisco: Disability Statistics Center, University of California, San Francisco.

Twamley, E. W., Jeste, D. V., & Lehman, A. F. (2003). Vocational rehabilitation in schizophrenia and other psychotic disorders: A literature review and meta-analysis of randomized controlled trials. *Journal of Nervous & Mental Disease, 191,* 515–523.

Unger, D. D. (2002). Employers' attitudes toward persons with disabilities in the workforce: Myths or realities? *Focus on Autism & Other Developmental Disabilities, 17,* 2–10.

U.S. Department of Education. (2004). *Projects with industry.* Retrieved January 20, 2005, from http://www.ed.gov/about/reports/annual/2004plan/edlite-projectindustry.html.

U.S. General Accounting Office. (1993). V*ocational rehabilitation: Evidence for federal program's effectiveness is mixed.* (Publication PEMD-91–19.) Washington, DC: Author.

Vandergoot, D. (1987). Review of placement research literature: Implications for research and practice. *Rehabilitation Counseling Bulletin, 6,* 243–272.

Vogel, L., Bishop, E., & Wong, M. (1998). Using the Functional Assessment Inventory (FAI) to measure vocational rehabilitation outcomes. *Journal of Rehabilitation Outcomes Measurement, 2*(2), 48–54.

Wagner, C. C., & McMahon, B. T. (2004). Motivational interviewing and rehabilitation counseling practice. *Rehabilitation Counseling Bulletin, 47,* 152–161.

Wehman, P., Revell, W. G., & Kregel, J. (1998). Supported employment: A decade of rapid growth and impact. *American Rehabilitation, 24,* 31–43.

Young, J., Rosati, R., & Vandergoot, D. (1986). Initiating a marketing strategy by assessing employer needs for rehabilitation services. *Journal of Rehabilitation, 52*(2), 37–41.

Zadny, J. (1980). *Employer reactions to efforts to place disabled and disadvantaged workers.* (Studies in Placement monograph #4.) Portland, OR: Portland State University. (ERIC Document Reproduction Service No. ED199474.)

Zadny, J., & James, L. F. (1977a). A review of research on job placement. *Rehabilitation Counseling Bulletin, 21,* 150–157.

Zadny, J., & James, L. F. (1977b). Time spent on placement. *Rehabilitation Counseling Bulletin, 21,* 31–35.

Zuckerman, D. (1993). Reasonable accommodations for people with mental illness under the ADA. *Mental and Physical Disability Law Reporter, 17*(3), 311–320.

SECTION IV

Assistive Technology and Design

INTRODUCTION TO
SECTION IV: ASSISTIVE
TECHNOLOGY AND DESIGN

This section on Assistive Technology poses several challenging questions to rehabilitation psychology researchers and practitioners. Perhaps the most interesting question is one of application and acceptance of assistive technology to communities and large populations. Fong Chan and his coauthors highlight the potential for the Internet to enhance participation among persons with disabilities. The U.S. labor market increasingly demands skills in technology and service, and is developing proportionally fewer jobs that require physical labor. Potentially, this shift should reduce barriers to employment among persons with physical disabilities. Also, the Internet as a medium of communication may allow for improved social activities among persons with disabilities. Juxtaposed against the potential to improve employment and social interaction is the growing recognition that persons with disabilities have, by and large, the least access to the Internet. The "digital divide" persists and there is no large-scale effort to reduce this disparity in access to the Internet. Furthermore, Chan and colleagues point out that the Internet, as much as any tool, has the potential to be misused and could contribute to the social isolation of persons with disabilities.

Marcia Scherer and her colleagues emphasize the importance of consumer participation in the application of assistive technology. They frame their discussion within the International Classification of Functioning, Disability, and Health (ICF) model (World Health Organisation [WHO], 2001). Just as with population-focused assistive technology, individually based applications have the potential to enhance the quality of life, health, and participation of persons with disabilities. But, the success of assistive technology depends largely on the use of a "person-centered" approach to research and intervention. Scherer and colleagues point to the high rate of abandonment of assistive devices, the result, they assert, of prescription without adequate consideration of consumers' goals, expected outcomes, living situation, personal skills, and preferences. Ecological validity is critical to assistive technology research and application.

The theme of ecological validity in rehabilitation research is also prominent in Thomas Seekins' chapter. Seekins credits this evolution toward an ecological model of rehabilitation to the Independent Living movement. With this movement came a demand for research that is relevant to the lives and goals of persons with disabilities and for research that involves consumers. Seekins makes a case that rehabilitation research is beginning to adapt its questions, theories, and methodologies to address problems of participation and control among persons with disabilities. He states that participation is seen as "an outcome of a dynamic interaction between the individual and a mutable environment over time." It is this mutable environment that rehabilitation research is beginning to explore. Seekins describes a voucher program for rural transportation as one example of a contextually appropriate, ecologically valid research-based intervention.

CHAPTER NINE

Policy Issues in Evaluating and Selecting Assistive Technology and Other Resources for Persons With Disabilities

Marcia J. Scherer
Franklyn K. Coombs
Nancy Hansen Merbitz
Charles T. Merbitz

Legislation and policy directions for persons with disabilities is typically led by federal initiatives and indirectly by the federal funding guidelines for medical, educational, and vocational programs. A primary example of federal initiatives is the Americans with Disabilities Act (ADA), which directed national attention toward the attainment of equal access to public facilities by persons with disabilities. The Rehabilitation Services Administration (RSA), Office of Special Education and Rehabilitation Services (OSERS), U.S. Department of Education, oversees educational and vocational programs addressing goals of independent living and access to educational, vocational, and avocational pursuits. The focus of this chapter is on these programs. Many of the federally funded health care programs for medical rehabilitation already have begun to use evidence-based practice guidelines, whereas the educational and vocational programs have been moving toward evidence-based practices more slowly.

Accessible forms of information, accommodations in the built or physical environment, appropriate health care, available personal assistance, and reasonable accommodations in public areas and work sites are all key resources essential for persons with disabilities to participate in society and fulfill desired social roles. A major focus of this chapter, however, is on assistive technology (AT), even though people with disabilities typically require an array of accommodations and resources as well as individualized blends of AT and personal assistance.

DEFINITION OF ASSISTIVE TECHNOLOGY

Assistive technology was first defined in the 1988 Technology-Related assistance for Individuals with Disabilities Act (or Tech Act, Pub. L.

TABLE 9.1   Examples of Assistive Technologies Within Major Product Categories

Recreation

Products in this category enable persons to participate in social activities, team sports, and other forms of indoor and outdoor recreation.

- Adapted games
- Gardening aids
- Sports wheelchairs

Sensory Disabilities

Devices in this category assist persons with vision and/or hearing loss.

- tactile and auditory mobility aids
- auditory signaling devices
- print and computer screen magnification devices
- audiotapes
- vibrating pagers and alarm clocks

Communication

Products for communication center on the ability to send and receive messages in spoken and written form.

(Continued)

TABLE 9.1 Continued

- adapted telephones
- captioned television
- voice-controlled computer input
- writing aids
- speech output devices

Personal care

These devices enable independence in such fundamental areas as grooming, bathing, dressing, eating and accessing home appliances.

- eating utensils with angled or built-up handles
- razor holders
- reachers
- non-slip placemats under dinner plates
- bath sponges
- book holders
- transfer boards
- commode chairs

Mobility

Devices in this category provide support for persons to get around in their environments of choice.

- walkers
- canes
- crutches
- manual and power wheelchairs, scooters

Note.: These product categories represent only a partial list from the ABLEDATA classification system. ABLEDATA [www.abledata.com] is a compilation of over 19,000 assistive devices organized by functional activities.
Source: Scherer, M. J. (Ed.). (2002a). Introduction. *Assistive technology: Matching device and consumer for successful rehabilitation.* Washington, DC: American Psychological Association Books.

100–407), which was reauthorized as Pub. L. 105–220 in 1998 as the Assistive Technology Act and was reauthorized in 2004 as Pub. L. 108–364. This definition of AT has been used in most subsequent legislation related to persons with disabilities, such as the Individuals with

Disabilities Education Act (IDEA), and the Americans with Disabilities Act (ADA):

> any item, piece of equipment, or product system, whether acquired commercially off the shelf, modified, or customized, that is used to increase, maintain, or improve functional capabilities of individuals with disabilities.

Examples of assistive technologies are listed in Table 9.1 according to major product categories and commonly used devices within them. Categorizing AT according to the functional purpose of a device is common and is used, for example, by the International Organization for Standardization as ISO/DIS 9999, "Technical Aids for Disabled Persons" [http://www.iso.org/iso/en/CatalogueListPage.CatalogueList?COMMID= 4129&scopelist = ALL]. According to the data collected by the National Center for Health Statistics, Centers for Disease Control and Prevention (2005):

- Approximately 7.4 million Americans use assistive technology (AT) devices to accommodate mobility impairments.
- Approximately 4.6 million Americans use ATs to accommodate orthopedic impairments.
- Approximately 4.5 million Americans use ATs to accommodate hearing impairments.
- Approximately 500,000 Americans use ATs to accommodate vision impairments (Advance Data 292, http://www.cdc.gov/ nchs/fastats/disable.htm).

While AT for mobility is the largest single group of AT products, there are many other types of products as well beyond those listed in Table 9.1. As of August, 2002, ABLEDATA (www.abledata.com) lists currently available assistive technology products (as well as many that are no longer available) from hundreds of different companies. This large number of devices can make the process of choosing the most appropriate one for a particular user seem overwhelming and complex.

The key to an individual obtaining devices is the availability of AT providers and services. The Tech Act of 1988 defined an assistive technology service as:

> Any service that directly assists an individual with a disability in the selection, acquisition, or use of an assistive technology device, including . . . evaluation of the needs of an individual . . . ; Purchasing, leasing, or otherwise providing for the acquisition by an individual with a disability of an assistive technology device; Selecting, designing, fitting,

customizing, adapting, applying, maintaining, repairing, or replacing assistive technology devices; . . . Training and technical assistance.

With legislation like the Tech Act, ADA, and advances in technology, persons with control over just their arms and shoulders can expect to live independently, travel, and work in a competitive job even though the technology they require is more complex and expensive than that required by persons with less severe disabilities. Levels of need for personal assistance and other accommodations also differ.

Often, people tend to think of AT as high-tech gizmos. However, simple low-tech devices such as grab-bars in the home bathroom can promote independence and improve the individual's quality of life (QOL). Environmental accommodations and products made universally accessible to all regardless of ability contribute additively to enhanced QOL.

While the Rehabilitation Act Amendments of 1998 reinforce the mandated order of selection requiring vocational rehabilitation agencies to serve people with the most severe disabilities first, it also allows serving elderly persons with age-related impairments. This means that Vocational Rehabilitation (VR) programs can consider homemaker status equivalent to employment. Under this provision, Georgia VR, for example, provides AT support, including accessibility and bathroom modifications, through its Assistive Work Technology Team. Georgia VR also includes AT for sensory loss, such as vision-related AT devices like Closed Circuit Television (CCTV), when prescribed by the vision health care provider.

Given such a wide range of service provision, measures of AT outcome cannot be limited to just employment or education goals. AT should be evaluated in the context of the whole person and the person's environment, which is in keeping with the World Health Organization's International Classification of Functioning, Disability, and Health (ICF) and includes home, recreation, work, school, and community. While this chapter emphasizes vocational and educational applications of AT services, we certainly do not mean to imply that life satisfaction and QOL issues of the home, community, or recreation are of less importance; in fact it is these that give life its richness.

AT RESOURCES WITHIN A PERSON-CENTERED PERSPECTIVE

Individuals with the most severe disabilities usually require customized, computerized, and complex devices to achieve enhanced independent functioning. In fact, if these technologies were not available, individuals with severe or multiple disabilities would face nearly insurmountable obstacles to productive activity at school and work. Individuals with less severe disabilities use different assistive devices to enable a productive workday. Of course, individuals without disability also use a wide constellation of devices (ranging from commuter trains to cell phones, and computers to cultivators) to work productively. Technology is useful only when it matches personal needs and desires better than alternatives (Scherer, 2003).

This general-population model of regular technology has several lessons for AT policy, and so bears more intense examination. Recall that marketers expend advertising resources to target consumers who purchase their products; higher sales result, which in turn mean lower unit costs of these items. Now let us consider some corollaries. First, technology is frequently discarded. Think of things you purchased that you thought would meet your needs but didn't fulfill your expectations. Second, consumers frequently procure multiple items that are functionally similar (redundant, even) in the engineering sense, but are utilized in different ways or different times, such as shoes. Third, consumers become sophisticated after some iterations of a need-buy-use—evaluate-discard cycle, and an experienced consumer wisely uses resources and carefully balances nonequivalent trade-offs among competing choices of consumer goods. Finally, the individual consumer and business bears the cost of unused or unusable technologies, and makers of technology that do not meet the needs of enough consumers eventually improve their products or go out of business.

AT development however, cannot rely strictly on market forces for several reasons. First, although the numbers of people with disabilities is large, the market for any one device or design is limited to the persons for whom it exactly meets a need; a smaller market means less economy of scale and higher prices. Second, this market is demographically and geographically dispersed because disabilities are visited upon members of every social class and area. The dispersion makes advertising and marketing efforts less cost-effective, and raises the unit cost again. Third, as with regular technology items, it can take several iterations of the "need-buy-use" cycle to develop an educated consumer. However, consumers with disabilities face a very different set of constraints when purchasing AT as opposed to regular technology items. The higher unit cost means that for any given number of dollars, consumers can afford to buy and test fewer items in search of the ones that work well. Fourth, policy limitations may come into play when resources toward AT purchase are contributed by governmental or institutional (e.g., insurance) entities.

For example, consider your shoes and a wheelchair. Both are mobility enhancers, and Medicare policy dictates that wheelchairs are replaced only every 5 years. Consider the care with which you would have to approach a shoe purchase if similar constraints were applied. Now imagine that you just arrived here and this is your first pair of shoes . . . think of the bewildering choices available, and the demand that you buy one pair for the next five years—and they had better fit correctly, too! Luckily, in many areas skilled AT service providers are available to help consumers navigate the maze of funding and different AT types. Obviously, though, the AT provider must learn both the AT and your lifestyle constraints and choices to help you make a good fit, and communicating sufficient information about your goals and potential activities within the clinical minutes which are funded may be a real challenge.

The key element in achieving successful AT use and satisfied users is making sure there is a person-focused program within which the person with a disability, or the responsible adult for a child with a disability, is the primary consideration and that consumer-desired outcomes are identified. This focus requires a comprehensive evaluation which helps identify desired outcomes and detects both facilitators and barriers to the achievement of those outcomes (Scherer, 2003).

One means of assessing a consumer's "stake" or perspective is to have individuals prioritize their desired outcomes and then rate over time the progress in achieving them. This is the approach used in the Matching Person & Technology (MPT) process as well as other measures such as Goal Attainment Scaling (e.g., Donnelly &Carswell, 2002). In this way, outcomes are measured in terms of changes in the person's satisfaction in being able to get to where they want to go, whether by walking or some other means, rather than just by the functional capability to do so. This is an idiographic approach (the person is the unit of analysis and serves as his or her own control) versus a normative one (the person is compared to a group standard); idiographic approaches best capture a consumer-directed and social model perspective of outcomes assessment (e.g., Punch, 1996).

Both for the assessment of AT needs and the evaluation of AT outcomes, the typology developed by the World Health Organization in its International Classification of Functioning, Disability, and Health (ICF) (WHO, 2001) provides an overview of important life domains to be considered. Body Functions and Structures; Activities and Participation (which include Activities of Daily Living, or ADLs, and Instrumental Activities of Daily Living, or IADLs), and educational, vocational, and recreational events; and the Environmental and Personal Contextual Factors comprise the basic elements of the ICF model of functioning. This ICF typology is intended for use in classification and research on health and the effects of health conditions and health services. According to the WHO,

> ICF describes how people live with their health condition. ICF is a classification of health and health related domains that describe body functions and structures, activities and participation. The domains are

classified from body, individual and societal perspectives. Since an individual's functioning and disability occurs in a context, ICF also includes a list of environmental factors. ICF is useful to understand and measure health outcomes. It can be used in clinical settings, health services or surveys at the individual or population level. (WHO, 2001, p. 3)

The ICF denotes positive health and functioning through the terms *Integrity of Body Structures and Functions*, *Activity*, and *Participation*, and applies the term *Facilitators* to any contextual factors that promote health and functioning. The ICF denotes problems in health and functioning through the terms *Impairment*, *Limitation*, and *Restriction*, and applies the terms *Barriers/Hindrances* to any contextual factors having a negative impact. Assistive Technology is intended to facilitate health and functioning, and is a Contextual Factor of the Physical Environment; lack of resources to purchase AT constitutes a Barrier. Lack of trained personnel to assist in choosing and obtaining AT constitutes a Barrier within the Social Environment (as do policies that set a low priority on resource allocation for AT). The failure of a service provider to require a comprehensive assessment of consumer needs, priorities, and AT preferences at the beginning of the AT and support selection process is also a Barrier within the Social Environment. Finally, a personal history of perceived failure with AT may hinder future use of AT (an example of a negative Personal Contextual Factor).

In the most straightforward conceptualization, Body Functions and Structures can be considered the substrate that enables Activities to occur, and in turn the capability to perform Activities enables Participation in social, vocational, civic, and other broader pursuits. Contextual factors (Environmental and Personal) facilitate or hinder Participation. A more comprehensive conceptualization of the ICF model recognizes the interconnectivity among all of these elements. Environmental factors can include access to health care and rehabilitation, access to assistive technology and personal assistance, and access to information—all of which could affect Body Functions, Activities, and Participation. Activities and Participation can affect Body Functions through exercise of joints and muscles, acquisition of skills (and synaptic branching), and improvement of mood. Contextual factors likewise are dynamic and subject to influence. For example, considering Personal Contextual factors, an individual may initially have negative attitudes toward assistive technology, but upon further experience with using well-matched assistive technology to carry out desired Activities, may change those attitudes so that additional AT could more readily be considered. In a less successful example, a person with memory deficits (Body Function) might have difficulties with IADLs (Activities) and thus not be able to move to his own apartment (Participation). A pager system (Environmental facilitator) might be programmed to prompt certain necessary activities, thus potentially enabling IADLs and independent living. But Contextual factors might be a barrier to its implementation, such as the attitudes of the person toward technology, or the family's fears about the individual's independence, or there might be financial limitations. Limits of the technology may prevent its successful use, that is, it may not be well matched to the sensory and cognitive characteristics of potential users with brain injury, such that the pager screen and font are too small, the pager sound too brief, and/or the programming too complex. As tools are developed for a preacquisition evaluation of person-technology match and an evaluation of AT outcomes, the ICF promotes consideration of relevant features to assess across these domains, and consideration of their interrelationships (e.g., Federici & Micangeli, 2003).

The person-focused model in Figure 9.1 has at its center AT use and is designed to provide the consumer with more control over the process of resource selection, use, and satisfaction in order to assure that the person's goals, desired lifestyle, and needs and preferences are served. This model is equally applicable to the use of other resources by persons with disabilities. It has been operationalized by the Matching Person and Technology assessment process (Scherer, 1998). The essential considerations in this model include:

- Assurance that the consumer receives a comprehensive and individualized evaluation by a qualified provider. The evaluation can include a focus on the ICF domains of Body Function and Structure, Activities and Participation in society, and Contextual factors (environmental barriers or facilitators, and current attitudes, interests, and preferences of the person).
- Adopting the perspective that consumers have a right to choose the technologies and other resources and should be involved in the processes of needs evaluation, selection, and outcomes evaluation.
- Recognition that a technology must be adapted to the individual's needs and preferences, rather than an individual adapting to technology's features.
- Discussing different consumer-professional perspectives and priorities openly. Professionals should not presume to know all the answers and then impose their view of what is best on the consumer.
- Focus on factors other than the cost of technology when selecting AT.
- Selecting relevant features across the ICF domains and monitoring them for desirable and undesirable changes.
- Avoiding failure by following up on how well needs are met.

Each of these steps will be discussed in the following sections.

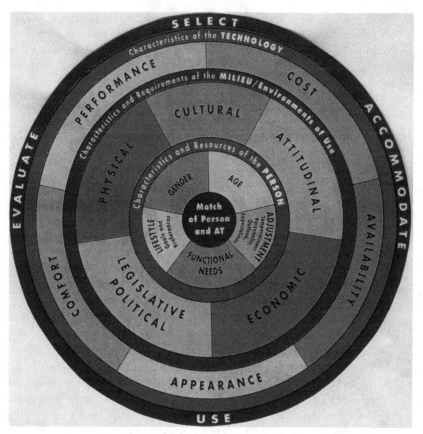

FIGURE 9.1 Influences to be considered when trying to achieve a good match of person and technology

Source: Institute for Matching Person & Technology, Inc.

ASSURING THAT THE CONSUMER RECEIVES A COMPREHENSIVE AND INDIVIDUALIZED EVALUATION BY A QUALIFIED PROVIDER

In spite of the assistance and promise of independence offered by many technologies and the growth in AT options, the rate of AT nonuse, abandonment, and noncompliance remains high (e.g., Scherer, 2002, 2005). Studies reveal that on average, approximately one third of all devices provided to consumers end up stored in the closet, basement, or drawer. While many AT products go into disuse because they are no longer needed, a lack of consumer involvement in selection is regarded by consumers themselves as an important reason devices are not used or used optimally (e.g., Scherer, 2002, 2005). This issue can be addressed appropriately in a comprehensive evaluation process. Individuals with disabilities, when involved in the decision in a meaningful way, generally will be more satisfied with AT services overall. There should be advance planning when an assistive device is being considered for (or by) a person with a disability of Body Function and/or Structures, to assist with Activities and ultimately Participation in social roles. Consideration must be given to the methods used by the therapist or other service providers to assess the match between person and device, as these methods are critical to the successful adoption (or informed rejection) of the device (e.g., Gray, Quatrano, & Lieberman, 1998).

It is crucial that the person's Body Functions and Structures are considered in the choice of device and instruction in its use. However, it is equally important that an evaluation is made of the person's attitudes, knowledge, and comfort with respect to assistive technology in general and the device in particular. An evaluation for person-technology matching should also include information on the person's Environment (both physical and social/cultural) and preferred goals within the domains of Activities and Participation. In order to reduce the likelihood of technology abandonment, the AT evaluation should facilitate prediction of how the person will respond to a given technology, what methods of teaching will facilitate the person's acceptance of it, or what alternative devices/resources might be better accepted and/or more appropriate for other reasons.

Figure 9.1 includes under "Characteristics and Requirements of the Milieu/Environments of Use" the need to take into account cultural and attitudinal influences on resources selection and use, as well as economic, physical, and legislative/political considerations. People with disabilities vary in their desire for AT versus personal assistance versus help from family members. Often, this is an outcome of one's cultural mores and expectations. Family members may resent the use or presence of an AT in the home. To use a truly idiographic, person-centered approach requires understanding such influences and pressures, level of program/professional trust, as well as language differences (a person who is deaf may require an ASL interpreter; a Native American may only communicate in his or her native language). Therefore, it is imperative that the consumer be involved in a dialogue that identifies such needs and preferences.

The Matching Person and Technology (MPT) assessment process is one means of initiating such a dialogue (Scherer, 1998). As mentioned earlier, it is an idiographic, person-focused process that can be used as an interview guide or the consumer can complete the forms independently.

It is divided into parts beginning with a general worksheet exploring limitations/strengths in many functional domains and then surveys users regarding their experiences with technologies in the past. The Assistive Technology Device Predisposition Assessment explores consumers' subjective ratings of their functioning in regards to Body Functions, subjective well-being/quality of life (Activities and Participation), and such Personal Factors as self-esteem, mood, and motivation for technology use (Scherer & Sax, 2005). It is designed to be used at the beginning of the AT selection process so that consumer preferences and goals drive the matching process, obstacles to optimal AT use and the need for additional supports/resources can be identified, and strategies for training in use can be implemented. When administered after AT acquisition and use, second form administration provides outcome data. The forms can be completed by consumers and providers in partnership, thereby offering the opportunity to explore particular areas in more depth and to ensure that the items have meaning to the consumer in keeping with their primary language and cultural background. What follows is a quote from a report by a rehabilitation professional on her experiences with using the MPT process, which exemplifies the value of using an idiographic measure and adapting it to the consumer's culture and language:

> Through this project, a Native American consumer was able to be an active part of the decision making process for his AT devices and as a result, will be more likely to utilize them and be successful in gaining more independence. My consumer is a male with a C6 spinal cord injury. He has limited use of his hands and arms and no use of his legs. He has greatly depended on others to do things for him. I knew from the start that it would be important to have everything translated into his traditional language if he was going to feel at ease during this interview process. Regarding the Matching Person & Technology assessment forms, the initial Worksheet was not difficult since he was able to list his limitations and think of goals for each area. He seemed to like this worksheet because it was positive and allowed him to look at the future and what he could do for himself with additional assistive technology. The Survey of Technology Use was not as easy because many of the English words could not be translated into his traditional language and the concept was hard for him to comprehend. For example, he struggled with the concept of childhood technology experiences because he grew up in a home that did not have running water, electricity or any modern devices. It took several minutes of conversation in his traditional language to arrive at something that made sense to him. In addition, he is an older man and had difficulty discussing personal things—feelings of success, creativity, satisfaction, etc. When we began asking the questions on the Assistive Technology Device Predisposition Assessment that describe an individual's personal characteristics, it

took more than 30 minutes to complete this section. It is very inappropriate for a male in the Native American culture to discuss these
things in front of women. Each time he had to give a negative response,
you could see the shame on his face. It was obvious that he wanted to
answer accurately, but he struggled immensely with those items that he
described as being weak in character. I told him that we did not have to
complete this form if he was too uncomfortable. He stated that he was
uncomfortable but also knew that his responses would be important
for this project. On several of his answers, he began to cry and we had
to give him time to recover and talk about the emotion before moving
on. At one point all four of the tech team members were in tears from
the emotion that the consumer had shared with us. I struggled with the
process of completing the surveys because I felt that they were violating
a very private part of this consumer. I don't recall exactly when the rev-
elation hit me, but I do remember the insight that I suddenly had—even
though the consumer had experienced emotional pain during the process, it was an avenue that had allowed this Native American to release
his feelings and talk about deep rooted issues that had been a part of
him for years. It was actually cathartic in nature and was moving him
from a place of despair to a place of hope. When I finally realized this,
I understood the importance of the MPT process. It isn't just about
finding the right assistive technology for a consumer, it is about a person centered process that takes a consumer through a progression of
steps to become more comfortable with his/her disability and more
independent in all areas of his/her life. (Holland, 2002)

As the above quote indicates, the Environmental Factors of attitudes
and culture are important, as well as characteristics of the individual's
built, or physical, environment. Within the ICF, the interface with the built
environment for a person with disabilities or an older person with diminished physical or cognitive function is part of Environmental Factors. It
is sometimes difficult to relate issues with the built environment to AT,
and yet resolving the environmental issues is a critical element in promoting independence. For example, Mann, Ottenbacher, Frass, Tomita,
and Granger (1999) reported that making minor modifications to the
residence of frail elderly people produced more independence. Mann and
colleagues reported that these changes in the residence allowed older, frail
persons to remain more functional in their homes, rather than being institutionalized. This resulted in a slower rate of decline of the person's IADL
activities and cost savings in terms of fewer nursing home placements.

For the consumer to receive a comprehensive evaluation, training dollars and time need to be devoted to educating professionals about available
technologies and strategies and measures which they can employ to assess
with consumers the most appropriate technologies for their use. This education has to be at the pre-service, field, and in-service levels. It also needs to

be across different disciplines and include health care (inpatient and outpatient), and social, educational, and vocational services.

AT practitioners require a means of determining consumer preferences and priorities and having consumer input guide AT selection and targeted outcomes. Examples of outcomes can be: performance in education or employment, performance of activities of daily living, and consumer satisfaction or subjective quality of life (e.g., DeRuyter, 1995, 1997, 1998; Fuhrer, 2001; Jutai, Ladak, Schuller, Naumann, & Wright, 1996; Scherer, 1996). The latter encompasses the person's sense of well-being, health, comfort, happiness, and satisfaction with such specific areas of functioning as work, social relationships, and finances. Providers need to assess and document the outcomes and impact of the AT services they provide to consumers in terms of social participation and quality of life rather than externally imposed educational or vocational goals.

Professionals in the AT field recognized the need for credentialing practitioners or providing certificates of specialty in AT. Rehabilitation Engineering and Assistive Technology Society of North America (RESNA), as a professional society, has established an AT credentialing exam for AT practitioners and AT suppliers (vendors and product trainers) who provide and service AT products (www.resna.org), and rehabilitation engineering technologists. Several universities (e.g., California State University, Northridge) offer certificate training in AT service delivery (www.csun.edu/cod). Other AT professionals have called for AT practitioners to support the need for and routine use of outcome measures in AT products and service delivery (e.g., DeRuyter, 1995).

Unfortunately, there has not been agreement on terminology or on outcomes to measure. The National Institute on Disability and Rehabilitation Research (NIDRR) announcement of Final Funding Priorities for FY 2001–2003, which came out on June 26, 2001, and which called for two Disability and Rehabilitation Research Projects on AT Outcomes and Impact (Notice of Final Funding Priorities for Fiscal Years 2001–2003 for Four Disability and Rehabilitation Research Projects, 2001), stated:

> Outcomes indicators are measures of the amount and frequency of those occurrences, and include service quality. Within this perspective, some analysts use the word "impacts" to distinguish between long-term or end results that occur on a societal versus an individual level. Still others use the term "impact" more strictly to refer to estimates of the extent to which the program actually "caused" particular outcomes.

This background statement provides an excellent overview of the issues and needs for AT outcome measurement. The NIDRR projects are to develop stakeholder support for AT outcomes, to develop methods for evaluating existing instruments, and to promote instruments that interact with the consumer and the other stakeholders. To do this requires consensus-building. One consensus-building process is based on reaching agreement among stakeholders in the process. In the AT consensus-building process, the primary stakeholders are the users of AT and other resources, and service practitioners and health care providers (including physicians, nurses, therapists, and allied health professionals). Secondary stakeholders are family members or caregivers for AT users, provider agencies (medical, educational, or vocational rehabilitation agencies), third-party payers (federal and state agencies and public and private insurers), and AT vendors and manufacturers.

CONSUMERS HAVE THE RIGHT TO CHOOSE THE TECHNOLOGIES THEY RECEIVE AND USE

When we consider the individual with a disability as the central element of resource selection, by logical extension the service provider ideally would choose an evaluation process and outcome measure that corresponds to such an individualized perspective. We know that consumers select their assistive technologies based, first, on how well the technologies satisfy their needs and preferences, then according to attractiveness and appeal (Temkin et al., 1999). If the device meets the person's performance expectations and is easy and comfortable to use, then a good match of person and technology has been achieved. Thus, the driving force in device selection is the perspective of the user, not which technology the service provider thinks is best, or which is most affordable or quickest to obtain. It is not acceptable to point to technological solutions before the prospective user's goals are fully defined and the individual's needs and preferences are apparent.

The real message is, consumers want "a voice in the choice" (Coombs, 2000). For example, a person being discharged with a recent spinal cord injury will still be adjusting and may be indecisive about the AT services being offered; questions about what wheelchair, what cushion, or what home or vehicle modifications are better than another, or why, can be overwhelming. However, six months to a year later, this consumer is likely to have a clear idea about what satisfies his or her needs—what works and doesn't work. This is the point where the dialogue can allow for different points of view between all of the stakeholders.

AT users' perspectives on AT develop and change over time. A consumer who is not ready for technology use initially may be ready in a few months. Professionals must raise the topic of technology again, when it appears the consumer may be more receptive to alternative approaches.

A TECHNOLOGY MUST BE ADAPTED TO THE INDIVIDUAL'S NEEDS AND PREFERENCES; CONSUMERS SHOULD NOT HAVE TO ADAPT TO A TECHNOLOGY'S FEATURES

Twenty-five years ago it was common to have one style of wheelchair prescribed for many people. Options and choices in wheelchairs and other assistive technologies, if they existed at all, were not vast. Manufacturers of products or devices did not think it worth their while or cost-effective to uniquely shape devices or craft them to fit individual needs and preferences, particularly in the wheelchair industry (Team Rehab Report, 1993). Then in the late 1980s, a new wheelchair company, Quickie, became established because it offered a range of colors in light-weight models instead of the bulky, chrome-plated models from two major manufacturers. The consumer's choice of colors, styling, lighter weight, and durability literally took a major market share away from the bigger, slower to change, former market leaders. This change in market dynamics demonstrates the power and influence of consumer choice. AT products should be refined to conform to the varied preferences and needs of the individual who will use them. It is precisely this need for the availability of varied choices in technology features that has led to over 20,000 products listed in ABLEDATA.

The wheelchair industry sales in North America have been estimated to be $750 million per year and growing at about 10% per year (Coombs, 1999). On the other end of the sales spectrum, Sonic Pathfinder, an ultrasonic electronic travel aid for the blind, is manufactured in Australia and has worldwide sales of less than 12 units a year (A. Heyes, owner, Sonic Pathfinder, personal communication, May 5, 2001). The Sonic Pathfinder is marketed without profit. Many other small manufacturers and vendors of AT products also operate without making a profit.

Unfortunately, good works alone will not keep a marginal product on the market. There are many AT products that break down too often and cost too much to repair. Just as the rigor of accountability demands quality performance measures for AT practitioners, it also demands AT manufacturers and their vendors to apply quality performance measures to reduce the cost and improve the reliability and durability of their AT products.

While computers are not in themselves assistive technology, the use of adapted computers by people with disabilities and older adults has increased dramatically as society has become more accepting of computer-based information and communication. The listserv maintained by RESNA can be a barometer of AT service provision by AT practitioners, suppliers, and technologists, and regularly lists information requests for ideas or resources for modifying the ways users input information into computers, navigate through programs and Web sites, and receive output. Reduced-cost and nearly-free computers are available through the efforts of programs like the National Cristina Foundation [www.cristina.org] and numerous regional programs, such as REBOOT (funded as part of the Georgia Tech Act program) and Tools For Life (TFL). REBOOT rebuilds and recycles used computers for persons with disabilities, provides training opportunities for the person to learn how to operate the computer, and has adapted computers to accommodate needs. REBOOT provides persons with disabilities and older adults with a place to perform community service to "pay" for their computer; this arrangement fosters dignity and independence as the computer is something a person has earned and was not given through charity. These programs reduce or eliminate the digital divide that can separate the haves from the have-nots in education, job preparation and opportunities, and recreation.

DIFFERING CONSUMER-PROFESSIONAL PERSPECTIVES AND PRIORITIES NEED TO BE DISCUSSED OPENLY

Rehabilitation professionals tend to define outcomes of their services, or goals achieved (e.g., improved range of motion or increased strength), in terms of physical functioning, whereas consumers more often equate independence with social and personal participation (e.g., Cushman & Scherer, 1996). In a social model of rehabilitation, outcome variables can be selected according to the person's priorities, and measured in terms of their satisfaction with changes in those selected variables (Scherer, 2002b). For example, getting out of the house quickly and efficiently via a wheelchair and ramp may bring more satisfaction than going down steps more slowly and with greater effort on foot using a quad cane. An observer may place greater value on the latter outcome, judging it to reflect more independence, but perhaps the person chooses to apply the savings in time and energy to work or recreation. Those following a social model of rehabilitation view it as essential to define the consumer's perspectives of the most desired outcomes. There also is a need to evaluate the AT service delivery process and its costs, efficiency, and effectiveness (Craddock, 2002a, 2002b; Ripat & Booth, 2005). Different stakeholders have different needs, which may be why no single outcomes instrument is accepted across stakeholders. Outcome instruments should be oriented toward the consumer's perspective if they are to gain credibility with the primary stakeholders. This approach is consistent with efforts to achieve evidence-based practices in rehabilitation.

PROFESSIONALS SHOULD NOT IMPOSE THEIR
VIEW OF WHAT IS BEST

Many health care professionals, in keeping with their training, define disability in a normative manner using a normal distribution curve of abilities and, thus, view disability as a health problem that requires treatment and cure (Cushman & Scherer, 1996; Scherer, 2002b)

Consumers with disabilities who are active in the independent living movement have advocated for the right of self-determination. They do not define people with disabilities as belonging in the lower tail of the normal distribution of health status, requiring treatment and designation as a separate group ("ill," "disabled," etc.). A focus of the independent living movement considers assisting the person with a disability to learn how to eliminate or minimize obstacles so as to achieve self-actualization, life satisfaction, and QOL associated normally with living in the middle (or higher end) of the normal curve. Using this perspective, "a healthy person with a disability" is not a contradiction in terms.

The independent living advocacy movement supports federal legislation for the creation of trust funds or credit unions to fund the needs of people with disabilities, including the purchase of AT devices and services. The Tech Act programs have served people with disabilities well and have been proactive in developing funding sources. *Dollars and Sense: A Guide to Solving the Funding Puzzle and Getting AT in Georgia* is an example of advocacy by the Tech Act programs. *Dollars and Sense* is available on CD from Tools For Life, the Georgia Tech Act program. Thirteen states have obtained a federal grant to create a credit union for people with disabilities to purchase AT with low-interest loans. These excellent programs are examples of advocacy at work to assist people with disabilities to overcome obstacles.

The expectation that consumer preference should be assessed in every aspect of service delivery is new to many professionals. A contemporary perspective of professionals is that consumers understand their disabilities well and that they have valuable insights into what will work for them and what doesn't. For this dialogue to be most effective, the practitioner and the consumer must have time, skills, and readiness to communicate and reach a consensus with consumers. The need for consumer agreement has been included in the Rehabilitation Act amendments of 1998 as a requirement for informed consumer choice. In today's time-managed programs, whether managed clinical care or agency case management, the professional's time with clients is limited, and yet it is a critical element of effective service delivery. The lack of time and funds to provide a full-service assessment and intervention frustrates all parties, although each for a different reason. Many practitioners do not have the flexibility to take the time to establish rapport and to listen to the underlying concerns of their clients. The ethical issue for AT practitioners of having the time necessary to interact with the consumer is the same issue facing other professionals in health care service delivery, whether the consumer is a person with a disability or not.

COST OF A TECHNOLOGY SHOULD NOT BE THE DECIDING FACTOR IN WHICH TECHNOLOGY A CONSUMER SELECTS AND RECEIVES

Cost issues are not unique to serving people with disabilities. In AT purchase decisions, these discussions must move beyond charity considerations because the person has a disability, and beyond the idea that they are deserving because of having a disability. The assessment process should look beyond judgments about the perceived role or value of the person in society and should not be focused solely on employment. Yet, there must be some cost containment, and achieving a balance between the "unfettered choices" and "informed choice" required in the Rehabilitation Act has yet to be accomplished.

The passage of the ADA legislation established the policy that people with disabilities are an equal part of American society, and have the right to equal access to public areas and services. The recent amendments to the Rehabilitation Act include electronic accessibility, which is to include access to cell phones, automatic teller machines, automated information kiosks, and the Internet.

American society has affirmed the right of people with disabilities to have public access to places, spaces, jobs, and information. The question for American society is: Now that people with disabilities have a right to access, will society pay for the means (i.e., AT) to allow them to use it?

A word of caution is needed when painting with such broad brushstrokes. ADA accommodations are the responsibility of the owners of public access places, spaces, and information. This is the difference between publicly available systems (e.g., assisted listening devices at the symphony hall) versus private use devices (e.g., hearing aids). Although the person with a hearing impairment must have a recent-model hearing aid to benefit from most of the public accommodation systems, to be ADA compliant, the public space or facility is required only to have a "reasonable accommodation," not one of every type.

At present these are separate issues, yet it is clear that these issues are related and that giving a person the equal right to access does not give them equal means to access. This argument is not to imply that every person with a disability should be given a wish list of every item available. It does say there should be a process by which a person with a disability can apply to receive the AT that will allow them public and electronic access.

An ethical issue to consider with cost is the quality of the AT services. The typical response of some government and managed care systems is, "We have so many customers waiting for service that we have to limit the cost to serve them all." It appears as though the message from these organizations is, "It is better to serve 100% of the patients in a cavalier manner, than to serve only 75% (in the same time/cost) in a controlled, quality manner." The managers of such service delivery organizations and the third-party payers will vigorously deny this allegation; however, careful review of the evidence of poor-quality services in any one of a number of public services belies their contentions. As an example of poor services, state-funded VR counselors, in numerous states, report case loads of 150 to 250 clients. The concerns of overburdened counselors is not limited to VR, nor should the need for AT service provision be viewed as related to vocational needs only. There are myriad federal, state, and local social programs where counselors, case managers, social workers, and psychologists are overburdened, and effective service delivery is compromised.

Human professionals play a major role in service provision for people with disabilities and older Americans. Those who fill the administrative ranks are required to understand the AT needs of these special populations as well as the needs of children with disabilities.

Individuals with cognitive disabilities, including people with Traumatic Brain Injury (TBI), Mental Retardation (MR), and some people with Learning Disabilities (LD) and Attention Deficit Hyperactivity Disorder (or ADHD), form another distinct segment of the disability community. AT has had its biggest impact in serving the educational needs of this population. However, portable devices like Palm Pilots (for memory cueing) or automated pillboxes (for taking medications on schedule) have had little success. The unique needs of these consumers makes generalized AT devices unhelpful while specialized AT devices are often too complicated. Thus, these populations are underserved. More interaction is required between AT professionals, consumer advocacy groups, and those with specialized training in serving individuals with mental health, developmental, or cognitive disabilities. A multidisciplinary team approach combining certified or licensed professionals, vocational evaluators, psychologists, social workers, physical or occupational therapists, speech and language pathologists, and technologists would be ideal. NIDRR funded in 2004 a Rehabilitation Engineering Research Center on Advancing Cognitive Technologies (RERC-ACT, 2005) that will address these issues.[1]

Many states are exploring different approaches to the AT service delivery. Georgia has the largest AT service delivery program in VR with 29 full-time employees statewide. Each of the 12 VR regions in Georgia has one technologist and a team consisting of an occupational therapist, rehabilitation engineer, and technician. An extra team and technologist serves the Atlanta-Macon metroplex, which accounts for almost one half of Georgia's population. The Georgia program is called Assistive Work Technology to emphasize its "return to work" orientation. The Georgia program provides a unique test bed for evaluating outcomes of effectiveness and efficiency of AT devices and services. It can also be used to model the multidisciplinary team approach in a VR setting.

Managers of AT service delivery programs and administrators of funding agencies (both public and private) have limited resources compared to the need, which makes it all the more critical that their programs are cost-effective and efficient. The stakeholders in the AT process must work together to balance (a) consumers' basic needs and preferences with (b) quality service delivery and (c) cost containment; these can be considered the three legs of a stool comprising the AT process—shorten any one leg and the stool is unstable. It would be ideal if a set of outcome instruments could measure each of these efforts, leading to a consumer-centered, balanced, cost-effective AT service system.

If there is an effort to improve quality by reducing the caseload, it must be recognized that this will result in a backlog of people waiting for service, so that the question becomes, is expediency a justification for poor service delivery? In the case of AT for people with disabilities, the AT is typically not considered to be life-supporting or life-sustaining. Just as there is triage in an emergency room for order of selection to the patient in most urgent need, there would be a process for order of selection in AT service delivery. Those with the most critical need are served immediately, while those with a less critical need are served in turn. In this case, the agency providing the service (or paying the costs) determines the order of selection as part of a quality assurance program. For example, the order of selection process could use, as one approach, a priority list with an additional drop-in clinic time. The Rehabilitation Act amendments of 1999 require states that receive block grants for VR services to have a plan for order of selection. Unfortunately, many of these plans are vague and inconsistent, which makes them difficult for VR staff to understand and enforce. In an evidence-based approach to service delivery, changes in outcomes measured before, during, and after implementation of a coherent plan for order of selection would allow a rational evaluation of such an approach.

FAILURE TO FOLLOW UP IS, INDEED, A FAILURE

Feedback is essential to improving quality of services. The term means to return or "feed" information about the output "back" into the input to improve or correct the output. When this process is applied to AT service delivery, there must be information given to the provider (i.e., input) on how well a service is working (i.e., output) in order to arrive at the desired result (i.e., performance).

Follow-up in AT service delivery is the feedback that closes the loop for achieving the desired result. Without the feedback (follow-up), the AT practitioner could miss the target, and the consumer (patient, client, AT user) suffers. Worse yet, without feedback the whole effort of the AT service provision may be wasted, as there is a high probability the AT will not meet the consumer's need and will be abandoned. Technology abandonment results in a waste of provider and consumer time as well as product and money. The available time for follow-up is small when compared to the original time expended on the selection and initial evaluation of the AT products. Follow-up must be an integral part of the process from the initial referral until the completion or release as agreed to by the consumer.

FUTURE DIRECTIONS NEEDED TO FILL GAPS

The primary stakeholder regarding AT selection and outcomes is the person who is expected to use a particular AT. Other primary stakeholders are the AT practitioner and health care providers who need outcome measures to assure quality and cost-effective service delivery. Family members and caregivers are primary stakeholders as they may be affected by the success or failure of an AT (i.e., it could affect how many hours they work and the nature of their tasks). Secondary stakeholders include provider agencies, third-party payers, and AT manufacturers and vendors. It is not only important that AT outcomes measurement focus on the individual (U.S. Department of Education, 1999) but to realize that AT outcomes are established at the beginning of the selection process. The adage "garbage in, garbage out" applies well to the AT service delivery process when a comprehensive, up-front assessment of consumer needs and preferences—a priority—is omitted. Diversity among persons with disabilities should be a central factor guiding assessment and not treated as error and noise to be obscured and ignored. The achievement of individual participatory preferences and priorities needs to be promoted, not solely functional standards (e.g., ability to feed oneself), by looking at subjective measures (e.g., quality of life) and more objective, but individualized, measures of more comprehensive desired changes such as changes in the person's activities and participation in society. AT outcomes should evaluate the service delivery process and its effectiveness according to individual levels of satisfaction and resource utilization, which may include cost-effectiveness.

AT outcomes research has lagged behind that in other fields. In part for this reason, in 2001 the National Institute on Disability and Rehabilitation Research awarded two Disability and Rehabilitation Research Project grants on Assistive Technology Outcomes and Impacts. The two projects have the shared purpose to develop AT outcome measures and measurement guidelines, which will be fundamental to establishing evidence-based practices for AT service delivery and funding.

While these Outcomes Centers have effectively developed and disseminated their results to date, there is still a cry for information available for special education teachers and administrators as to what AT devices work best for supporting children's educational needs. Similarly, information is needed for vocational rehabilitation counselors as to what AT devices work best for vocational needs. A problem with such global needs is they can tend to lead to a one-size-fits-all solution, which should be avoided. One fundamental approach recommended for quality evaluation and service delivery is to recognize the role of the person with disabilities as an individual with unique needs, preferences, and information to contribute during the resource selection and matching process. For example, people with SCI as a group may be characterized as needing wheelchairs for mobility; however, each individual person with a SCI does not need the same wheelchair. Yet, though a person's individual needs may vary, it is possible to develop guidelines for determining those individual needs and preferences.

The evolution of more enlightened policy will involve understanding the features and aims of person-focused programs. The first step is to develop process models that guide the evaluation of AT needs in educational and vocational programs. This simple statement masks the complexity of the task, as is apparent by examining Figure 9.1.

In studying outcomes of AT use, consideration of the interactive nature of the ICF model could promote logical as well as creative idiographic research designs. For one example, suppose a wheelchair evaluation is carried out for an individual with SCI, diabetes, and deconditioning, taking into account Body Function and Structure, as well as the Environment of his home and his intended Activities. A particular wheelchair is selected and provided. Outcomes to be monitored could include changes in number and type of Activities (e.g., exercise, pressure lift-offs, self-care including skin checks, exiting his home) and Participation (e.g., recreational activities, attending school, shopping).

Changes in Body Function and Structure also could be monitored (e.g., mood, blood sugar, range of motion, heart rate, upper body strength, skin condition). These body function and structure changes might result from a synergy that combines the benefits of a well-matched wheelchair plus the changes across other domains. In a second example, an individual who acquires an Environmental facilitator such as a service dog might experience changes in other features of the Environment, such as the social behaviors of strangers, that could be assessed as an outcome (Sachs-Ericsson, Hansen, & Fitzgerald, 2002; Zapf & Rough, 2002).

The complex interactions of the ICF Domains and Contextual Factors are indecipherable until one considers timelines. For example, time since injury or condition onset is a crucial factor in planning services for someone with an acquired disability. If one does not limit consideration of outcomes to a final point of adaptation, a world of possibilities opens up for outcomes measurement applied to the process of adaptation. At each point in a lifetime, what was considered as an outcome at an earlier point may now be a predictor of other outcomes. In the language of science, what was a dependent variable (outcome) in one equation may now be an independent variable in the prediction of another, later outcome. Every skill and habit and attitude acquired by the individual affects the acquisition of future skills and habits and attitudes. People respond to and shape their social environments. In the language of applied behavior analysis, the consequences of one behavior become part of the antecedent conditions for future behaviors.

In an example: A person sees a rehabilitation professional who has the time and skill to assess for technology matching (Social Environmental facilitation), and the resources are available to obtain useful AT (Physical Environmental facilitation). The individual uses this well-matched AT to exit her home several times per week (an Activity outcome). She is still unable to find a job due to Social/Physical Environmental barriers, but with increasing experience living in her community, her confidence and interpersonal assertiveness increase (an outcome in a Personal Contextual factor). This Personal factor, in turn, facilitates her involvement in community affairs, namely, she learns about and joins a consumer advocacy group (a Participation outcome). She also notices changes in how her family treats her; they make fewer assumptions about her abilities and start helping her locate leads for jobs (an outcome in the Social Environment that may facilitate an outcome in Participation).

How could the consideration of adaptation as a timeline facilitate outcomes measurement and allocation of resources to promote better outcomes? When adaptation is construed in this way, we realize the need for measures that can be applied and analyzed in a universal manner and for a variety of purposes. If key indicators are measured in terms of number of occurrences over a period of time, they can be examined in any context for any relevant purpose (Merbitz, 1996). For example, a question about the effects of caseload size on the success of AT matching can be examined by asking: How does the number of clients seen per week by rehabilitation professionals affect the number of clients who acquire and use their new AT? For one of these clients, the success of a mobility device might be measured in terms of how many times per week she exits her home, pre- versus post-AT acquisition. Among a sample of people with mobility impairments, number of home exits per week could be examined for its relationship to changes in the frequency of other events such as telephone calls from friends per week (Social Environmental outcome), spending of health care dollars per year for health complications (Physical Environmental outcome), number of times per day the person notices a positive mood (a Body outcome resulting from the Activity of directing one's thoughts, which might be facilitated by Social support encountered during increased Participation in interpersonal relationships), and so forth.

Ultimately, it is likely that a person-focused approach to assistive technology will demand an optimal blend of qualitative and quantitative evaluation. With the use of qualitative methods, individual, familial, and cultural variations can be detected, explored, and accommodated; these may include variations in the experience and perceptions of a disability, in preferred technology options, and in desired communication patterns with health service providers. Quantitative methods can be employed with each individual, to track in a time-series the occurrence of personally relevant details of daily life and how they may change as a new technology is introduced and used. Data on selected variables can be aggregated in larger studies employing group designs. The particular level of analysis will vary according to the needs of each stakeholder, but data that captures the flow of events in individual lives provides the best foundation for any analysis of AT impact.

A person-focused assessment of assistive technology needs will result in the exploration and accommodation of individual, familial, and cultural factors that impact the quality of the match of an individual and the device(s) recommended and adopted for use. As rehabilitation emphasizes evidence-based practices and places a research priority on randomized controlled trials (RCT), there is a danger that the reality of individual lives will be lost. This may ultimately take us backwards to a "one-size-fits-all" solution, which should be avoided. Further, this would work against the emphasis of the International Classification of Functioning, Disability, and Health (ICF) on the barriers and enablers to individual activity performance and societal participation. Yet, though a person's individual needs may vary, it is possible to develop scientifically solid guidelines for determining those individual needs and preferences. The evolution of more enlightened policies will involve understanding the features and aims of person-focused programs.

QUESTIONS FOR DISCUSSION AND/OR FURTHER STUDY

Service Domain

1. What makes attitudinal and cultural factors so important when working with individuals with disabilities? How does this influence the use or nonuse of AT?
2. There are three major factors that directly influence use and nonuse of AT: characteristics of the milieu of use, the person, and the technology itself. Why is it important that each factor be addressed with the consumer?
3. How does the definition of *quality of life* affect decisions about the use of AT?
4. Is it essential that a comprehensive assessment be completed before providing an individual with an assistive technology? What circumstances may affect the decision to complete a comprehensive assessment?

Research Domain

5. What are some of the key differences between the traditional medical and person-centered models of rehabilitation? How do these differences affect the research questions that are asked and the methodologies used in studies?

Policy Domain

6. How do the factors that influence the use of AT map with the ICF? What are the implications for use of the ICF in policy development?

NOTE

1. For more information on RERC-ACT (Advancing Cognitive Technologies), see http://www.uchsc.edu/atp/RERC-ACT (retrieved June 28, 2005). For more information on RESNA, an interdisciplinary association for the advancement of rehabilitation and assistive technologies (AT), see http://www.resna.org (retrieved June 22, 2005).

REFERENCES

Americans with Disabilities Act of 1990. Pub. L. No. 100–633. [On-line] Retrieved March 8, 2006, from http://www.jan.wvu.edu/links/ADAtam1.html.

Cook, A., & Hussey, S. (2002). *Assistive technologies: Principles and practice* (2nd ed.). St. Louis, MO: Mosby.

Coombs, F. K. (1999). *Development of an ultra-lightweight manual wheelchair from engineered resins.* Proceedings of the RESNA 1999 Annual Conference, June 25–29, 1999, Long Beach, CA (pp. 291–293). Arlington, VA: RESNA.

Coombs, F. K. (2000). *Outcomes measures in assistive technology service delivery.* Annual Conference of the American Congress of Rehabilitation medicine, October 5. Hilton Head, SC.

Craddock, G. (2002a). Partnership and Assistive technology in Ireland. In M. J. Scherer (Ed.), *Assistive technology: Matching device and consumer for successful rehabilitation* (pp. 253–266). Washington, DC: American Psychological Association Books.

Craddock, G. (2002b). Delivering an AT service: A client-focused, social and participatory service delivery model in assistive technology. *Disability & Rehabilitation, 24*(1/2/3), 160–170.

Cushman, L. A., & Scherer, M. J. (1996). Measuring the relationship of assistive technology use, functional status over time, and consumer-therapist perceptions of ATs. *Assistive Technology, 8*(2), 103–109.

DeRuyter, F. (1995). Evaluating outcomes in assistive technology: Do we understand the commitment? *Assistive Technology,. 7,* 3–16.

DeRuyter, F. (1997). The importance of outcome measures for assistive technology service delivery systems. *Technology and Disability, 6*(1,2), 89–100.

DeRuyter, F. (1998). Concepts and rationale for accountability in assistive technology. In *RESNA resource guide for assistive technology outcomes: Vol. 1. Measurement tools* (pp. 2–14). Arlington, VA: RESNA.

Donnelly, C., & Carswell, A. (2002). Individualized outcome measures: A review of the literature. *Canadian Journal of Occupational Therapy, 69*(2), 84–94.

Federici, S., & Micangeli, A. (2003). *Psicotecnologie per la salute e le disabilità.* Trento: Erickson.

Fuhrer, M. J. (2001). Assistive technology outcomes research: Challenges met and yet unmet. *American Journal of Physical Medicine and Rehabilitation, 80*(7), 528–535.

Gray, D. B., Quatrano, L. A., & Lieberman, M. L. (Eds.). (1998). *Designing and using assistive technology: The human perspective.* Baltimore, MD: Paul H. Brookes.

Holland, R. L. (2002, August 29). Unpublished raw data. Tech team project report for Applications of Rehabilitation Technology course (ARP 607), San Diego State University. A course final project integrating knowledge of AT devices and services and means of involving the consumer in the AT selection process.

Jutai, J., Ladak, N., Schuller, R., Naumann, S., & Wright, V. (1996). Outcomes measurement of assistive technologies: An institutional case study. *Assistive Technology, 8*(2), 110–120.

Mann, W. C., Ottenbacher, K. J., Frass, L., Tomita, M., & Granger, C. V. (1999). Effectiveness of assistive technology and environmental interventions in maintaining independence and reducing home care costs for the frail elderly: A randomized controlled trial. *Archives of Family Medicine, 8*(3), 210–217.

Merbitz, C. T. (1996). Frequency measures of behavior for assistive technology and rehabilitation. *Assistive Technology, 8*(2), 121–130.

National Center for Health Statistics, Centers for Disease Control and Prevention. (2005). Disabilities/limitations. Retrieved from http://www.cdc.gov/nchs/fastats/disable.htm.

Punch, K. F. (1996). *Introduction to social research: Quantitative and qualitative approaches.* Thousand Oaks, CA: Sage.

Ripat, J. & Booth, A. (2005). Characteristics of assistive technology service delivery models. *Disability and Rehabilitation, 27,* 1461–1470.

Sachs-Ericsson, N., Hansen, N., and Fitzgerald, S. (2002). Benefits of assistance dogs: A review. *Rehabilitation Psychology, 47*(3), 251–277.

Scherer, M. J. (1996). Outcomes of assistive technology use on quality of life. *Disability and Rehabilitation, 18*(9), 439–448.

Scherer, M. J. (1998). *Matching Person & Technology (MPT) model manual and assessments* (3rd ed.). Webster, NY: Institute for Matching Person & Technology. Retrieved from http://members.aol.com/IMPT97/MPT.html

Scherer, M. J. (Ed.). (2002a). *Assistive technology: Matching device and consumer for successful rehabilitation.* Washington, DC: American Psychological Association Books.

Scherer, M. J. (2002b). The change in emphasis from people to person: Introduction to the special issue on assistive technology. *Disability & Rehabilitation, 24*(1/2/3), 1–4.

Scherer, M. J. (2005). *Living in the state of stuck: How technology impacts the lives of people with disabilities* (4th ed.). Cambridge, MA: Brookline Books.

Scherer, M. J., & Sax, C. (2005, June 22). *Cross mapping the ICF to a measure of assistive technology (AT) predisposition and use.* Eleventh World Health Organization (WHO) North American Collaborating Center (NACC) Conference on the International Classification of Functioning, Disability, and Health (ICF): Mapping the Clinical World to ICF, Mayo Clinic, Rochester, MN. Retrieved from http://www.icfconference.com/abstracts/Batch%20A/1_Scherer.doc.

Team Rehab Report. (1993, June). *Mobility Focus.* Culver City, CA: Cannon Publications.

Temkin, T., Kraus, L., Galvin, J., Carlson, B., Hanson, S., Jans, L., et al. (1999). *Needs assessment and resource analysis for the Family Center on Technology and Disability* (Final Report). Berkeley, CA: InfoUse.

World Health Organization. (2001). *International classification of functioning, disability, and health.* Switzerland: WHO.

Zapf, S. A., & Rough, R. B. (2002). The development of an instrument to match individuals with disabilities and service animals. *Disability & Rehabilitation, 24*(1/2/3), 47–58.

CHAPTER TEN

Contextually Appropriate Design in Rural Community Disability and Rehabilitation Science

Tom Seekins

After the discovery had been assimilated, scientists were able to account for a wider range of natural phenomenon. . . . But that gain was achieved only by discarding some previously standard beliefs or procedures and, simultaneously, by replacing those components of the previous paradigm with others. . . . (*Often*) The awareness of anomaly had lasted so long and penetrated so deep that one can appropriately describe the fields affected by it as in a state of growing crisis. Because it demands large-scale paradigm destruction and major shifts in the problems and techniques of normal science, the emergence of new theories is generally preceded by a period of pronounced professional insecurity.

—T. S. Kuhn (1962)

In the early 1970s, the fields and disciplines that conduct research in disability began experiencing what Kuhn (1962) describes as a crisis (DeJong, 1979, 1983). The crisis in disability and rehabilitation came when conventional research designs and approaches no longer provided satisfying answers to people with disabilities (e.g., Brooks, 1983; National Council on Independent Living, 2002). A primary feature of this crisis involves tension between the so-called medical model that views disability as an individual defect and an ecological model. The ecological model, recently referred to as the New Paradigm (NP) of disability (Seelman, 2000), emphasizes the role individuals play in shaping their world and the role the environment plays in limiting participation of individuals in their community (e.g., Fougeyrollas & Beauregard, 2001). This crisis in disability and rehabilitation science has left researchers and academics struggling to create new theories and new science. Researchers have continued to apply scientific methods to important issues in the absence of such theories but, while some of that research may be relevant and satisfying, there is a need to organize these efforts in a more coherent fashion that can focus research efforts more efficiently and effectively. Fortunately, the ideas behind this criticism contain the seeds of the solution to the crisis in science they created.

The recent publication of the International Classification of Function, Disability, and Health (ICF) highlights these tensions (World Health Organization, 2001). The ICF presents an expanded view of disability that significantly increases the role accorded the environment and focuses on participation as the primary outcome. More recently, some researchers have suggested that participation is becoming a gold-standard construct in disability science (e.g., Berland, 2003). These developments underscore the need for models to organize research in a way that leads to useful, empirically derived practices.

This chapter briefly reviews the history of the ongoing paradigm shift, provides an analysis of the community context of disability research, describes strategies for designing contextually appropriate interventions, and provides an example of such an intervention by describing a voucher model for rural transportation. The brief historical review emphasizes the relationship between social goals, and between theories and methods (i.e., research tools, methods, and design).

A BRIEF HISTORY OF DISABILITY AND PSYCHOLOGY

Psychology has a long history in the fields of disability and rehabilitation. Several subfields specifically incorporate a strong role for the environment.

In the 1950s, the community mental health movement emerged with a vision of community service and justice for those with mental illness, but its primary techniques involved office-based therapy and counseling (Bloom, 1977). Prevention and community integration were goals and became social policy, but the tools for achieving that vision did not yet exist (Albee, 1986). While the social goals were consistent with what we now see as the NP, the science was rooted in a model that focused on treating the individual to increase his or her ability to adapt to an environment that was seen as relatively immutable. Drug therapy contributed substantially to the possibility and practicality of deinstitutionalization, but focused on controlling individual symptomatology. In many cases, the critics of the deinstitutional movement were correct: people were being moved "out of their beds and into the streets" with little or no real support or community integration (Torrey, 1997). Little progress was made in developing environmental measures, methods, principles, and practices that could be tested or implemented on any scale.

At the same time, ecological concepts were emerging in other sciences and were applied to psychology (Barker, 1968). Ecological psychologists developed measurement systems and several important concepts, but stopped short of methods or practices. Nevertheless, they began tying psychology to the environment with concepts such as environmental press, over-manned and under-manned settings, and behavior within context (Barker & Gump, 1964). Similarly, even with its focus on the individual, developmental psychology contributed by also emphasizing that the environment shapes behavioral outcomes (Horowitz, 1987).

Beginning in the 1960s, researchers and practitioners in the field of developmental disabilities were influenced by principles of normalization that emphasized the effect of the environment on the adjustment of those with mental retardation (Wolfensberger, 1972). The goal of social advocates was to normalize institutions and to move people out of institutions into community-based programs. This movement found a friend in the field of applied behavior analysis that provided both a conceptual system (i.e., principles, measures, methods, and techniques) and tools for modifying the environment to manage behavior (Wolery, Bailey, & Sugai, 1988). These tools included the theoretical orientation that the environment determined behavior. Social advocates used this success to support their argument for deinstitutionalization and the development of community-based supports.

THE EMERGENCE OF THE INDEPENDENT LIVING MOVEMENT

The IL movement is more than a grassroots effort on the part of the disabled to acquire new rights; it is also intent on reshaping the thinking of disability professionals and researchers . . . and on encouraging new directions in research. Independent living (is) an analytic paradigm which aims to redirect the course of disability policy, practice, and research.

—Gerbon DeJong (1983)

One of the challenges of applied science is balancing rigor with relevance; balancing theory and practicability to advance a science. In the field of disability and rehabilitation, the current crisis was brought on by several factors, including social change and scientific advancements. One starting place, however, is the emergence of the Independent Living (IL) movement. Early forms of this movement emphasized dissatisfaction with the ability of the current treatment and research models to produce outcomes desired by people with disability (Brooks, 1983; National Council on Independent Living, 2002). Even when rehabilitation practice—defined as techniques to restore function and help people with disabilities adjust to their condition—was applied well, many people with disabilities were left in institutions, segregated from and unable to participate in their community.

The IL movement emerged in the 1970s. While this movement was organized primarily by those with disabilities related to physical impairments, its view was much broader and encompassed individuals with any disability. Gerben DeJong (1979, 1983) captured the essence of the importance of the IL movement. He described people with disability as creating and taking control of a social movement and an analytic paradigm intent on changing things, including research in disability and rehabilitation.

Researchers who sought to improve rehabilitation techniques, or sought to focus on promoting individual adjustment or to use theories of intrapsychic adjustment to explain the experience of people with disabilities, found their work being criticized as irrelevant (Brooks, 1983; National Council on Independent Living, 2002). In terms of the concepts of social validity outlined by Wolf (1978), the customary practice of science and research was no longer addressing issues of importance to a key constituency, no longer addressing issues in a manner they judged as appropriate, and no longer producing meaningful results. From Kuhn's perspective, this is the essence of a science in crisis. Fortunately, the ideas behind the criticisms contain the seeds of a solution.

THE FUNCTION AND FEATURES OF THEORY AND SCIENCE

Theory is important because it has function and influences the conduct of research. Science, while it often rests on theory, involves the process of systematically classifying and organizing observations and the methods of discovery within a domain. Science provides the measures and methods for conducting research in an area both to test expected relationships and to produce useful practices. This view of theory suggests that it provides an organizing framework for research by defining categories of interest, identifying key variables, and outlining their expected relationships.

Theory, simply defined, is a scheme or system of ideas that categorizes observations and experiences in a way to explain or account for them. Further, theories suggest the key variables of interest and how they are expected to be related. Theory is an organized collection of principles involving statements of facts on which a science depends.

If the dominant disability and rehabilitation theory is in crisis, researchers might begin considering potential new theories more consistent with the emerging New Paradigm. So, what can researchers learn about needed theory from the New Paradigm and people with disability?

The Emerging Outline of a Science for the New Paradigm

The outlines of a "normal science" within the New Paradigm are beginning to emerge. There are several depictions of this outline. For example, Brandt and Pope (1997), Horowitz (1987), Litvak and Enders (2001), and White (2002) present models that depict outcome as an interaction between the individual and his or her environment over time. Figure 10.1 depicts one such framework within the context of disability and independent living. Here, an individual's IL outcome

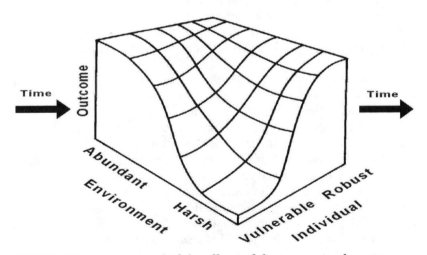

FIGURE 10.1   A portrayal of the effects of the interaction between individual and environmental characteristics on independent living outcome over time. Individuals are portrayed as varying along a dimension from vulnerable to robust. Environments are portrayed as varying along a dimension from harsh to abundant

is portrayed as a function of the interaction of specific individual characteristics with specific environmental features at a specific point in time. Environments can vary from harsh to abundant and supportive. Individuals can vary along a continuum of vulnerable to robust. This framework accommodates the observation, for example, that an individual with vulnerable characteristics within a specifiable context can still have positive outcome, if the environment is abundant and supportive. It also accommodates the observation that people with similar impairments can have dramatically different outcomes, depending on the cultural context in which they live.

The New Paradigm shifts attention away from simply examining physiological and functional states, and away from explaining individual adjustment to those states and their consequences in an environment assumed to be relatively static. Rather, it points to a focus on participation as an outcome of a dynamic interaction between the individual and a mutable environment over time. It calls on researchers to consider how the environment contributes to creating disability or accommodating impairment. Perhaps more important, it calls on researchers to examine the ecological interactions as unique unto themselves— identifiable phenomena—and their effects on the individual and the environment.

Regardless of the level of analysis, disability is now being defined as a normal part of the human condition. Advocates want to be integrated into the community, to participate equally in daily life, and to feel like a part of their community.[1] Indeed, participation is becoming a gold standard of measurement in disability research (Berland, 2003; World Health Organization, 2001).

In a review of rural public health, Elder, Ayala, Zabinski, Prochaska, and Gehrman (2001) found that the accepted view in the field of public health is that health is an outcome of the interaction between the individual and his or her environment. They identified 11 theories used as the foundation of public health research reports in the literature. However, only 4 could be said to be interactional (i.e., applied behavior analysis, social learning theory, social ecology model, and theories of community self-control). These researchers further commented that, despite the dominance of models that view health as interactional across multiple levels, most health promotion efforts continue to focus on the individual. It seems likely that reports in the field of disability and rehabilitation are in a similar state.

Generally, the environment may be viewed as nested layers, including such major levels as the physical world, culture, and social structures (e.g., political, market, religious, and civic structures) that influence a wide range of activities. Similarly, the individual can be analyzed as a parallel set of nested levels, including physiology, values, knowledge, skills, and abilities. Figure 10.2 suggests how these come together at the point of ecological transaction between the individual and the environment.

At this ecological intersection, individuals organize physical and social resources into behavioral settings to create niches and achieve goals. Behavioral settings include four components: architectural spaces, social structures, assistive technologies, and behavioral technologies within those spaces. An individual's engagement constitutes participation in ways that include observable behavior and subjective consequences (e.g., psychological sense of community). Such frameworks provide tools for organizing observations and identifying potential causal variables associated with the experience of people with disabilities.[2]

Table 10.1 organizes selected features of the three main elements of the New Paradigm across levels of theory and science. For example, it shows that, at the level of worldview, the individual feature includes physiology, the environmental feature includes the physical and social world, and the ecological feature is recursive. It is at the level of measures and methods, values and practices, that the design of interventions occurs.

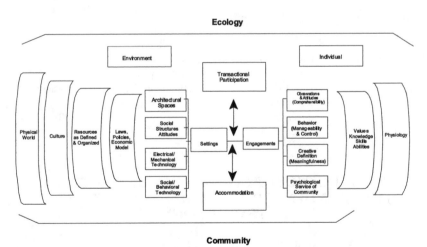

FIGURE 10.2   A portrayal of layers of the environment, the individual, and the point of ecological transaction between the two. The central feature of this figure involved individual engagements in environmental settings. These engagements involve transactional participation in which the environment changes to accommodate an individual or the individual changes to match existing circumstances

TABLE 10.1 Examples of Key Concepts of Theory Across Elements of The New Paradigm

Levels of Theory	Individual Capacity	Environmental Factors	Ecology
Worldview or Paradigm	Physiological, Developmental, and Active Agent	Physical, Social, Cultural, Contextual, Malleable, Varied	Interactive, Recursive, Reciprocal
Concepts and Key Variables	Limitation, Behavior, Sense of Community, Secondary Conditions, Creativity Capacity	Accessible, Options, Contingencies of Reinforcement	Participation, Accommodation, Fit
Categories and Relationships	Knowledge, Skills, and Abilities	Laws, Regulations, Models, Programs	Ecological, Interactive, Recursive
Measures and Methods	Self-report, Direct Observation, Permanent Product Traces	Universal Design, Classification, Impacts	Appropriate Design, Grounded, Behavioral Analysis
Values and Practice	Rehabilitation, Treatment, Assistive Technology, Behavioral Intervention	Public Policy, Support Systems, Contingency Management, Advocacy	Consumer Choice, Community Development, Participatory Action Research

CONVERGENCE OF COMMUNITY DEVELOPMENT, INDEPENDENT LIVING, AND REHABILITATION PSYCHOLOGY

A great deal of applied research involves using scientific methods to develop and evaluate new means for social change. While social change can be viewed in different ways (e.g., treatment intervention, service models, programs, resource allocation decisions, or new policies and laws), the creation of interventions requires specific design elements. Design reflects all elements of theory (implicit or explicit). It is influenced by measures and methods, as well as values and practices.

When one considers participation, it implies participation in a community. As disability may be seen as a social construct, community is an ecological concept. Participation involves intricate and sometimes simultaneous events that occur as a result of other events. It can be defined by individuals in a wide variety of ways leading to diverse responses affecting the environment, and that affect one another in reciprocal and recursive ways.[3] The following sections provide an analysis of community context, outline strategies for designing contextually appropriate interventions, and give an example of such design in rural transportation.

A Functional Analysis of Community

In ecology, community is a natural population of organisms occupying a common area. For humans, there are communities of place, communities of interest, and communities of blood. They all share the characteristic of people interacting in a definable context. The behavior of individuals within any community is determined by their history, setting events, antecedent stimuli, and consequent events, including contingencies of reinforcement, and individual capacity (Skinner, 1981). Individuals actively organize resources in the community's environment to increase the likelihood of achieving their goals (i.e., reinforcing events). The community environment has identifiable features that can be measured, such as distributive equity, availability, accessibility, distance, and slope. These features can be assessed independently or as a product of behavior. Similarly, behavior has measurable features such as frequency and rate. The ecological interactions of the two, environment and behavior, also have definable and measurable features, including engagement, participation, reasonable accommodation, and others, but these features are less well understood.

In transportation, "rides" is an ecological event that includes behavior in interaction with physical and social resources. As such, transportation represents ecology.

Contextually Appropriate Design

The fields of behavioral and community psychology, and community development offer a range of methods, measures, and practices that are consistent with the emerging outline of a science for the New Paradigm. Both IL philosophy and community development practice emphasize the interdependence of individuals living in communities, including empowerment, environmental determinants of life quality, inclusion, and civil rights. They both also incorporate a strengths orientation to theory, research, and practice.

While IL and community development provide values and practices, the field of appropriate technology provides criteria for contextually appropriate design (e.g., Fawcett, Mathews, & Fletcher, 1980; Schumacher, 1999).[4] These criteria suggest that interventions should be effective, simple, flexible and adaptable, inexpensive, decentralized, sustainable with local resources, and compatible with the social context. From a scientific perspective, researchers should be developing innovations that meet these criteria. Measures used should also address these dimensions.

These values, principles, and design criteria can be brought together through methods of Participatory Action Research (Whyte, 1991). Community ecologies can be extremely complex. Participatory Action Research (PAR) is a particularly useful method in designing ecological research because it increases knowledge of the range of variables and their intricate relationships. Any one event can be influenced by many others. In turn, a purposeful change in some arrangement can have multiple collateral and often unintended consequences. By involving individuals from a given environmental context, researchers call on the knowledge and experience of those imbedded within it. Involvement increases awareness of available resources, the intricacies of variables interacting within a context that must be considered and accommodated in contextually appropriate design, options, and appropriate research and development procedures. By applying the criteria for appropriate design, researchers can also increase the likelihood that the results of research will be relevant and used. As such, the process protects research from threats to its social validity (Seekins, 2002).

Rural Community Disability and Rehabilitation

The study of *rural* disability and rehabilitation is particularly well suited for developing a science for the NP of disability. First, rural is a context. That context is community and community is social ecology. Further, unlike cities, where community can be hard to find, most rural places clearly define community boundaries. Second, while the structures and relationships in rural communities are often more tightly knit, there are somewhat fewer of them and they are often clearer. In short, concern for rural is a concern for rural communities. Community is environment.

Problems—discrepancies between desired goals and actual outcomes—emerge when people interact with a context. Rural communities have certain features that can create problems when individuals with disability attempt to achieve goals within that context. As a problem-solver applying scientific methods, one can attempt to change the features of the context or environment: building resources, removing barriers, increasing equitable distribution of resources, and expanding on strengths so more can experience their benefits. This is typically called rural community development.

Values, Principles, and Methods of Resource Management

A concern for equity and efficiency is at the heart of many of the problems identified by rural Americans (DeFries & Ricketts, 1989; Flora & Christenson, 1991). Researchers and rural advocates consistently marshal evidence that rural populations receive disproportionately less of society's resources to address problems that are often greater than those experienced in urban areas. In general, rural areas have a more limited range of services and their residents must use more informal and lower specialized services, travel farther, and use more of their own income to get lower quality assistance than their urban counterparts.

Our research and development is based on rural resource management practice (Jackson, Seekins, & Offner, 1992). A resource management approach assumes that it is unlikely that enough resources will ever be allocated by government to solve these problems. Rather, in the rural tradition, this approach asks how available resources can be redefined, reorganized, extended, linked, or supplemented to support the efforts of people with disabilities to live healthy lives and participate in their communities. This makes a tight fit with the interactive model of independence and the ecological perspective.

The Example of Rural Transportation

Transportation provides a good example of the features described above, in the effort to manage resources in order to promote participation. A simplistic view of transportation involves four major variables: money, vehicles, riders, and an organizational model for bringing the other three together. In this framework, rides are an ecological event that involve resource management (Jackson et al., 1992). A key question is, what resources exist and who manages them? Our programmatic line of research has attempted a multilevel approach, including addressing issues involved in resource allocation at the federal level, contracting policy at the state and local level, resource organization and management, transactional mechanisms, consumer control, and psychological sense of community.

Resource environment. There are approximately 12.5 million people with disabilities living in rural areas of the United States, 6 million of whom have a severe disability (Seekins, 1995). People with disabilities and disability service providers in rural areas cite the lack of transportation as one of their most frequent, significant, and persistent problems (Arnold, Seekins, & Nelson, 1997; Bernier & Seekins, 1999; Jackson et al., 1992; Kidder, 1989; Nosek, Zhu, & Howland, 1992; Tonsing-Gonzales, 1989).

Historically, federal public transportation funds have been inequitably allocated between urban and rural areas—an inequity with a particularly significant, deleterious impact on people with disabilities and disability service providers in rural areas. Clearly, this lack of transportation is a serious obstacle to achieving the independent living and employment goals that are central to the mission of the Rehabilitation Services Administration (RSA), and its state vocational rehabilitation (VR), independent living (IL), and tribal partners.

The 1998 authorization of the Transportation Equity Act for the 21st Century (TEA-21) increased the total funding for public transportation, and increased the funding for rural transportation and transportation for the elderly and individuals with disabilities. Still, the discrepancy between urban and rural transportation allocations remains significant. Over 94% of transportation funds subsidize transportation for the 75% of the population living in urban areas, while only about 6% goes to support transportation for the 25% of the nation's population living in rural areas (Transportation Equity Act for the 21st Century, 1998).

The Rural Transit Assistance Program (1994) reports that one out of six households in large urban areas doesn't own a vehicle. Urban public transportation provides an average of 955 trips annually for such households, which translates to an average of nearly 20 rides for each work week. In contrast, Rucker (1994) reports that 1 out of 13 rural households doesn't own a private vehicle and 41% of rural residents live in the nation's 1,200 counties with no public transportation at all. People living in rural areas who don't own a vehicle average only about 38 publicly-subsidized rides per *year*, fewer than *one* ride per work week. Obviously, this discrepancy can make independent living and working relatively more difficult in rural areas.

We estimate that an additional $523 million in federal rural transportation allocation would be required to equalize funding between urban and rural areas on the basis of population alone (RTC: Rural, 1999). The magnitude of this discrepancy suggests why transportation has been a consistent problem in rural areas. However, it is unlikely that this discrepancy will soon change significantly. As such, there is a tremendous need to develop and demonstrate cost-effective innovative models of rural transportation for people with disabilities using readily available resources (Jackson, et al., 1992).

While the funding for general rural transportation, and for rural transportation of people with disabilities, is unlikely to change quickly, a model showing how funds can be used effectively is an important support for efforts to secure such funding. It may also suggest ways to address the poverty which many people with disabilities experience.

Transportation resource management. Transportation problems can be seen as stemming from individual-level variables and from environmental factors. Each might suggest a different target and approach to research. Along the individual dimension, one could define the transportation problem as involving individuals who lack physical, sensory, or cognitive capacity to drive their own car. This analysis might suggest research and development in educational, behavioral, and technological strategies to compensate for functional discrepancies between needed and actual capacity. In fact, quite a few services are based on this analysis (e.g., Kessler Medical Rehabilitation Research and Education Corporation, 2003).

Alternatively, one might focus analysis along the environmental and ecological dimensions. At the environmental level, one might consider the distribution of public transportation resources such as funding and vehicles, the associated public policies, and various resource management models.

Along the ecological dimension, one might examine the individual's role in creating and managing his or her own transportation resources and strategies. We asked, what are the resources available and how can they be organized to increase participation in rural communities? What is the role of individuals with disabilities in creating and managing these resources?

In one form of PAR, community members directed our attention to a transportation program that had emerged in one rural community. The program consisted of a small allocation of funds ($1,500 annually) by the county commission to a CIL serving the county for consumers to use for transportation in the way they thought best. They created a common pool of resources from which they could draw. Consumers arranged for rides themselves, relying on friends, neighbors, family, and other volunteers. Not only were the participants satisfied with this arrangement, there was money left over at the end of each year that carried forward.

There are many elements of this program but, for us, it suggested that, in an environment that did not provide a socially organized structure for transportation, individuals with disabilities could (and do) manage their own resources effectively. Further, by supplementing their personal resources and allowing them the freedom to use their creative talents and personal resources to meet their needs as they saw fit, a substantial portion of their concern over transportation was solved. Importantly, this practice had emerged from a rural context and had what might be called contextual validity.

From these lessons and observations, we derived a program based on a voucher model for rural transportation (Bernier & Seekins, 1999). The key element of the program addresses resources. That is, the program is designed to place resources (money in the form of vouchers) into the hands of consumers and, with minimal support, to allow them to organize and manage these and their own resources to achieve their goals. In brief, a local sponsoring agency identifies and recruits consumer participants, allocates resources in the form of vouchers, works with consumers to help them develop strategies to use the vouchers effectively, identifies any public transit providers and negotiates with them to accept the vouchers in lieu of payment, and reimburses providers who submit vouchers for payment.

We have examined the voucher model in four rural areas serving over nine frontier counties in three states (Bernier & Seekins, 1999). Figure 10.3 portrays the commutative number of trips by type of ride in one such application over 18 months. We also collected data on the extent of participation and its effects on perceived sense of community, but variables outside of the researchers' control reduced response rate and precluded analysis.

The voucher model, now called the Traveler's Cheque model, meets many criteria or features of appropriate technology. It is simple, flexible, inexpensive, decentralized, sustainable with local resources, and compatible

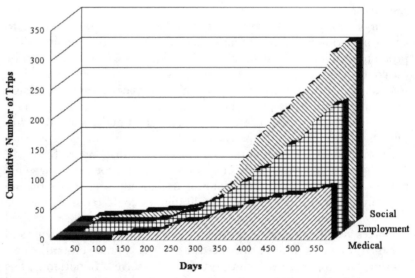

FIGURE 10.3   The cumulative number of trips by type of ride over time in Yankton, South Dakota

with IL philosophy and rural community traditions of self-help. This research is analytic and scientific across individual, environmental, and ecological factors. Further, meeting the criteria of appropriate design is helping lead the way to impact, defined as changes in the way others do their work; and outcomes, defined as the consequences of new approaches experienced by individuals with disabilities.

There are now many variations of this approach that have begun to emerge spontaneously from various community contexts and systematically in an effort to determine their utility in practice. For example, RSA funded two demonstrations of this model. One is a state-level effort being conducted by the Arkansas vocational rehabilitation program in the form of the DELTA Cadet model and the second is a national demonstration by our collaborators, the Association of Programs for Rural Independent Living (APRIL).

A POSTSCRIPT ON TRANSFORMATIONS

The New Paradigm (NP) of disability emerged, in part, from a recognition that there was a paradigm shift occurring in disability and rehabilitation (DeJong, 1979). This major shift in perspective was to focus on the environment as a contributing factor to disability rather than focusing on the individual alone. This perspective transformed the research paradigm in disability and rehabilitation.

Another transformation that accompanied the IL paradigm was a shift in the understanding of how research questions should be developed, who should be in charge of research, and who the audience was for applied research in disability and rehabilitation. Variously termed participatory action research (PAR), constituency-oriented research and development (CORD), and market-oriented research in disability and rehabilitation, the focus shifted away from theory-driven, disciplinary-oriented research toward applied research that addressed issues of importance to people with disabilities.

A third transformation taking place is in basic assumptions about the nature of disability experienced in the context of community. Rather than simply viewing disability as a problem to be solved through various forms of rehabilitation, it views disability as part of the natural course of life, and recognizes the strengths of people with disabilities and the contributions they make to their community.

Transformational Research

Transformational research may be defined as research that by the way it frames questions and reports results literally transforms an audience's perspective on disability and people with disabilities. It is consistent with IL philosophy and is consistent with a positive psychology or a strengths orientation and may be contrasted with deficits-oriented research.

Seligman and Csikszentmihalyi (2000) describe positive psychology as focusing on achievements and possibilities of normal and exceptional people rather than focusing solely on individual deficits experienced by those with mental illness. Others have articulated the need for strengths-based research as compared to deficit-oriented research (e.g., Rappaport, 1977). These approaches share an orientation that views individuals as full of creative possibilities, and as contributors to community, and ask how such talents, and personal and community resources, can be maximized.

Much research on disability has taken a deficit-oriented approach. Questions are typically framed in a way that defines people with disabilities or their lives as problematic, limited by the disability. In essence, a physiological characteristic (i.e., an impairment) or its functional consequences (within environments that are typically restrictive) may come to define individuals. The purpose of such research is often stated as seeking a solution or cure to these problems or deficits.

Alternately, if a strengths orientation is applied to studies of disability, the questions are framed in such a way as to ask: What do people with disability contribute to their community? How can their contribution be understood and maximized? What lessons can be learned from the accumulated wisdom of life experiences of people with disabilities? What personal resources and talents do people with disabilities bring to their life's task and to their community?

When research questions are framed in this way and research results report on the extent of contributions and strengths, the research audience's view of disability in general, and of people with disability, may undergo a dramatic shift in orientation. The research may literally transform the audience's perspective on disability and on people with disability. The impairment and associated difficulties may recede in this gestalt, to be replaced by creative perspectives. In the context of the NP of disability, such work may be said to be transformational research. Giving individuals with disabilities the resources to control their own transportation represents one small example of a strengths-oriented study.

Another example involves a series of studies of business ownership among people with disability (e.g., Arnold & Seekins, 1994; Arnold, 2001). When these researchers report their findings that nearly as many people with disabilities are self-employed as work for federal, state, and local governments combined, and that people with disabilities are nearly twice as likely to report being self-employed as the general population, audiences are often puzzled—even stunned. Most had never thought of people with disabilities as acquiring the status of owning their own business—never thought of people with disabilities as creating jobs and hiring others. They had usually viewed most people with disabilities as supplicants for jobs created by others. These data were literally helping audiences through a transformation of how they thought of disability and people with disabilities.

SUMMARY

The emerging outlines of a science for the New Paradigm of disability require that research be grounded in the daily experience of individuals within their context. It should respect and build upon the resources and intricacies of that context and can do so most effectively by using methods of Participatory Action Research. Further, it should recognize and respect the skills, capacities, and values individuals bring to creating their own choices, as well as creating opportunities for others.

QUESTIONS FOR DISCUSSION AND FURTHER STUDY

Service Domain

1. What is the relationship between rural community development, and disability and rehabilitation research?
2. What are the design criteria suggested by the appropriate technology movement, and how might they be applied to disability and rehabilitation research?

Research Domain

3. How does T. S. Kuhn's view of the structure of scientific revaluations apply to disability and rehabilitation research?
4. What does the International Classification of Function, Disability, and Health set as a gold standard for outcome measurement? How does it affect disability and rehabilitation research?
5. What is transformational research and how is it related to positive psychology?

Policy Domain

6. What has been a primary criticism of disability and rehabilitation research by members of the disability movement? What policies and other approaches might address that criticism?

7. What is at the heart of many of the problems identified by rural Americans with disabilities? How does a resource management approach help address these basic concerns? Explain how the problem of rural transportation provides an example of both the core problem and the use of resource management.

ACKNOWLEDGMENTS

Preparation of this manuscript was supported, in part, by grants from the National Institute on Disability and Rehabilitation Research and the Centers for Disease Control and Prevention. The author wishes to thank his many colleagues and collaborators for their contributions to the ideas represented in this chapter, in particular: Craig Ravesloot, Meg Traci, Nancy Arnold, and Glen White. He also wishes to acknowledge Kathy Dwyer for assistance in preparing the figures.

NOTES

1. Interestingly, Putnam (2000) has documented that people with disabilities are not the only ones feeling alienated from community. He points out that civic engagement has been on a decline for decades.
2. Such general levels provide an outline for theory but do not represent theory. That requires much more specific statements about variables and their relationships. For example, one might specify the features of universal design and articulate their relationship to engagement or participation in a given context. These statements can then be phrased as hypotheses. For example, a hypothesis in this framework might be stated like so: "The availability of universally designed transportation and accessible places within a given community is positively related to the frequency, duration, and variability of engagement and participation in the community."
3. The ways in which a given group of people define various elements and link them conceptually may be described as culture. These systems act recursively. For example, in some cultures, having an impairment may elevate one's status within the community. The ways in which an individual with an impairment responds to being a valued-as opposed to a devalued-wmember of a community are likely to be very different.
4. It is important to distinguish notions of appropriate technology emerged from the field of international economic development (Taylor-Ide & Taylor, 2002) from those of assistive technology as is understood in rehabilitation. The concept of universal design may be the closest disability concept to appropriate technology as used in community development. Some would argue that much assistive technology violates criteria of appropriate technology.

REFERENCES

Albee, G. (1986). Toward a just society: Lessons from observations on the primary prevention of psychopathology. *American Psychologist, 41*(8), 891–898.
Arnold, N. (2001). *First national study of people with disabilities who are self-employed.* Missoula, MT: RTC: Rural, Rural Institute, University of Montana.

Arnold, N., & Seekins, T. (1994). Self-employment as a vocational rehabilitation closure: An examination of state policies. *Journal of Disability Policy Studies, 5,* 65–80.

Arnold, N., Seekins, T., & Nelson, R. (1997). A comparison of vocational rehabilitation counselors: Urban and rural differences. *Rehabilitation Counseling Bulletin, 41*(1), 2–14.

Barker, R. G. (1968). *Ecological psychology: Concepts and methods for studying the environment of human behavior.* Stanford, CA: Stanford University Press.

Barker, R. G., & Gump, P. V. (1964). *Big school, small school.* Sanford, CA: Stanford University Press.

Berland, B. J. (2003). *Comments on the long range plan of the National Institute on disability and rehabilitation research.* Paper presented at the annual meeting of the National Association of Rehabilitation Research and Training Centers, Washington, DC.

Bernier, B., & Seekins, T. (1999). Rural transportation voucher program for people with disabilities: Three case studies. *Journal of Transportation and Statistics, 2*(1), 61–70.

Brandt, E. N., & Pope, A. M. (1997). *Enabling America: Assessing the role of rehabilitation science and engineering.* Washington, DC: National Academy Press.

Bloom, B. L. (1977). *Community mental health: A general introduction.* Monterey, CA: Brooks/Cole Publishing Company.

Brooks, N. A. (1983). Using field research to gain subjective insight. In N. A. Crewe and I. K. Zola (Eds.), *Independent living for physically disabled people: Developing, implementing, and evaluating self-help rehabilitation programs* (pp. 292–310). San Francisco: Jossey-Bass Publishers.

DeJong, G. (1979). Independent living: From social movement to analytic paradigm. *Archives of Physical Medicine and Rehabilitation, 60,* 435–446.

DeJong, G. (1983) Defining and implementing the independent living concept. In N. A. Crewe and I. K. Zola (Eds.), *Independent living for physically disabled people: Developing, implementing, and evaluating self-help rehabilitation programs* (pp. 4–27). San Francisco: Jossey-Bass Publishers.

Elder, J. P., Ayala, G. X., Zabinski, M. F., Prochaska, J. J., & Gehrman, C. (2001). Theories, models, and methods of health promotion in rural settings. In S. Loue & B. E. Quill (Eds.), *Handbook of rural health* (pp. 295–314). New York: Kluwer Academic/Plenum Publishers.

Fawcett, S. B., Mathews, R. M., & Fletcher, R. K. (1980). Some promising dimensions for behavioral community psychology. *Journal of Applied Behavior Analysis, 3,* 319–342.

Horowitz, F. D. (1987). *Exploring developmental theories: Toward a structural/behavioral model of development.* Hillsdale, NJ: Lawrence Erlbaum Associates.

Jackson, K., Seekins, T., & Offner, R. (1992). Involving consumers and service providers in shaping rural rehabilitation agenda. *American Rehabilitation, 18*(1), 23–29, 48.

Kessler Medical Rehabilitation Research and Education Corporation. (2003). *The use of virtual reality technology for assessment of driving skills following acquired brain injury.* Documents indexed in REHABDATA :H133G000073. Lanham, MD: National Rehabilitation Information Center.

Kidder, A. (1989). Passenger transportation problems in rural areas. In W. R. Gillis (Ed.), *Profitability and mobility in rural America* (pp. 3–4). University Park, PA: Pennsylvania State University Press.

Kuhn, T. S. (1962). *The structure of scientific revolutions.* Chicago, IL: University of Chicago Press.

Litvak, S., & Enders, A. E. (2001). Support systems: The interface between individuals and environments. In G. L. Albrecht, K. D. Seelman, & M. Bury (Eds.), *Handbook of disability studies* (pp. 711–733). Thousand Oaks, CA: Sage.

Nosek, M., Zhu, Y., and Howland, C. (1992). The evolution of independent living programs. *Rehabilitation Counseling Bulletin, 35*(3), 174–189.

Putnam, R. D. (2000). *Bowling alone*. New York: Simon & Schuster.

Rappaport, J. (1977). *Community psychology: Values, research, and action*. New York: Holt, Rinehart, and Winston.

RTC: Rural. (1999). *Rural facts: Inequities in rural transportation*. Missoula, MT: Research and Training Center on Rural Rehabilitation, University of Montana.

Rucker, G. (1994). *Status report on public transportation in rural America*. Washington, DC: Community Transportation Association of America.

Rural Transit Assistance Program. (1994). Washington, DC: Federal Transit Administration.

Schumacher, E. F. (1999). *Small is beautiful: Economics as if people mattered—25 years later with commentaries*. Point Roberts, WA: Hartley & Marks Publishers Inc.

Seelman, K. D. (2000). The new paradigm on disability: Research issues and approaches. In National Institute on Disability and Rehabilitation Research, *The new paradigm on disability: Research issues and approaches* (pp.3–6). Washington, DC: Office of Special Education and Rehabilitative Service, National Institute on Disability and Rehabilitation Research, U.S. Department of Education.

Seekins, T. (1995). Rural rehabilitation. In A. E. Dell Orto & R. P. Marinelli (Eds.), *Encyclopedia of disability and rehabilitation* (pp. 643–651). New York: Simon and Schuster Macmillan Library Reference USA.

Seekins, T. (2002) *Participatory action research designs in applied disability and rehabilitation science: Protecting against threats to social validity*. Missoula, MT: Research and Training Center on Rural Disability and Rehabilitation, University of Montana.

Seligman, M.E.P., & Csikszentmihalyi, M. (2000). Positive psychology: An introduction. *American Psychologist, 55,* 5–14.

Skinner, B. F. (1981). Selection by consequences. *Science, 213,* 501–504.

Taylor-Ide, D., & Taylor, C. E.. (2002). *Just and lasting change: When communities own their futures*. Baltimore: Johns Hopkins University Press.

Tonsing-Gonzales, L. (1989). Rural independent living: Conquering the final frontier. In G. Foss (Ed.), *Meeting the rehabilitation needs of rural Americans* (pp. 3–6). Missoula, MT: Rural Institute on Disabilities.

Torrey, E. F. (1997). *Out of the shadows: Confronting America's mental illness crisis*. New York: John Wiley.

Transportation Equity Act for the 21st Century, P.L. 105-178. (1998).

White, G. W. (2002). PAR and the new paradigm of disability: Implications for rehabilitation. Paper presented at the 15th Annual William A. Spencer Lectureship, the Institute for Rehabilitation Research, Houston, TX.

Whyte, W. F. (1991). *Participatory action research*. Newbury Park, CA: Sage.

Wolery, M., Bailey, D. B., & Sugai, G. M. (1988). *Effective teaching: Principles and procedures of applied behavior analysis with exceptional students*. Boston: Allyn and Bacon.

Wolf, M.M. (1978). Social validity: The case for subjective measurement or how applied behavior analysis is finding its heart. *Journal of Applied Behavior Analysis, 11,* 203–214.

Wolfensberger, W. (1972). *The principle of normalization in human services*. Toronto, Ontario: National Institute on Mental Retardation.

World Health Organization (2001). *International classification of functioning, disability, and health*. Geneva: World Health Organization.

CHAPTER ELEVEN

Internet Resources for People With Disabilities: Applications and Research Directions

Fong Chan
Steven R. Pruett
Susan M. Miller
Michael Frain
Kacie Blalock

The Internet has and will continue to have a profound impact on our lives. It is at once a worldwide broadcasting mechanism, an instrument for information dissemination, and a medium for collaboration and interaction between individuals and their computers regardless of geographic location (Leiner et al., 2002). In order to function effectively in our increasingly wired social and work worlds, it is important that we become computer and Internet literate. It is also important that we conduct research that will help facilitate the use of the Internet by people with disabilities, as it could potentially have a profound effect on the quality of life of these individuals.

The advent of microprocessor technology over the past three decades has led to an information revolution, which has in turn led us away from a manufacturing-based to an information- and service-based economy.

Interestingly, the information-based economy might actually be better for people with physical disabilities. As we move from muscle power to brainpower, barriers such as the physical demands of many jobs, the physical confines of the work environment, and the need for transportation to and from work are reduced for people with physical disabilities (Chan, McCollum, & Parker, 1985). However, although an estimated 54 million Americans have disabilities (Gould, 2002), the preparedness of people with physical disabilities to function in the information technology world remains relatively unknown. To what extent people with disabilities have benefited from information technology, especially the Internet, and how much more it can benefit them, by improving their physical, social, psychological, and vocational well-being, warrants systematic research investigations.

The focus of this chapter is on the Internet and people with physical disabilities. Specifically, we review several issues, including computer/Internet literacy, social-environmental barriers, utilization rates, and Internet services that can help improve the quality of life of people with disabilities. In addition, we identify and discuss rehabilitation research issues and determine research directions related to optimal use of computer/Internet technology by people with physical disabilities.

UTILIZATION RATES AND PATTERNS OF PEOPLE WITH AND WITHOUT DISABILITIES

According to a U.S. Department of Commerce National Telecommunication and Information Administration (NTIA) Report (2000), a digital divide exists between those who have access to digital technologies and those who do not have access. This gap between the digital haves and have-nots is defined by income, education, and ethnicity.

A recent study found that 57% of American adults use the Internet from home (Taylor, 2003). According to the NTIA report, as of 2000, computers were found within 51% of the homes in the United States. The share of households with Internet access was estimated to be 42% (NTIA, 2000). Thus, more than 80% of households with computers also have Internet access. Virtually every demographic group has participated in the sharp upward trend of Americans connecting their homes to the Internet.

Internet penetration rates are greatly affected by education level, household income, and age. According to a survey commissioned by the National Organization on Disability and conducted by the Harris Poll (Taylor, 2000b), people with disabilities have lower educational levels and incomes than people without disabilities. Approximately 22% of people with disabilities have not completed high school, in comparison with 10% of people without disabilities. Only 12% of people with disabilities have graduated from college whereas 23% of people without disabilities have graduated from college. In addition, this survey found that 43% of people with disabilities are unable to work due to disability or health-related reasons. Likewise, 29% of people with disabilities have a household income of $15,000 or less versus 10% of people without disabilities. People with disabilities tend to be older, as well. Since there are a higher proportion of people with disabilities in the categories that the NTIA report indicates have reduced access to the Internet, it is reasonable to conclude that people with disabilities are less likely to go online (Taylor, 2000a).

The digital divide between people with and without disabilities is alarming. Approximately 60% of people with disabilities have never used a computer, compared with 25% of people without a disability. People with disabilities are only half as likely to be Internet users as people without disabilities: 22% compared to 42% (NTIA, 2000). Differences also exist in Internet access rates among people with different disabilities. For example, people with visual impairments have access rates of less than 20% while people with learning disabilities have a 40% access rate.

People with disabilities often need accommodation with devices such as key guards, voice controls, and magnifying screens. Ironically, it is people with physical disabilities who can benefit from the digital economy, perhaps more so than people without disabilities. The Internet has the potential to negate environmental barriers (such as transportation problems) that hinder full community participation.

INTERNET APPLICATIONS FOR PEOPLE WITH DISABILITIES

Communication is a key way that people without disabilities use the Internet. According to the 2000 NTIA report, 85% of Internet users send and receive e-mails, 58% search for information (e.g., check news, weather, sports), 34% shop and pay bills, 32% take courses, 28% perform job related tasks, and 8% use the Internet to search for jobs. Grimaldi and Goette (1999) found that people with physical disabilities who use the Internet have a higher perceived level of independence than those that do not. The Internet may be used to gain access to information, increase general fund of knowledge, interact with government agencies, shop, pay bills, look for jobs, perform job tasks at home, receive telehealth care services, receive cybercounseling services, receive education and training, and socialize with people regardless of disability status. Summarized below are several major Internet applications that are relevant to people with disabilities.

Government Services

Gould (2002) reported that the United States government is moving towards increasing citizen access to government services and participation in the democratic process through an e-government agenda. E-government is a means for government to use new technologies to provide citizens with convenient access to public sector information and services, to improve the quality of services, and to provide greater opportunities to participate in democratic institutions and processes.

For people with disabilities, the e-government services can improve their ability to advocate for and access government services. For example, people with disabilities may receive more effective and integrated services because government agencies will be more integrated and able to communicate more efficiently. For example, case files can be shared instantly among the social security specialist, the vocational rehabilitation counselor, and the job placement specialist in a one-stop career center (Gould, 2002). The possibility of applying for social security benefits online is another convenience for people with physical disabilities. E-government also has the potential of allowing people with disabilities to be more informed citizens. Gould suggests that people with disabilities can efficiently access the federal government through a one-stop portal (http://www.firstgov.gov/), follow public legislation affairs through the Internet (http://thomas.loc.gov/), and obtain comprehensive statistical information about the United States through the FedStat website (http://www.icsp.gov/). The Internet can enhance active participation by people with physical disabilities in the democratic process. For example, people with disabilities can provide input to the myriad of interagency committees or advisory commissions to address telecommunication, employment, and education issues, as well as disability and rehabilitation topics through electronic testimony.

Telehealth Services

Clinical services such as health care, counseling, and rehabilitation services can be provided through the Internet to augment conventional face-to-face clinical services. *Rehabilitation Psychology* recently published a special issue on telehealth, addressing the use of the Internet to help people with chronic illness and disability manage their health issues at home. Glueckauf, Nickelson, Whitton, and Loomis (2004) defined telehealth as "the use of telecommunication and information technology to provide access to health information and services across a geographical distance, including (but not limited to) consultation, assessment, intervention, and health maintenance." Glueckauf and colleagues cited several reasons for the growth of telehealth services. One major factor is related to the need to increase access to rehabilitation and other specialty care services for underserved populations, including people with disabilities with mobility limitations and those who lack adequate transportation. Telehealth services can be provided using multiple modalities (e.g., telephone, videoconferencing, and the Internet). Several studies have demonstrated the positive effect of telehealth services for people with chronic illness and disability. Gustafson and colleagues (1999) published an experimental study regarding the use of the Comprehensive Health Enhancement Support System (CHESS) with people with HIV-AIDS in Wisconsin. Individuals use CHESS to communicate with others in a chat room, consult with experts, read articles related to health concerns, monitor their health status, and learn coping skills. Patients with HIV-AIDS who had access to CHESS reported higher quality of life, fewer hospitalizations, and spent less time at medical visits than their counterparts without access to CHESS. McKay, Glasgow, Feil, and Barrera (2002) reported that Internet-based information and support have a positive impact on health promotion behaviors of patients with Type 2 diabetes.

Concerns about telehealth were expressed by Reed, McLaughlin, and Milholland (2000). They note that the telehealth technology is neither inherently good nor bad. However the power that technology offers to expand access to services can also be used to restrict it. The same means that promote the freedom of patients and providers can also be used to exploit them. They offer 10 ethical principles for interdisciplinary professional practice within telehealth. These principles specify that the same guidelines for clinical competence, ethics, and confidentiality are maintained in the realm of telehealth as in traditional health services (Reed et al., 2000).

Cybertherapy

Research has demonstrated that persons with disabilities are at a higher risk for anxiety, depressive symptoms, and major depression. For example, Turner and McLean (1989) found the prevalence of affective disorders among persons with disabilities in the general community was three times higher compared to a nondisabled group matched for age, gender, and area of residence. Similarly, several studies have identified a high prevalence of depression among persons with spinal cord injury, clients with multiple sclerosis, and elderly persons with Alzheimer's disease (Chan & Leahy, 1999). Social isolation and loneliness are frequent concerns of people with physical disabilities (Livneh & Antonak, 1999). Cybertherapy can be used by people with disabilities as an adjunct to face-to-face therapy.

Cybertherapy, Behavioral eHealth, eTherapy, Technology-Assisted Distance Counseling, Cybercounseling, Online Counseling, and Internet Counseling are terms that specify that a client is using a computer and the Internet to communicate with a therapist or counselor rather than by face-to-face communication (National Board for Certified Counselors, 2001). Cybertherapy has been compared to telephone and Internet based general health services, which allow for assessment, diagnosis, treatment, and other services across distance (Nickelson, 1998).

Therapist-client interactions can occur synchronously or asynchronously in cybertherapy. Interactions are synchronous in chat-rooms, using instant messaging, Internet Relay Chats (IRC), or a video-based Internet meeting. Asynchronous therapeutic interactions occur with Web-page based information, bulletin boards, and e-mail.

A survey of approximately 600 doctoral-level practitioner members of the American Psychological Association found that only 2% had provided services over the Internet, satellite, or closed-circuit television (VandenBos & Williams, 2000). It is likely that the percentage of psychologists using cybertherapy will grow in the near future (Stamm, 1998). An expert panel of psychologists has predicted that a growing percentage of psychotherapy will be offered over the Internet, telephone, or other electronic mediums (Norcross, Hedges, & Prochaska, 2002). Over 200 websites offering therapy and/or counseling online with access to approximately 350 practitioners have been identified (Sampson, Kolodinsky, & Greeno, 1997; Segall, 2000). The results of an Internet survey designed to determine who is providing cybertherapy and what services they offer, indicated that the highest frequency service offered to clients is educational information, followed by advice, counseling, therapy, and crisis intervention (Maheu & Gordon, 2000). The types of problems addressed most frequently through cybertherapy include mood disorders, anxiety disorders, family problems, and relationship problems (Carlbring, Westling, Ljungstrand, Ekselius, & Andersson, 2001; Cook & Doyle, 2002; Maheu &Gordon, 2000). Sexual disorders and grief and bereavement issues were the least frequently treated with cybertherapy (Maheu & Gordon, 2000). In one of the first of its kind, a study by Jacobs and colleagues (2001) compared a computer-based psychotherapy approach to traditional, individual therapy. The authors found that clients receiving computer-based therapy demonstrated improvement over the course of therapy and that these changes were maintained over a six-month follow-up period. The computer-based therapy generated similar effects on most of the evaluative measures as the traditional therapy and involved less than half the therapist time provided with traditional therapy. However, clients receiving traditional therapy reported a higher level of satisfaction and had higher scores on several outcome measures compared to clients receiving the computer-based approach.

It is not known whether cybertherapy is effective for people with severe psychiatric illnesses. The Jacobs and colleagues (2001) study recruited subjects who had minor mental health problems and may not have met any diagnostic criteria according to the American Psychological Association's *Diagnostic and Statistical Manual of Mental Disorders* (4th ed.). Other studies have demonstrated success with clients with panic disorders and family problems. Most cybertherapy adopts a cognitive or cognitive behavioral approach.

Patterson (2000) advocated for the use of the Internet in the rehabilitation counseling process. She suggested that rehabilitation consumers could use the Internet to search for medical and occupational information, take psychological or educational tests, join support groups, and pursue online education.

The use of the Internet has introduced new ethical issues into the practice of psychotherapy. The American Psychological Association (APA) asserts that its ethics code is applicable for all psychologists regardless of the context in which services are delivered, including electronic media such as the Internet (APA, 2002). The preponderance of ethical issues surrounding cybertherapy concern confidentiality and practitioner competence (Maheu & Gordon, 2000; Sampson et al., 1997).

Confidentiality may be compromised by confidential e-mail that is intercepted or left on an Internet Service Provider server (Maheu & Gordon, 2000; Sampson et al., 1997). Good risk management includes the use of encryption software for e-mail communications with clients. Informing clients that Internet communications may not always be secure is also recommended (Commission on Rehabilitation Counselor Certification, 2001; Humphreys, Winzelberg, & Klaw, 2000; Maheu & Gordon, 2000; National Board for Certified Counselors [NBCC], 2001).

Frequently, the credentials of a cybertherapist are not listed in a professional manner. Thus, the education and qualifications of a cybertherapist may not be obvious to a client (Gold, 1998; Maheu & Gordon, 2000; Segall, 2000). The Internet reaches across all state and national borders, making it difficult to ascertain whether a cybertherapist is licensed to practice in the state where the client is. Thus, there may be violations of state and/or national laws if a cybertherapist is not licensed to practice in the state or country where the client is located (Sampson et al., 1997; Koocher & Morray, 2000; Maheu & Gordon, 2000; NBCC, 2001; Nickelson, 1998). Therapists using the Internet should verify that professional liability insurance covers provision of services over the Internet (Koocher & Morray, 2000; Segall, 2000).

Since there is no physical presence, the cybertherapist generally has no paralinguistic communication with the client. Hence there is a greater risk of misunderstandings between the client and cybertherapist than in face-to-face encounters (Sampson et al., 1997). It is also important for the cybertherapist to know exactly who the client is. There must be verification of the client's age. If the client is a minor, written consent from the client's guardian must be secured (Segall, 2000).

Cybertherapy has not been recommended for individuals requiring crisis management. Cybertherapists should have arrangements with local emergency services and crisis hot-lines for clients who are at risk for suicide or other emergencies (NBCC, 2001).

Benefits of cybertherapy include improved access to services in remote or rural areas, monitoring of client progress via computer documentation, and administration of assessments online with less counselor involvement (Nickelson, 1998; Sampson et al., 1997). The use of e-mail as a means of communication allows a client to review previous messages from a counselor when such advice or information is needed (Segall, 2000). Other advantages to cybertherapy relate to the reduced cost of counseling services (Jacobs et al., 2001; Nickelson, 1998; Segall, 2000) when compared to face-to-face counseling, and the time effectiveness associated with e-mail and Internet-based communications (Maheu & Gordon, 2000).

The major criticisms of cybertherapy are low client satisfaction (Jacobs et al., 2001), the limited number of empirically based studies on its effectiveness (Barak, 1999; Maheu & Gordon, 2000), and credentialing issues related to service providers.

Social Support and Skill Training

A consequence of mobility limitations and lack of transportation among many people with disabilities is social isolation. Social isolation can hinder the development of social skills and reduce social interactions and support. However, the positive effects of social support groups on the psychological and physical health of people with chronic illness, especially for those with stigmatizing diseases (e.g., AIDS and alcoholism) are well established (Davison, Pennebaker, & Dickerson, 2000). Since people with physical disabilities frequently struggle with deficits in social skills, coping skills, interpersonal support, and health care management, skill training is central to the rehabilitation of many people with disabilities. It helps persons who lack basic social and coping skills learn adaptive behaviors so they can reinforce their support network and cope with the demands of everyday life. The Internet access may help people with physical disabilities who lack real-world support gain information, support, and skill training through the use of online education and social support groups. In fact, several theorists have suggested that Internet use increases social interaction and support (Silverman, 1999).

Research on the impact of Internet use and social support, however, is mixed. For example, several studies have found only marginal relationships between computer use and social support (e.g., Swickert, Hittner, Harris, & Herring, 2002), while other studies suggest heavy Internet use may even lead to isolation, loneliness, and depression among its users (e.g., Kraut et al., 1998). Research results from samples of people with chronic illness and disabilities (e.g., HIV-AIDS and diabetes) are more positive, suggesting that the use of the Internet for health care information and support significantly improved psychosocial well-being and reduced hospitalizations and clinic visits (Gustafson et al., 1999; McKay et al., 2002). A recent Harris Poll (Taylor, 2000a) of online users supports the positive effect of Internet use by people with disabilities. The Harris poll reported that people with disabilities spent twice as much time online as people without disabilities (20 hours per week versus 10 hours per week) and people with disabilities are more likely to report that the Internet has significantly improved their quality of life (48% versus 27%). People with disabilities also reported that the Internet has helped them to better connect to the world and reach out to people with similar interests and experiences. Interestingly, a higher percentage of people without disabilities reported the Internet has helped them to communicate and socialize with close friends, relatives, or neighbors (49% versus 42%).

RESEARCH DIRECTIONS AND OTHER RECOMMENDATIONS

The Internet has enormous potential for improving the quality of the personal, social, and work lives of all people, but perhaps has greater potential for improving the lives of people with physical disabilities. Through the Internet, physical barriers to face-to-face communication encountered by people with disabilities who have mobility limitations, speech impediments, and/or transportation problems can be minimized. Yet, it may be difficult for people with disabilities and professionals to obtain up-to-date information about research, health services, intervention techniques, and community resources by using the Internet. Among these areas where research is needed are employment and training, health services, counseling, psychosocial development, and education and training of counselors.

Research into the digital divide between people with and without disabilities is basic to many of these areas of interest. Some of the factors affecting the lower rate of Internet access among people with disabilities are known (e.g., education, income, age, and employment status) and affect the have-nots without disabilities. However, barriers such as attitudes toward information technology, computer and Internet literacy, computer hardware and software designs, and Web site accessibility that are specific to people with disabilities have not yet been studied in a systematic manner. It is imperative that research be conducted to fully examine the digital divide between people with and without disabilities. It will be easier to bridge the digital divide by exploring research questions such as: What factors cause the lower Internet participation rates of people with disabilities? And: What is the effectiveness of different intervention strategies for improving the Internet utilization rates of people with disabilities?

Employment and Training

People with disabilities will continue to be left behind in terms of accessibility and participation in the digital economy if they do not have the skills and tools to use new technologies. Innovative instructional approaches should be implemented in educational and public training and career programs to help people with disabilities use these new technologies.

The digital economy has created new jobs that require more cognitive and less muscle power. People with physical disabilities can fill many of these jobs. However, many computer jobs require skills in mathematics and familiarity with computers and Internet resources. Stoddard and Nelson (2001) reported that the average math score for state vocational rehabilitation (VR) clients is at the 7.7th grade level. The relatively low math and science skills of many individuals severely limit their opportunities to participate in the information technology jobs created by the digital economy. One important research question concerning employment and training is: What are the best ways to help students with disabilities develop appropriate math and science skills to be competitive in the digital economy? Once individuals with disabilities have the skills and resources needed to utilize the Internet, distance learning might become a cost-effective method for continued education and job training. At this point, clinicians and researchers might ask: What is the effectiveness of different online training approaches for people with disabilities? Which occupations are more conducive to online training?

The advent of the Americans with Disabilities Act and requirements for reasonable accommodations has caused many individuals to look at telecommuting as an employment opportunity for people with disabilities.

President Bush's New Freedom Initiative (Bush, 2001) is a proposal for continued reduction of barriers that people with disabilities face in the United States. Its purpose is fourfold: (a) to improve access to assistive and universally designed technologies; (b) create greater educational opportunities for people with disabilities; (c) increase employment for people with disabilities; and (d) ensure that there are matching federal funds to states for low-interest loans so that people with disabilities are able to purchase equipment for telecommuting. In order for these developments to occur, government policies and regulations to entice the information technology industries to develop computer hardware as well as software products that are easy to use and accessible to people with disabilities must be strengthened and reinforced. Section 508 of the Workforce Investment Act of 1998 prescribed new accessibility standards for six areas of information and electronic technologies:

- Software applications and operating systems
- Web-based information or applications
- Telecommunication products
- Video or multimedia products
- Information appliances, such as fax machines and kiosks
- Desktop and portable computers

In light of President Bush's New Freedom Initiative, research funding should be made available to rehabilitation researchers who conduct research in the area of assistive technology, augmentative communication devices, and human-computer interface designs to extend their research from making personal computers accessible to people with disabilities to increasing the accessibility of the Internet. Funding should also be made available to people with disabilities to access the Internet. Likewise, monies are needed for people with disabilities to secure these new technologies. The Internet may be used to improve educational programming for people with disabilities. The Internet may also allow for educational opportunities for individuals with severe mobility restrictions or who live in rural areas. President Bush's program supports telecommuting for people with disabilities. The Bush Administration has also proposed tax incentives for companies that contribute to computer and Internet access for employees with disabilities, so that they might be able work from a home office. Research completed at Virginia Commonwealth University's Rehabilitation Research and Training Center on Workplace Supports found that telework was instrumental in providing industrially injured individuals the chance to begin second careers (West, 2002).

Future research might seek answers to questions such as: What percentage of teleworkers have a physical disability? What percentage of workers with a physical disability telecommute? How successful are the New Freedom Initiative incentives in helping people with disabilities obtain or maintain employment? What are employers' attitudes toward hiring people with disabilities for telecommuting jobs versus jobs requiring a physical presence within the company? Do virtual applications for tele-commuting jobs (e.g., through an Internet job placement company like Monster.com) make it easier to hire a person with a disability?

Some research questions that are relevant to assistive technology include: What are the barriers and solutions to the development of a universal Internet service that is affordable, available, user-friendly, and interoperable for all users, specifically for persons with disabilities? What are the barriers and solutions to affordable, available, user-friendly, and interoperable devices to access this system?

Health Services

Clinical applications of the Internet for people with disabilities are encour-aging. The Internet has been used successfully in several self-help activi-ties including health care management, counseling and psychotherapy, and social support. However, many research questions remain, including: How can people with disabilities be helped to navigate the medical and rehabilitation information resources available through the Worldwide Web? How can they be helped to develop efficient information-gathering strategies? How can the validity of information obtained be evaluated? How can the information and social support portals for people with dis-abilities be best organized?

Additional research questions regarding health services and the Internet include: What are the most effective ways to provide Internet-based medical and rehabilitation services? How active should the Internet portal be, as designed for people with disabilities? When should Internet services be used in conjunction with face-to-face ser-vices? What are the preferences and utilization patterns of people with different disabilities? What factors influence the decision of people with disabilities to use the Internet for services and social interactions? What are the benefits of Internet use to the psychosocial adjustment of people with different disabilities?

Counseling

Cybercounseling has been criticized because of the lack of empirically based research on its effectiveness (Barak, 1999; Maheu & Gordon, 2000). Surveys of cybercounselors have shown how the Internet has been used for persons with various psychological and psychosocial disorders.

Yet, there have been just a few studies into the effectiveness of the Internet in therapy. Some examples of research questions that might be addressed in this domain include: Is asynchronous or synchronous communication more useful in treating depression? Can the improved data-keeping potential of the Internet facilitate assessment, diagnosis, and treatment of people with psychological problems? Can cybercounseling be effective in assisting people with disabilities to adjust to their condition and/or society? Are all psychotherapeutic approaches effective online? If not, which approaches are effective and which are not? Is e-mail more effective than a chat-room? Are face-to-face sessions better than video conferencing? Questions regarding the effectiveness of psychotherapy have been addressed by 50 years of research (Chan, Thomas, & Berven, 2004). The advent of cybercounseling provides new opportunities to extend this field of research.

Psychosocial Issues

The use of the Internet by the general public has led to concerns over Internet addiction and depression. It is not evident whether these concerns are also pertinent to individuals with disabilities. Research should be conducted on the association between Internet use and loneliness and depression among people with disabilities. Research could also focus on the extent to which Internet addiction is a problem among people with disabilities.

Research into the Internet activity patterns of users with disabilities could assist in identifying how the Internet might promote greater autonomy, empowerment, and psychosocial well-being, as well as determining how the Internet has not helped achieve these goals. More research questions include: How frequently are online support groups used? Do chat rooms offer individuals with mobility impairments greater opportunities to socialize? How does chat room use affect well-being, connectedness, and locus of control? Research into patterns of Internet activity could also be conducive to research into new devices, software, regulations, and procedures that would be designed to improve the Internet's use for people with disabilities.

CONCLUSION

The potential research directions related to Internet resources and use of the Internet by people with disabilities are vast and diverse. This chapter has highlighted research questions related to the Internet and disability. It is vital for the disability policies of the federal and state governments to be grounded in empirical research. The intention of this chapter is to promote the use of the Internet for improving the lives of people with disabilities and to outline the scope of research needed to explore this topic.

QUESTIONS FOR DISCUSSION AND/OR FURTHER STUDY

Service Domain

1. Describe the benefits of Internet use for people with disabilities.
2. What are the major ethical considerations related to cybertherapy?

Research Domain

3. Why is research related to Internet use and people with disabilities important?
4. Summarize the existing research about Internet use and social support.

Policy Domain

5. What are the factors that contribute to the "digital divide"? How can these factors be addressed by policy or legislation?
6. How is the Internet increasing access to government services and democratic participation in individuals with disabilities?

REFERENCES

American Psychological Association. (2002). *Ethical Principles of Psychologists and Code of Conduct 2002*. Washington, DC: Author.

Barak, A. (1999). Psychological applications on the Internet: A discipline on the threshold of a new millennium. *Applied and Preventive Psychology, 8,* 213–246.

Bush, G. W. (February, 2001). *New Freedom Initiative*. Retrieved August 18, 2004, from the United States White House Web site: http://www.whitehouse.gov/news/freedominitiative/freedominitiative.pdf

Carlbring, P., Westling, B. E., Ljunstrand, P., Ekselius, L., & Andersson, G. (2001). Treatment of panic disorder via the Internet: A randomized trial of a self-help program. *Behavior Therapy, 32,* 751–764.

Chan, F., & Leahy, M. (1999). *Healthcare and disability case management*. Lake Zurich, IL: Vocational Consultants Press.

Chan, F., McCollum, P. S., & Parker, H. J. (1985). Computer assisted job placement: Selected applications. *American Rehabilitation, 11,* 18–21.

Chan, F., Thomas, K., & Berven, N. (2004). *Counseling theories and techniques for rehabilitation health professionals.* New York: Springer Publishing Company.

Commission on Rehabilitation Counselor Certification. (2001). *Code of professional ethics for rehabilitation counselors.* Rolling Meadows, IL: Author

Cook, J. E., & Doyle, C. (2002). Working alliance in online therapy as compared to face-to-face therapy: Preliminary results. *CyberPsychology and Behavior, 5,* 95–105.

Davison, K. P., Pennebaker, J. W., & Dickerson, S. S. (2000). The social psychology of illness support group. *American Psychologist, 55,* 205–217.

Glueckauff, R. L., Nickelson, D. W., Whitton, J., & Loomis, J. S. (2004). Telehealth and health-care psychology: Current development in telecommunications, regulatory practices, and research. In T. Boll, R. G. Frank, A. Baum, & J. Wallender (Eds.), *Handbook of health psychology* (Vol. 3, pp. 377–411). Washington, DC: American Psychological Association.

Gold, J. (1998). Mental health and the Internet. *Computers in Nursing, 16,* 85–86, 89.

Gould, M. (2002). Building an inclusive e-government agenda for all Americans. In L. R. McConnell (Ed.), *Systems change: Emerging service delivery model. A report on the 23rd Mary E. Switzer Memorial Seminar* (pp. 29–35). Alexandria, VA: National Rehabilitation Association.

Grimaldi, C., & Goette, T. (1999). The Internet and the independence of individuals with disabilities. *Internet Research, 9,* 272–280.

Gustafson, D. H., Hawkins, R., Boberg, E., Pingree, S., Serlin, R. E., Graziano, F., et al. (1999). Impact of patient-centered, computer-based health information/support system. *American Journal of Preventive Medicine, 16,* 1–9.

Humphreys, K., Winzelberg, A., & Klaw, E. (2000). Psychologists' ethical responsibilities in Internet-based groups: Issues, strategies, and a call for dialogue. *Professional Psychology: Research and Practice, 31,* 493–496.

Jacobs, M. K., Christensen, A., Snibbe, J. R., Dolezal-Wood, S., Huber, A., & Polerok, A. (2001). A comparison of computer-based versus traditional individual psychotherapy. *Professional Psychology: Research and Practice, 32,* 92–96.

Koocher, G. P., & Morray, E. (2000). Regulation of telepsychology: A survey of State Attorneys General. *Professional Psychology: Research and Practice, 31,* 503–508.

Kraut, P., Patterson, M., Lundmark, V., Kessler, S., Mukopadhyay, T., & Scherlis, W. (1998). Internet paradox: A social technology that reduces social involvement and psychological well-being? *American Psychologist, 53,* 65–77.

Leiner, B. M., Cert, V. G., Clark, D. D., Kahn, R .E., Kleinrock, L., Lynch, D. C., et al. (2002). *A brief history of the Internet.* Reston, VA: The Internet Society.

Livneh, H., & Antonak, R. (1999). Psychosocial aspects of chronic illness and disability. In F. Chan & M. Leahy (Eds.), *Healthcare and disability case management* (pp. 121–168). Lake Zurich, IL: Vocational Consultants Press.

Maheu, M. M., & Gordon, B. L. (2000). Counseling and therapy on the Internet. *Professional Psychology: Research and Practice, 31,* 484–489.

McKay, H. G., Glasgow, R .E., Feil, E., Boles, S. M., & Barrera, M. (2002). Internet-based diabetes self-management and support: Initial outcomes from the Diabetes Network Project. *Rehabilitation Psychology, 47,* 31–48.

National Board for Certified Counselors. (2001). The practice of Internet counseling. Retrieved from http://www.nbcc.org/ethics/webethics.htm

National Telecommunication and Information Administration. (2000). *Falling through the net: Toward digital inclusion.* Washington, DC: Author.

Nickelson, D. W. (1998). Telehealth and the evolving health care system: Strategic opportunities for professional psychology. *Professional Psychology: Research and Practice, 29,* 527–535.

Norcross, J. C., Hedges, M., & Prochaska, J. O. (2002). The face of 2010: A Delphi Poll on the future of psychotherapy. *Professional Psychology: Research and Practice, 33,* 316–322.

Patterson, J. B. (2000). Using the Internet to facilitate the rehabilitation process. *Journal of Rehabilitation, 66,* 4–10.

Reed, G. M., McLaughlin, C. J., & Milholland, K. (2000). Ten interdisciplinary principles for professional practice in telehealth: Implications for psychology. *Professional Psychology: Research and Practice, 31,* 170–178.

Sampson, J., Kolodinsky, R., & Greeno, B. (1997). Counseling on the information highway: Future possibilities and potential problems. *Journal of Counseling and Development, 75,* 203–212.

Segall, R. (2000). Online shrinks. *Psychology Today, 33*(3), 38–43.

Silverman, T. (1999). The Internet and relational theory. *American Psychologist, 54,* 780–781.

Stamm, B. H. (1998). Clinical applications of telehealth in mental health care. *Professional Psychology: Research and Practice, 29,* 536–542.

Stoddard, S., & Nelson, J. (2001, Spring/Summer). Math, computers and the Internet: Better employment opportunities for people with disabilities. *American Rehabilitation,* 9–14.

Swickert, R. J., Hittner, J. B., Harris, J. L., & Herring, J. A. (2002). Relationships among internet use, personality, and social support. *Computers in Human Behavior, 18,* 437–451.

Taylor, H. (2000a, June 7). *How the Internet is improving the lives of Americans with disabilities* (Harris Poll #30). Washington, DC: Harris Poll.

Taylor, H. (2000b, October 7). *Conflicting trends in employment of people with disabilities 1986– 2000* (Harris Poll #59). Washington, DC: Harris Poll.

Taylor, H. (2003, February 5). *Those with Internet access to continue to grow but at a slower rate* (Harris Poll #8). Washington, DC: Harris Poll.

Turner, R. J., & McLean, P. D. (1989). Physical disability and psychological distress. *Rehabilitation Psychology, 34,* 225–242.

VandenBos, G. R., & Williams, S. (2000). The Internet versus the telephone: What is telehealth, anyway? *Professional Psychology: Research and Practice, 31,* 490–492.

West, M. D. (2002). Profiles of teleworkers with disabilities. Retrieved March 8, 2006., from the Web site of Virginia Commonwealth University, Rehabilitation Research and Training Center on Workplace Supports, http://www.worksupport.com/research/viewContent.cfm/389.

Index

SPRINGER / PUBLISHING COMPANY

Rehabilitation Caseload Management
2nd Edition, Concepts and Practice

Lee Ann Grubbs, PhD, CRC, CFLE
Jack L. Cassell, PhD
S. Wayne Mulkey, PhD, CRC

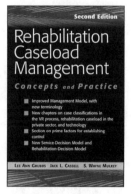

Newly organized with more comprehensive information and over 55 illustrative tables and figures, the second edition of *Rehabilitation Caseload Management* provides valuable caseload information in one resource-filled volume. Whether you're new to rehabilitation counseling or an experienced professional in the field, this is the ultimate desk reference. It fills a much-needed void in the management arena of rehabilitation counseling and expands beyond both public and private rehabilitation caseload management.

Benefits of the 2nd Edition:
- Improved Management Model, including new terminology
- Redeveloped section on prime factors for establishing control
- Two new rehabilitation models: Service-Decision Model and Rehabilitation-Decision Model
- New chapters on case classifications in the VR process, rehabilitation caseload in the private sector, and technology

Partial Contents:

Part I: Conceptual Aspects of Rehabilitation Caseload Management • A Management Model for Rehabilitation Counselors • Establishing Effective Control in the Rehabilitation Caseload Management Process • Elements of Effective Decision Making • The Understanding and Management of Time

Part II: Practical Aspects of Rehabilitation Caseload Management • Case Classifications in the Vocational Rehabilitation Process • Case Recording and Documentation in Rehabilitation • Rehabilitation Caseload Management in the Private Sector • Using Technology in Caseload Management

Springer Rehabilitation Series
2005 · 352pp · 0-8261-5165-5 · softcover

11 West 42nd Street, New York, NY 10036-8002 • Fax: 212-941-7842
Order Toll-Free: 877-687-7476 • Order On-line: www.springerpub.com

Medical Aspects of Disability
3rd Edition

A Handbook for the Rehabilitation Professional

Herbert H. Zaretsky, PhD
Edwin F. Richter III, MD
Myron G. Eisenberg, PhD

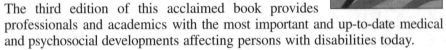

Medical
Aspects
of Disability

3rd Edition

A Handbook for
the Rehabilitation
Professional

HERBERT H. ZARETSKY, PhD
EDWIN F. RICHTER III, MD
MYRON G. EISENBERG, PhD
EDITORS

"A comely arrangement of...the salient medical and physiological features of the disease processes and syndromes that rehabilitation professionals will encounter in their clinical practices."
—**Physical Therapy,** from review of first edition

The third edition of this acclaimed book provides professionals and academics with the most important and up-to-date medical and psychosocial developments affecting persons with disabilities today.

With the field's increasing move toward evidence-based practice, a need for information in the areas of accreditation and outcome measurement has arisen. In response, the editors have added an essential special topics chapter detailing the importance of the accreditation process as a fundamental component of the quality assurance and improvement process. Because this information can be used by current or future clinicians, the volume continues to be the most comprehensive handbook available for the dynamic world of rehabilitation and medical science.

New to the Third Edition:
- Innovative perspectives by new co-editor
- Updated references representing advances in evaluation and treatment of disabling conditions and health care systems
- Up-to-the-minute information on accreditation based on feedback from teachers who have used previous editions in the classroom
- Consultations with Primary Care Physicians

Springer Series on Rehabilitation
2005 • 944pp • 0-8261-7973-8 • hard

11 West 42nd Street, New York, NY 10036-8002 • Fax: 212-941-7842
Order Toll-Free: 877-687-7476 • Order On-line: www.springerpub.com